Advanced
Endovascular
Therapy of Aortic
Disease

Advanced Endovascular Therapy of Aortic Disease

EDITED BY

Alan B. Lumsden, MD, ChB

Professor of Surgery, Division of Vascular Surgery and Endovascular Therapy
Michael E. DeBakey Department of Surgery, Baylor College of Medicine
Houston, TX, USA

Peter H. Lin, MD

Chief of Vascular Surgery, Michael E. DeBakey Veterans Affairs Medical Center
Chief of Interventional Radiology, Michael E. DeBakey Veterans Affairs Medical Center
Associate Professor of Surgery, Division of Vascular Surgery and Endovascular Therapy
Michael E. DeBakey Department of Surgery, Baylor College of Medicine
Houston, TX, USA

Changyi Chen, MD, PhD

Professor of Surgery & Molecular and Cellular Biology, Director, Molecular Surgeon Research Center
Vice Chairman, Surgical Research, Division of Vascular Surgery and Endovascular Therapy
Michael E. DeBakey Department of Surgery, Baylor College of Medicine
Houston, TX, USA

Juan C. Parodi, MD

Professor of Surgery
Chief of Endovascular Surgery
Division of Vascular & Endovascular Surgery Department of Surgery
University of Miami Medical School
Miami, FL, USA

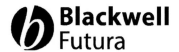

Blackwell
Futura

© 2007 by Blackwell Publishing
Blackwell Futura is an imprint of Blackwell Publishing

Blackwell Publishing, Inc., 350 Main Street, Malden, Massachusetts 02148-5020, USA
Blackwell Publishing Ltd, 9600 Garsington Road, Oxford OX4 2DQ, UK
Blackwell Publishing Asia Pty Ltd, 550 Swanston Street, Carlton, Victoria 3053, Australia

First published 2007

1   2007

ISBN: 978-1-4051-5570-0

Library of Congress Cataloging-in-Publication Data

Advanced endovascular therapy of aortic disease / edited by Alan B. Lumsden ... [et al.].
       p.   ; cm.
    Includes bibliographical references and index.
    ISBN-13: 978-1-4051-5570-0 (alk. paper)
    ISBN-10: 1-4051-5570-1 (alk. paper)
    1. Blood-vessels – Endoscopic surgery.   2. Aorta–Diseases.   3. Aorta–Surgery.
I. Lumsden, Alan B.
    [DNLM: 1. Aortic Diseases – surgery.   2. Angiography.   3. Angioplasty. WG 410
A244 2007]

    RD598.5.A384 2007
    617.4'130597 – dc22

                                                                        2006031411

A catalogue record for this title is available from the British Library

Commissioning Editor: Gina Almond
Editorial Assistant: Victoria Pittman
Development Editor: Beckie Brand
Set in 9.5/12 Minion and Frutiger by TechBooks, New Delhi, India
Printed and bound in Singapore by C.O.S. Printers Pte Ltd

For further information on Blackwell Publishing, visit our website:
www.blackwellcardiology.com

The publisher's policy is to use permanent paper from mills that operate a sustainable forestry
policy, and which has been manufactured from pulp processed using acid-free and elementary
chlorine-free practices. Furthermore, the publisher ensures that the text paper and cover
board used have met acceptable environmental accreditation standards.

Contents

v

Acknowledgments

We would like to thank all the faculty contributors for their tireless efforts in the preparation of the chapters. We are indebted to Yvette Whittier, our administrative coordinator, for her countless hours of hard work in bringing this project together. Last, but not least, we are grateful to our families, Cathy, Aaron, Amber, Donal, Sarah, Terry, Mark, Pete, and Cynthia, for their patience and support in making this book a reality.

Contributors

Jennifer L. Ash, MD
Department of Surgery
University of Illinois College of Medicine
Peoria, IL
USA

Jan D. Blankensteijn, MD
Department of Vascular Surgery
Radboud University Nijmegen Medical Centre
Nijmegen
The Netherlands

Jacob Buth, MD
Catharina Hospital
Eindhoven
The Netherlands

Lisandro Carnero, MD
Division of Vascular Surgery
Department of Surgery
Emory University School of Medicine
Atlanta, GA
USA

Jeffrey P. Carpenter, MD
Department of Surgery
Hospital of the University of Pennsylvania
Philadelphia, PA
USA

Elliot Chaikof, MD, PhD
Division of Vascular Surgery
Department of Surgery
Emory University School of Medicine
Atlanta, GA
USA

Jae-Sung Cho, MD
Division of Vascular Surgery
Department of Surgery
University of Pittsburgh School of Medicine
Pittsburgh, PA
USA

Frank J. Criado, MD
Division of Vascular Surgery
Department of Surgery
Union Memorial Hospital-MedStar Health
Baltimore, MD
USA

Michael D. Dake, MD
Professor of Radiology, Internal Medicine (Pulmonary
Disease), Surgery;
Chairman of the UVA Department of Radiology and the
Harrison Medical Teaching Professor of Radiology
Charlottesville, VA
USA

Edward B. Diethrich, MD
Arizona Heart Institute and Arizona Heart Hospital
Phoenix, AZ
USA

Kathryn Dougherty, RN
Department of Cardiology
St. Luke's Episcopal Hospital
The Texas Heart Institute
Houston, TX
USA

Hosam El Sayed, MD
Division of Vascular Surgery and Endovascular Therapy
Michael E. DeBakey Department of Surgery
Baylor College of Medicine
Houston, TX
USA

Ron Fairman, MD
Division of Vascular Surgery
Department of Surgery
University of Pennsylvania
Philadelphia, PA
USA

Mark A. Farber, MD
Division of Vascular Surgery
Department of Surgery
University of North Carolina
Chapel Hill, NC
USA

Richard G. Fisher, MD
Department of Radiology
Baylor College of Medicine
Houston, TX
USA

Nicholas J. Gargiulo III, MD
Division of Vascular Surgery
Department of Surgery
Montefiore Medical Center
New York, NY
USA

Shan-e-ali Haider, MD
Division of Vascular Surgery
Department of Surgery
University of Pittsburgh School of Medicine
Pittsburgh, PA
USA

Peter Harris, MD, FRCS
Regional Vascular Unit
Royal Liverpool University Hospital
Liverpool
UK

Kim J. Hodgson, MD
Division of Vascular Surgery
Department of Surgery
Southern Illinois University
Springfield, IL
USA

Brian R. Hopkinson, MD
Division of Vascular Surgery
Department of Surgery
University of Nottingham
Queen's Medical Centre
Nottingham
UK

Syed M. Hussain, MD
Vascular and Endovascular Surgery
HeartCare Midwest
Assistant Clinical Professor of Surgery
University of Illinois College of Medicine at Peoria
Peoria, IL, USA

Tam T. Huynh, MD
Division of Vascular Surgery and Endovascular Therapy
Michael E. DeBakey Department of Surgery
Baylor College of Medicine
Houston, TX
USA

Karthik Kasirajan, MD
Division of Vascular Surgery
Department of Surgery
Emory University School of Medicine
Atlanta, GA
USA

Panagiotis Kougias, MD
Division of Vascular Surgery and Endovascular Therapy
Michael E. DeBakey Department of Surgery
Baylor College of Medicine
Houston, TX
USA

Zvonimir Krajcer, MD
Department of Cardiology
St. Luke's Episcopal Hospital
The Texas Heart Institute
Houston, TX
USA

W. Anthony Lee, MD
Division of Vascular Surgery and Endovascular Therapy
University of Florida College of Medicine
Gainesville, FL
USA

Lina Leurs, MD
Catharina Hospital
Eindhoven
The Netherlands

Peter H. Lin, MD
Division of Vascular Surgery and Endovascular Therapy
Michael E. DeBakey Department of Surgery
Baylor College of Medicine
Houston, TX
USA

Evan C. Lipsitz, MD
Division of Vascular Surgery
Department of Surgery
Montefiore Medical Center
New York, NY
USA

Lars Lönn, MD, PhD
Departments of Radiology
Sahlgrenska University Hospital
Göteborg University
Göteborg
Sweden

Michel S. Makaroun, MD
Division of Vascular Surgery
Department of Surgery
University of Pittsburgh School of Medicine
Pittsburgh, PA
USA

Louis G. Martin, MD
Vascular and Interventional Radiology
Department of Radiology
Emory University School of Medicine
Atlanta, GA
USA

Kenneth L. Mattox, MD
Michael E. DeBakey Department of Surgery
Baylor College of Medicine
Houston, TX
USA

Ross Milner, MD
Division of Vascular Surgery
Department of Surgery
Emory University School of Medicine
Atlanta, GA
USA

Ali Mortazavi, MD
Department of Cardiology
St. Luke's Episcopal Hospital
The Texas Heart Institute
Houston, TX
USA

Kenneth Ouriel, MD
Division of Surgery
The Cleveland Clinic
Cleveland, OH
USA

Eric K. Peden, MD
Division of Vascular Surgery and Endovascular Therapy
Michael E. DeBakey Department of Surgery
Baylor College of Medicine
Houston, TX
USA

Bo Risberg, MD, PhD
Departments of Surgery
Sahlgrenska University Hospital
Göteborg University
Göteborg
Sweden

Hazim J. Safi, MD, FACS
Department of Cardiothoracic and Vascular Surgery
The University of Texas Medical School at Houston
Memorial Hermann Heart and Vascular Institute
Houston, TX
USA

Tae K. Song, MD
Division of Vascular Surgery
Department of Surgery
Harbor-UCLA Medical Center
Torrance, CA
USA

Randolph Statius-van Eps, MD
Catharina Hospital
Eindhoven
The Netherlands

S. William Stavropoulos, MD
Departments of Radiology
Hospital of the University of Pennsylvania
Philadelphia, PA
USA

Neil E. Strickman, MD
Department of Cardiology
St. Luke's Episcopal Hospital
The Texas Heart Institute
Houston, TX
USA

Frank J. Veith, MD
Department of Vascular Surgery
The Cleveland Clinic
Cleveland, OH
USA

Matthew J. Wall, Jr., MD
Michael E. DeBakey Department of Surgery
Baylor College of Medicine
Houston, TX
USA

Cliff Whigham, DO
Department of Radiology
Baylor College of Medicine
Houston, TX
USA

Rodney A. White, MD
Division of Vascular Surgery
Department of Surgery
Harbor-UCLA Medical Center
Torrance, CA
USA

David M. Williams, MD
Division of Interventional Radiology
Department of Radiology
University of Michigan
Ann Arbor, MI
USA

Wei Zhou, MD
Division of Vascular Surgery and Endovascular Therapy
Michael E. DeBakey Department of Surgery
Baylor College of Medicine
Houston, TX
USA

Preface

Since the concept of using an endovascular stent-graft to repair an abdominal aortic aneurysm was initially described by Dr. Parodi and Dr. Palmaz, this treatment strategy has undergone a dramatic technological evolution. This evolution is further fueled by the increased public acceptance of this minimally-invasive therapy, miniaturization of endovascular stent-grafts, and availability of multiple devices approved by the Food and Drug Administration (FDA). Growing evidence clearly supports the early treatment success of this treatment strategy, in terms of morbidity and mortality reduction, when compared to the conventional open repair in well-selected patient cohorts. Advances in this endovascular technology have also broadened the treatment armamentarium of thoracic aortic pathologies. Since the FDA has approved the use of endovascular repair of descending thoracic aneurysms, many researchers have found a beneficial role of using this technology in the treatment of other thoracic aortic pathologies, including dissection and traumatic transection.

Treatment outcome of endovascular repair of aortic diseases is highly dependent on the appropriate patient selection, physician's experience, and post-procedural device surveillance. Disseminating the clinical experiences from physician experts in this field will undoubtedly educate other endovascular interventionalists and potentially improve treatment outcome for all physicians who perform endovascular aortic procedures. The basis of this book "Advanced Endovascular Therapy of Aortic Disease" represents the collection of clinical experiences from a group of well-known endovascular interventionalists who participated in the 2006 Total Endovascular Aorta Symposium, sponsored by the Division of Vascular Surgery and Endovascular Therapy of the Baylor College of Medicine. A total of 26 chapters are included which cover four sections, including natural history and preoperative planning, thoracic aortic aneurysm, aortic dissection and traumatic aortic injury, and techniques, new devices, and surveillance.

It is our hope that the collection of these chapters provided by faculty experts in the field of endovascular aortic therapy as assembled in this symposium will help to enhance the practice of endovascular interventionalists. It is our sincere privilege to put forth this compendium book as a token of their contributions to the field of endovascular aortic therapy.

Alan B. Lumsden, MB, ChB
Peter H. Lin, MD
Changyi Chen, MD, PhD
Juan C. Parodi, MD

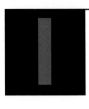

PART I

Natural history and preoperative planning

CHAPTER 1

Etiology and pathogenesis of aortic disease

Bo Risberg & Lars Lönn

The aorta can be affected by a variety of pathological conditions. Some of them have a clear genetic component and affect young patients or patients in the early adolescence. Most pathology is however encountered in the grown-up population and is caused by degenerative diseases. This chapter will focus on the following pathological conditions that affect the aorta: atherosclerosis, aneurysms, dissections, Marfan's syndrome, Ehlers–Danlos syndrome, and Takayasu's disease.

Atherosclerosis

Atherosclerosis is a systemic and generalized disease that is the main cause for premature death in the adult population in the Western world. Several vascular beds are affected simultaneously, the heart, brain, viscera, and extremities. The pathophysiology of atherosclerosis in large arteries, such as aorta, is not different from that in small vessels. The etiology of atherosclerosis is extremely complex. Despite intense research there is still a long way to go before we have a good understanding of the disease that is reflected in new preventive and therapeutic strategies. The atherosclerotic process involves predominantly the intimal and medial layers of the wall.

The response to injury hypothesis proposed by Ross has had a heavy input on atherosclerotic research [1, 2]. It has stimulated research on endothelial interaction with blood cells and signaling to smooth muscle cells. An initial event is some sort of injury to the endothelium leading to permeability alterations allowing passage of large molecules such as lipids. The injury may not be mechanical. Low-density lipoproteins in hypercholesteroemic patients can in itself cause endothelial injury.

The thromboresistance is lost with increased risk for thrombosis. Platelets adhere to the site of injury. They release growth factors, e.g. PDGF (platelet-derived growth factor) which is a strong mitogen for smooth muscle cell proliferation. This local stimulus leads to accumulation of smooth muscle cells within the intima and deposition of extracellular matrix proteins. Furthermore, there is deposition of lipids and infiltration of lipid-loaded cells. A proliferative lesion has been formed.

Fatty streak and fibrous plaque

The intimal layer with the endothelial cells is the first line of defense against atherosclerosis. The very first event is the fatty streak which consists of lipid accumulation in macrophages located in and beneath the endothelium [3]. Depending on genetics and life style, the fatty streak may either regress or progress into atheroma. Progression of lipid accumulation leads to focal intimal thickenings. Formation of fibrous plaques is usually not seen until in the fourth decade. Fibrotic tissue and smooth muscle cells form a *fibrous cap* surrounding the lipid core. There is a necrotic center of amorphous material, extracellular proteins, matrix fibers, lipid-containing cells, cholesterol crystals, and calcium salts. The plaques are infiltrated with vasa vasorum. The lipid-rich core is extremely thrombogenic due its high content of tissue factor. An intact fibrous cap prevents release of procoagulative activity.

The lesions can be characterized as soft or hard. The soft plaques are dominated by lipid deposition in the necrotic core. They are particularly prone to rupture leading to thrombotic complications. The hard sclerotic lesions are characterized by calcification. They cause stenosis and, depending on the degree of flow impairment, ischemia.

Inflammation and plaque

The involvement of inflammatory cells as well as their activation has put forward the hypothesis of inflammation as an initial event in atherosclerosis. The atheromatous plaque consists of a core of foam cells and lipids. The border regions, shoulders, of the plaque are made up of inflammatory cells such as T-cells, macrophages, and mast cells [4]. These cells produce cytokines as signs of activation [5]. The plaques are predominantly located in areas of flow disturbances such as branches. The macrophages produce PDGF as a mitogen, cytokines and growth factors. Interleukin 1 (IL-1), tumor necrosis factor α (TNF-α), transforming growth factor β (TGF-β), and several others factors are produced. Through these mediators, the macrophages can affect and regulate cellular organization in the plaque. The macrophages may be antigen presenting cells to T-lymphocytes that participate in the inflammatory process. Oxidized LDL is such an antigen that can trigger the inflammation [6].

Role of the endothelium

The integrity of the endothelium is essential in preventing the initial developments of the plaque. Perturbation of the endothelium causes expression of growth factors that stimulate proliferation of smooth muscle cells. Likewise adhesion molecules are expressed on the endothelial surface causing cellular interactions. Platelets adhere to the endothelium through expression of their surface glycoproteins Ib and IIb/IIIa. Specific adhesion molecules such as selectins are involved in leukocyte rolling on the surface followed by sticking and extravasation of the cells. VCAM-1, vascular cell adhesion molecule, adheres monocytes and lymphocytes and is upregulated by high cholesterol levels. Activated adhering cells and cells in the vessel wall release inflammatory mediators, e.g., cytokines. Proteolytic enzymes, metalloproteinases (MMPs), and their inhibitors are activated and contribute to the development of the plaque by facilitating migration and proliferation of cells.

Recent research has demonstrated the importance of a variety of immune cells in the atherosclerotic process. T-cells activated from antigens release cytokines, which trigger activation of macrophages and other vascular cells. The process is balanced by regulatory T-cells, which produce IL-10 and TGF-β, both anti-inflammatory mediators. Release of inflammatory cytokines especially IL-6 will stimulate production of CRP in the liver. An excellent and comprehensive review of inflammation and atherosclerosis was recently published [7].

Plaque rupture

There is an overwhelming body of knowledge on the role of plaque rupture to initiate thrombosis and ischemia [8]. Most of the data stems from coronary arteries but the process does not differ in other parts of the vascular system.

The lipid core of the plaque is highly thrombogenic due to its content of tissue factor. When the lipid is sealed in its fibrous cap, it is harmless but when released it initiates an immediate and very strong coagulation. Activated macrophages in the plaque express tissue factor, which further enhances the thrombotic state.

The shoulders of the plaque are at risk for rupture. Cytokine-mediated cell activation leads to proteolytic degradation of the matrix particularly in the shoulder region. MMPs are key players in these events. Functional polymorphism in several MMP genes is associated with atherosclerotic manifestations and complications such as coronary thrombosis, myocardial infarction, stenosis, arterial stiffness, and blood pressure [9]. MMP genotyping can probably be of importance in the clinical management of cardiovascular patients in the future.

In small arteries such as the coronaries, plaque rupture can lead to thrombotic occlusion. In larger arteries including the aorta, this can occur as well only if there is a pronounced stenosis. More often plaque rupture will cause ulceration with thrombotic depositions and subsequent risk for embolization.

Degeneration of the plaque

Degeneration of the plaques can occur from necrotic changes in the plaque. Insufficient circulation through the vasa vasorum causes ischemia. Activated MMPs degrade the extracellular matrix thereby contributing to the plaque destabilization. The plaque degeneration can lead to ulceration or other complications such as thrombosis or embolization of thrombotic or atheromatous material.

Plaque and flow

The likelihood of developing atherosclerotic lesions differs between arteries at various locations. Plaques develop in relation to branches, twists, and bends. Typically they are found in the proximal, upstream part of the orifice. One common feature is flow disturbances with turbulence, flow separation, and low shear stress. Shear stress influences directly the endothelium, which leads to increased permeability and altered cellular functions such as expression of nitric oxide and adhesion molecules. Plaques localize predominantly in areas with low shear stress while areas of high shear stress are relatively spared from atherosclerosis [10].

Formation of a stenotic plaque does not initially encroach on the luminal transverse area and volume. There is a compensatory enlargement of the artery to accommodate the plaque without affecting flow. Usually the plaque is eccentric in the vessel leaving a rounded lumen but an oval vessel. This has been demonstrated in different parts of the vascular tree. Large plaques may however encircle the whole circumference and cause a stenosis [11].

Constriction and dilatation, mediated through the endothelium, are means of keeping wall shear stress constant [12].

Infection and atherosclerosis

The strong inflammatory components of the disease have put forward the intriguing question of an infectious etiology to atherosclerosis. Virus and bacteria have been found in diseased vessel wall. Until now a causative role has not been established. *Chlamydia pneumoniae* is found in a large number of patients with atherosclerosis. About 60% of these patients are seropositive. No relations have been found between symptoms, degree of atherosclerosis, and extent of *C. pneumoniae* involvement [13]. Similarly, no correlation was found between plaque destabilization and herpes simplex or cytomegalovirus seroreactivity.

A few studies have been published on effects of antibiotics against *C. pneumoniae* for prevention of coronary events and with negative results [14, 15]. *Chlamydia* may not be the cause of atherosclerosis but can speed up the development and progression

of the disease [16], perhaps by enhancing the inflammatory reaction. Much of this basic research will of course have implications on the future therapeutic strategy.

Atherosclerosis in different parts of the aorta

The manifestations of atherosclerosis differ not only in different vascular regions such as carotid, coronary, and femoral arteries but also in various parts of the aorta.

The infrarenal abdominal aorta is a frequent site of plaques with or without ulcerations. Ulcerated areas are covered by thrombotic material. Embolization from these areas can cause focal ischemia in the lower extremities. Often there is a heavy calcification. The stenotic lesions can develop into total occlusions. The atherosclerotic process causes medial degeneration with risk for dilatation while the thoracic aorta is relatively spared these severe manifestations.

These findings could be due to different architecture in the thoracic and the abdominal aorta. The vascular nutrition differs in these two regions of the aorta. In the thoracic aorta, the main part of the vessel wall is supplied by vasa vasorum. The abdominal aorta lacks vasa vasorum and relies on diffusion of oxygen and nutrients from the lumen. The likelihood of ischemia in this part of the aorta is thus greater and this can contribute to the degeneration of the wall.

Risk factors for atherosclerosis

Several risk factors for atherosclerosis have been identified. Most are associated with the metabolic syndrome and they are all life-style associated. The metabolic syndrome is already a widespread condition affecting 10–25% of western populations and its prevalence is increasing. Adipositas, hypertension, hyperlipidemia, and type-2 diabetes are dominating components of this syndrome. The attractiveness of the metabolic syndrome as an entity lies in the assumption that the syndrome has greater power to predict morbidity and mortality than individual components themselves.

Smoking initiates the atherosclerotic process at an earlier stage and accelerates its progression. Smoking is probably the most important factor in the development of atherosclerosis. The mechanistic details are still unknown but it is likely that oxygen-free radicals play a role. Cessation of smoking decreases the risk for clinical manifestations of atherosclerosis probably by arresting the progression of the lesions.

The role of lipids

Disturbances in lipid metabolism have since long been associated with atherosclerosis. High cholesterol levels lead to accumulation of cholesterol esters in macrophages, which are turned into foam cells. High levels of LDL can change the endothelial barrier, particularly oxidized LDL can be noxious to the endothelium. Modified LDL can via scavenger receptors be taken up by macrophages leading to formation of foam cells.

The hydroxymethylglutaryl-coenzyme A (HMG-CoA) reductas inhibitors (statins) are effective in LDL lowering. The enzyme is the rate-limiting step in the cholesterol synthesis. Another action, probably of equal importance, is its anti-inflammatory effect. Through this mechanism, the very early events in atherogenesis can probably be prevented.

Another exciting approach to treat atherosclerosis is by using recombinant Apo-AI Milano that in animal experiments can cause regression of atherosclerosis. It is a variant of apolipoprotein A-I identified in an Italian subpopulation characterized by low HDL and low incidence of atherosclerosis. The drug was recently found to reduce the atheroma volume in coronary arteries in a controlled randomized trial in humans [17].

Aneurysms

Aneurysms develop in the degenerated aorta. Atherosclerosis is the most common cause for degeneration of the wall. Genetic components have been identified in Marfan's syndrome and Ehlers–Danlos disease. Even in the most common, degenerative, form of aortic aneurysms there is a genetic component. There is a clear familiar occurrence with a risk of about 25% for first-degree probands [18].

Degradation of elastin has been associated with dilatation while rupture of the wall is related to collagen degradation [19]. MMP-9 (gelatinase B) that degrades elastin, collagen type IV, fibronectin, and other matrix proteins has been linked to aneurysmal disease. High levels of MMP-9 and MMP-3 have been found in abdominal aortic aneurysmal tissue [20, 21]. Levels of MMP-9 are associated with aneurysmal size [22].

Of particular interest is the importance of mutations in the genes coding for MMPs. Single nucleotide polymorphism in the MMP-9 gene at location-1562 (1562 bases from the start of the gene) has been associated with atherosclerosis and intracranial aneurysms. The latter is however controversial [23]. This mutation has been linked to aortic aneurysms in one study [24] while this was not confirmed in another investigation [25]. The latter study furthermore indicated that genetic variations in inhibitors of MMPs, TIMPs, were involved in aneurysm formation. More research is clearly needed to establish details of the genetic interplay in aortic aneurysms.

The aneurysmal pathology is characterized by a chronic inflammation with destruction of the extracellular matrix, remodeling of the wall layers, and reduction in number of smooth muscle cells. The smooth muscle cells are essential for production of extracellular matrix proteins. Less supportive scaffold enhances the degradation. The balance between MMPs and their inhibitors, TIMPs, is pivotal in the degradation of the wall. As the process progresses, dilatation occurs. This leads to flow disturbances, changes in wall tension with reduced tensile strength, and finally rupture. Therapeutic trials with doxycycline, a MMP inhibitor, are ongoing and preliminary results are encouraging with less progression of aneurysmal size in treated patients [26].

Dissections

Acute dissection can occur following degeneration with weakening of the wall. The most common form is the atherosclerotic variety typically seen in hypertensive patients. Lipid deposition, intimal thickening, fibrosis, and calcification are seen. The extracellular matrix is degraded with lysis of elastin, collagen breakdown, and cellular apoptosis. Through the action of MMPs the intima and vessel wall become fragile. The elastin synthesis may be inefficient. Macrophages, which express the elastin gene and produce tropoelastin, may play an important role by producing a defective elastin [27]. The histology is characterized by media necrosis, scarcity of smooth muscle cells, and loss of elastin [28].

The polymerization of elastin is a very complicated process. Fibulin-5 is an extracellular protein expressed in the basement membrane in blood vessels. It is a key player in the synthesis of elastin. Patients with dissection in the thoracic aorta were recently found to have reduced levels of fibulin-5 [29]. This means that a low content of elastin in patients with dissection could be due to reduced synthesis, increased degradation or both.

Familial dissection in the ascending aorta (type A) was recently linked to a genetic mutation involving dysregulation TGF-β signaling. This suggests that TGF-β may have a critical role in this condition [30].

Obstruction of the vasa vasorum can cause local ischemia in the wall. The burden of mechanical stress in the hypertensive patient facilitates disruption.

The intramural hematoma is regarded as a special variety of a localized dissection even if this concept has been disputed recently [31]. The etiology may be disruption of a medial vasa vasorum causing a localized bleeding with hematoma. The intramural hematomas are particularly hazardous since approximately half of these patients go on to dissection or rupture [32].

Localized ulcers can occur in all parts of the aorta. They develop from plaque rupture and constitute weak points in the wall where a dissection can start.

There has been an interesting discussion on seasonal variation and the influence of atmospheric conditions on thoracic dissections. There seems to be a peak in wintertime [33, 34]. Atmospheric pressure and temperature seemed to be unrelated to aortic dissection in another recent study [35].

Marfan's syndrome

Marfan's syndrome is an autosomal dominant trait with main manifestations from the connective tissue with degeneration of the elastic fibers. The incidence is about 1/5000 inhabitants. Typically the main abnormalities are found in the cardiovascular, skeletal, and ocular systems.

Apart from mitral valve prolapse, dilatation of the aorta is typical for the cardiovascular involvement. The aortic dilatation is progressive and starts with enlargement of the sinuses of Valsalva. All parts of the aorta can be affected as the disease progresses distally. The most serious complications are dissection of the aorta or aneurysm formation with rupture. The patients are typically long and slender with arachnodactily (long fingers). They have pectus excavatus, flat feet, and scoliosis. The ocular abnormalities are mainly lens luxation and myopia.

The aortic wall is thin with fragmentation of the elastic fibers in the medial layer. There is also defective synthesis and crosslinking of elastin. Collagen metabolism is affected as well with signs of increased collagen turnover (elevated hydroxyproline secretion in the urine and low proline/hydroxyproline ratio) [36].

The genetic defect responsible for Marfan's syndrome has been localized to the fibrillin gene (FBN1) on chromosome 15. Fibrillin is a glycoprotein about 350 kD. A large number of mutations (>500) in the gene are found in Marfan patients. In the connective tissue there is a reduced fibrillin-1 deposition. This leads to defect fibrillin aggregation and crosslinking of elastin. Extracellular microfibrils are mainly made up of fibrillin. The defective microfibrils impair anchoring and structural maintenance in various tissues. The elastin formed is more easily degraded by MMPs. The weakness in the wall leads to aneurysmal dilatation and/or dissection.

Ehlers–Danlos syndrome

The Ehlers–Danlos syndrome is a genetically determined disease of the connective tissue. The main abnormalities are found in the described skin, joints, and arteries. Of all the 11 types of Ehlers–Danlos syndrome described, number IV is of particular interest from a cardiovascular point of view. This form is an autosomal dominant or recessive trait. The arterial manifestations make type IV particularly serious. The major cutaneous symptom is echymoses. Collagen type III synthesis is reduced in the arterial system. This renders the vessels thin and fragile. Especially the medial layer is thin with fragmentation of the internal elastic membrane.

Takayasu's disease

Takayasu described this disease in 1908 [37]. It is characterized by a chronic inflammation that is predominantly localized to the arch. Synonymous names are "pulseless disease" or "aortic arch syndrome," names that are quite descriptive of the nature of the disease. However, the disease is not limited to the aortic arch but is found in most other large vessels. Women are much more frequently affected than men with a ratio of 4:1. The disease always starts before 40 years of age with a mean onset around 30. The incidence is 2–3 per million inhabitants in the USA.

Macroscopic findings

Stenotic processes that can involve all parts of the aorta and its main branches characterize the disease. The walls are thickened with perivascular sclerosis. The external diameter of the vessel is not affected. The stenotic process intrudes into the lumen and reduces the luminal surface area. In advanced cases, there may be complete occlusion. Typically there is a poststenotic dilation in Takayasu's disease. Aortic aneurysms or dissection are not features of the disease. The supra-aortic branches are involved in 50% of the cases. The clinical symptoms depend on the extent and location of the lesions.

The typical lesions are usually seen in the arch and its branches but changes can occur in all other branches such as the visceral and the iliac vessels.

Microscopic findings

The most characteristic finding is that of a chronic inflammation. The most pronounced changes are seen in the adventitial and medial layers. The adventitia is site for a sclerotic collagenous dense tissue and with thickening of the vasa vasora. The media show breakage of the elastic fibers and with signs of neovascularization. The vessel wall is infiltrated with inflammatory cells, lymphocytes, histiocytes, and sometimes giant cells. The intima is grossly thickened with a loose connective tissue. The intimal changes are secondary to the pathological processes in the outer layers. Sometimes frank deposition of atherosclerotic material can be seen in the stenotic lesions. The histopathological changes can be related to the clinical stage. In the active phase, the findings of granulomas and infiltration with inflammatory cells are common. Later during the occlusive stage, the chronic inflammation with scarring is predominant.

The granulomatous appearance in the chronic stage has initiated speculations on tuberculosis being of etiological importance. Antigens from mucobacteria can cause granuloma. In recent clinical surveys, tuberculosis was found in 20% of the patients [38] and tuberculin test was positive in 47% [39]. The inflammatory component of the disease is further stressed by a correlation between IL-8 levels in plasma and degree of disease activity [40].

References

1 Ross R, Glomset JA. The pathogenesis of atherosclerosis. N Engl J Med 1976; **295**: 369–377.

2 Ross R. The pathogenesis of atherosclerosis: An update. N Engl J Med 1986; **314**: 488–500.

3 Stary HC, Chandler B, Glagov S et al. A definition of initial, fatty streak and intermediate lesions of atherosclerosis: A report from the committee on vascular lesions of the council on arteriosclerosis. Circulation 1994; **89**: 2462–2478.

4 Jonasson L, Holm J, Skalli O, Bondjers G, Hansson GK. Regional accumulation of T cells, macrophages, and smooth muscle cells in human atherosclerotic plaque. Arteriosclerosis 1986; **6**: 131–138.

5 Frostegård J, Ulfgren AK, Nyberg P et al. Cytokine expression in advanced human atherosclerotic plaques: Dominance of proinflammatory (Th 1) and macrophage-stimulating cytokines. Atherosclerosis 1999; **145**: 33–43.

6 Stemme S, Faber B, Holm J, Wiklund O, Witztum JL, Hansson GK. T lymphocytes from human atherosclerotic plaques recognize oxidized low density lipoprotein. Proc Natl Acad Sci USA 1995; **92**: 3893–3897.

7 Hansson GK. Inflammation, atherosclerosis and coronary artery disease. N Engl J Med 2005; **352**: 1685–1695.

8 Falk E, Shah PK, Fuster V. Coronary plaque disruption. Circulation 1995; **92**: 657–671.

9 Ye S. Influence of matrix metalloproteinase genotype on cardiovascular disease susceptibility and outcome. Cardiovasc Res 2006; Feb 15; **69**(3): 636–645.

10 Zarins CK, Giddens DP, Glagov S. Atherosclerotic plaque distribution and flow velocity profiles in the carotid bifurcation. In: Bergan JJ & Yao JST, eds. Cerebrovascular Insufficiency. Grune & Stratton, New York, 1983, pp. 19–30.

11 Glagov S, Weisenberg E, Zarins CK, Stankunavicius R, Kolettis GJ. Compensatory enlargement of human atherosclerotic coronary arteries. N Engl J Med 1987; **316**: 1371–1375.

12 Zarins CK. Adaptive responses of arteries. J Vasc Surg 1989; **9**: 382.

13 Muller BT, Huber RH, Henrich B, Adams O, Berns G et al. Chlamydia pneumoniae, herpes simplex virus and cytomegalovirus in symptomatic and asymptomatic high grade internal carotis artery stenosis. Does infection influence plaque stability? Vasa 2005; **34**: 163–169.

14 Grayston JT, Kronmal RA, Jackson LA, Parisi AF, Muhlestein JB, Cohen JD et al. Azithromycin for the

secondary prevention of coronary events. N Engl J Med 2005; **353**: 1637–1645.

15 Cannon CP, Braunwald E, McCabe CH, Grayston JT, Muhlestein B, Giugliano RP *et al*. Antibiotic treatment of Chlamydia pneumoniae after acute coronary syndrome. N Engl J Med 2005; **352**: 1646–1654.

16 Hu H, Pierce GN, Zhong G. The atherogenic effects of chlamydia are dependent on serum cholesterol and specific to Chlamydia penumoniae. J Clin Invest 1999; **103**: 747–753.

17 Nissen SE, Tsunoda T, Tuzcu EM, Schoenhagen P, Cooper CJ, Yasin M *et al*. Effect of recombinant ApoA-I Milano on coronary atherosclerosis in patients with acute coronary syndromes: A randomized controlled trial. J Am Med Assoc 2003; **290**: 2292–2300.

18 Powell JT, Greenhalgh RM. Multifactorial inheritance of abdominal aortic aneurysms. Eur J Vasc Surg 1987; **1**: 29–31.

19 Powell JT. Genes for hypertension. In: Halliday A, Hunt BJ, Poston J, & Schachter M eds. An Introduction of Vascular Biology. Cambridge University Press, Cambridge, 1998: 166–172.

20 Thompson RW, Parks WC. Role of matrix metalloproteinases in abdominal aortic aneurysms. Ann NY Acad Sci 1996; **800**: 157–174.

21 Newman KM, Ogata Y, Malon AM, Irizarry E, Ghandi RH, Nagase H. Identification of matrix metalloproteinases 3 (stromelysin-1) and 9 (gelatinase B) in abdominal aortic aneurysms. Arterioscler Thromb 1994; **14**: 1315–1320.

22 McMillan WD, Tamarina NA, Cipollone M, Johnson DA, Parker MA, Pearce WH. Size matters: The relationship between MMP-9 expression and aortic diameter. Circulation 1997; **96**: 2228–2232.

23 Krex D, Kotteck K, Konig IR, Ziegler A, Schackert HK, Schackert G. Matrix metalloproteinases-9 coding sequence single-nucleotide polymorphism in Caucasians with intracranial aneurysms. Neurosurgery 2004; **55**: 207–212.

24 Jones GT, Phillips VL, Harris EL, Rossak JI, van Rij AM. Functional matrix metalloproteinase-9 polymorphism (C-1526T) associated with abdominal aortic aneurysm. J Vasc Surg 2003; **38**: 1363–1367.

25 Ogata T, Shibamura H, Tromp G, Shina M, Goddard KA, Sukalihasan N *et al*. Genetic analysis of polymorphisms in biologically relevant candidate genes in patients with abdominal aortic aneurysms. J Vasc Surg 2005; **41**: 1036–1042.

26 Mosorin M, Juvonen J, Biancari F, Satta J, Surcel HM, Leinonen M *et al*. Use of doxycycline to decrease the growth rate of abdominal aortic aneurysms: A randomized, double-blind, placebo-controlled pilot study. J Vasc Surg 2001; **34**: 606–610.

27 Krettek A, Sukhova GK, Libby P. Elastogenesis in human arterial disease: A role for macrophages in disordered elastin synthesis. Arterioscler Thromb Vasc Biol 2003; **23**: 582–587.

28 Nakashima Y, Kurozumi T, Sueishi K, Tanaka K. Dissecting aneurysm: A clinicopathologic and histopathologic study in 111 autopsied cases. Hum Pathol 1990; **21**: 291–296.

29 Wang X, LeMaire SA, Chen L, Carter SA, Shen YH, Gan Y *et al*. Decreased expression of fibulin-5 correlates with reduced elastin in thoracic aortic dissection. Surgery 2005; **138**: 352–359.

30 Pannu H, Fadulu VT, Milewics DM. Genetic basis of thoracic aneurysms and aortic dissections. Am J Med Genet 2005; **139**: 10–16.

31 Nienaber CA, Sievers HH. Intramural hematoma in acute aortic syndrome: More than a variant of dissection? Circulation 2002; **106**: 284–285.

32 von Kodolitsch V, Csosz SK, Koschyk DH, Schalwat I, Loose R, Karck M *et al*. Intramural hematoma of the aorta: Predictors of progression to dissection and rupture. Circulation 2003; **107**: 1158–1163.

33 Manfredini R, Portaluppi F, Salmi R, Zamboni P, La Cecilia O, Kuwornu H *et al*. Seasonal variation in the occurrence of non-traumatic rupture of thoracic aorta. Am J Emerg Med 1999; **17**: 672–674.

34 Mehta RH, Manfredini R, Bossone E, Fattori E, Evangelista A, Boari B *et al*. The winter peak in the occurrence of acute aortic dissection is independent of climate. Chronobiol Int 2005; **22**: 723–729.

35 Repanos C, Chadha NK. Is there a relationship between weather conditions and aortic dissection? BMC Surg 2005; **5**: 21–27.

36 Nusgens B, Lapiere CM. The relationship between proline and hydroxyproline urinary excretion in human as an index of collagen metabolism. Clin Chim Acta 1973; **48**: 203–211.

37 Takayasu M. Case with unusual changes in the central vessels in the retina. Acta Soc Ophtalmol Jpn 1908; **12**: 554–555.

38 Mwipatayi BP, Jeffery PC, Beningfield SJ, Matley PJ, Naidoo NG, Kalla D. Takayasu arteritis: Clinical features and management. Report and angiographic features and a brief review of the literature. ANZ J Surg 2005; **75**: 110–117.

39 Sheikhzadeh A, Tettenborn I, Noohi F, Eftekharzadeh M, Schnabel A. Occlusive thromboaortopathy (Takayasu disease): Clinical and angiographic features and a brief review of the literature. Angiology 2002; **53**: 29–40.

40 Tripathy NK, Sinha N, Nityanand S. Interleukin-8 in Takayasu's arteritis: Plasma levels and relationship with disease activity. Clin Exp Rheumatol 2004; **22**: 27–30.

CHAPTER 2

Clinical consideration of aortic disease: atherosclerosis, aneurysm, dissection, and traumatic injury

Lars Lönn, & Bo Risberg

The thoracic and abdominal aorta carries various pathologies such as atherosclerosis, aneurysms, traumatic lesions, dissections, and penetrating ulcers which may be life-threatening and necessitate urgent treatment. Currently there is a change in treatment paradigm. More of aortic pathology is approached with endovascular techniques i.e. endovascular aortic repair (EVAR). It is used for the minimally invasive repair of the aorta for several disease states, such as aneurysms, penetrating ulcers, acute or chronic dissections, and contained or traumatic ruptures. EVAR is a solid alternative to open repair since many patients have serious comorbidities such as coronary artery disease, emphysema, high blood pressure, or diabetes. Open surgery, especially in the thorax, is a procedure that can lead to death in many frail and elderly patients. For patients, considered unfit for open repair, conservative medical management, or "watchful waiting," is often used as a treatment option but can lead to increased mortality and morbidity in many elderly patients due to the risk of rupture. This review of pathology in the thoracic aorta deals with the following conditions: atherosclerosis, thoracic aneurysms, dissections, and traumatic aortic injury.

Atherosclerosis

Comprehensive vascular anatomical, physiological, and pathophysiological information is the cornerstone of the management of patients with vascular disease, in order to provide an effective treatment plan. The appearance of atherosclerosis differs in the thoracic and abdominal aorta. Heavy stenotic lesions, calcification, or occlusions are seldom encountered in the thoracic aorta. Degeneration of abdominal aorta makes it prone to develop stenoses, heavy calcification, ulcers, and also aneurysms.

In the thoracic aorta *stenotic atherosclerosis* is located preferentially at the orifices of the large branches in the arch. Cerebrovascular thromboembolism is the most serious complication. Lesions in the carotid bifurcation were the most frequent findings (>40%) in patients with neurological symptoms. Lesions in the orifices at the arch accounted only for 5–15% [1]. Only when several vessels are involved cerebral blood flow may be a critical factor. Lesions at the orifices must be taken into account in the work-up of these patients even in the presence of a carotid stenosis.

The atherosclerotic patient is typically in the older age (>65 years) and has several risk factors such as hypercholesterolemia, diabetes, obesity, and smoking. The symptoms depend on the organs affected. Stenoses at the subclavian arteries impair the flow to the upper extremities. Because of retrograde flow through the vertebral arteries even occlusions at the origin of the subclavian arteries seldom cause severe ischemic symptoms. The term "subclavian steal" syndrome means that by heavy exercise of the arm, cerebral symptoms occur due to massive retrograde vertebral flow into the arm. Retrograde flow can fairly often be demonstrated radiographically but the clinical syndrome is a rare condition [2]. Surgical or endovascular interventions are only indicated in advanced cases.

Atherosclerotic degeneration of the wall predisposes for dilatation, elongation, and aneurysm

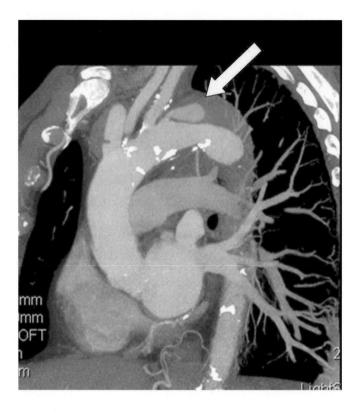

Figure 2.1 Penetrating aortic ulcer (PAU), shown on sagittal reconstructed tomaographic image (CT 3D MIP).

formation. There is an ongoing progressive increase in diameter of the aorta with age. The conditions in the thoracic aorta are probably similar to those in the abdomen. The diameter of the abdominal aorta increases by about 30% between the ages 25 and 70 years [3]. In a recent study, it was found that this progressive dilatation with age was counteracted by a compensatory thickening of the aortic wall in order to prevent an accompanying elevation of circumferential wall stress. Males were found to have a defective compensation as opposed to females, a finding that can help in explaining the higher incidence of aortic aneurysms in males [4]. The distensibility of the aortic wall is reduced with age, particularly in men, implying that degeneration of the wall is more pronounced and occurs at an earlier age in men than in women [5].

The dilatation of the wall with time can give a homogenous dilatation of the whole aorta or focal areas with increased diameter. Apart from widening there is also a progressive elongation particularly of the thoracic aorta. Once a bend in the aorta has started to form mechanical stress from blood flow continuously exaggerates the angulation. This can in advanced cases produce twists with over 90° angulation of the aorta in any plane, sagittal, coronar, and oblique views as shown on CT and MR images. The elongation and twisting can sometimes take grotesque proportions. It is often combined with aneurysm formation.

Atherosclerotic ulcerations can occur in the whole aorta but are more frequent in the thoracic part (Fig. 2.1). It is a matter of discussion if penetrating ulcers are variants of aortic dissection. Some ulcers may develop into saccular aneurysms or not. They can present either acute or chronic. In the acute form symptoms may resemble an acute dissection with severe chest pain. The chronic presentation can be in the form of distal microembolization. The subsequent workup will disclose the ulcer in the aortic wall. In a fair number of patients the size of the ulcer will increase and there is an association with development of intramural hematoma. Atherosclerotic ulcers are considered unpredictable. Patients presenting with atheroembolization represent a small but important group in the practice of vascular specialists. Men over 60 years old are most commonly affected and the embolization can occur spontaneously as well as due to arterial manipulations during endovascular or open interventions. Atheroembolism may originate anywhere in the arterial tree, but the aorto-iliac segment is the most common source. Microemboli consist of cholesterol or fibrinoplatelet aggregates or thrombus while macroemboli are considered parts of the atherosclerotic artery wall. Macroemboli cannot be distinguished from the clinical picture caused by cardiogenic emboli.

There is no consensus as to the best way of treating these patients, conservative or surgical–interventional. There are an increasing number of reports on endovascular stent-graft treatment. Recent surveys have indicated however that nonoperative management is safe in the acute situation [6–8]. Expansion or large ulcers and ulcers with other signs of complications e.g. saccular aneurysm formation, may probably benefit from surgical intervention, open or endovascular. A more aggressive approach has been recommended by other researchers based on the "virulent" appearance of penetrating ulcers and a progressive dilatation of the aorta.

Thoracic aneurysms

Thoracic aneurysms constitute about 20% of all aortic aneurysms. The incidence is 6 per 100,000 patient-years [9]. Aneurysms are characterized by degeneration of the media resulting in a weakness of all the layers of the aortic wall. One particular form of aneurysm develops after aortic dissection. Approximately 50% of the thoracic aneurysms originate in a dissection. These are truly pseudoanurysms since not all layers of the aortic wall are engaged. Early population-based studies demonstrated a 5-year survival rate for untreated thoracic aneurysms of only 13% [9] and for patients with degenerative aneurysm 3-year survival was 35% [10]. During a 15 follow-up period a clear increase in the incidence of degenerative aneurysms but with improved survival was noted [11]. Improved diagnostic accuracy and more frequent use of CT and echocardiography accounts for this relative increase. The incidence of ruptured thoracic aneurysms is 3.5–5/100,000 patient-years. The overall risk for rupture during a 5-year period was 20%.

The risk for rupture in women was approximately seven times that of men. This pattern may differ in various parts of the world. In Scandinavia an equal sex distribution in ruptured thoracic aneurysms was found [12].

Ascending and arch thoracic aneurysms

Thoracic aortic aneurysms do not differ etiologically in various parts of the aorta. They can be due to atherosclerotic degeneration, chronic dissections or caused by noninflammatory medial degeneration. The most common connective tissue disorder associated with aneurysm is the hereditary disorder Marfan's Syndrome, while Ehlers–Danlos syndrome and pseudoxanthoma elasticum are less frequent. More rarely, Osteogenesis imperfecta, Klipper–Feil syndrome, Turners syndrome among other syndromes may involve the aorta. Aortitis includes several diseases that can cause destruction of the medial layer in the aortic wall due to chronic inflammation. Aortitis can be divided into two categories, infective or noninfective. The latter can then be subdivided into luetic or nonsyphilitic disorder, while the former group can be classified into those diseases in which the aorta is mainly involved (Takayasu's disease) and those predominantly involving other organ systems than the aorta (Gaint Cell arthritis, rheumatoid arthritis) but may rarely involve the vascular tree. Aortic valvular insufficiency is of particular concern in aneurysms of the ascending aorta. The risk is proportional to the increase in size of the aneurysm.

The standard indication for intervention is an aneurysmal diameter of 6.0 cm or a growth rate 10 mm/y. In patients with Marfan's or chronic dissection the recommended limit is 5.0 cm due to the greater risk for rupture. Standard repair is an open replacement of the diseased segment of the aorta and if needed combined with a new valve insertion and reattachment of the coronaries.

In the present era of endovascular repair significant contributions have been made in mini-invasive replacement of the ascending aorta. The evolving technology often implies hybrid operations, combining open and endovascular approaches [13]. A variety of innovative techniques including transposition of the great arch vessels and elephant trunk reconstruction, have been published [14–17]. As with most endovascular techniques there is, for obvious reasons, a lack of proper long-term evaluation.

Descending thoracic aortic aneurysms

Aneurysms in the descending aorta have an incidence of approximately 30–50/million inhabitants/y [18]. The risk of rupture is related to the largest diameter of aorta [19]. Rupture causes a fatal outcome in 33–50% of the patients, while comorbidities are responsible for the remaining deaths [9, 10]. Although regular observation and medical management are indicated in many cases, surgical intervention is recommended if the sac diameter reaches 6 cm for asymptomatic aneurysms, and immediate treatment is recommended for symptomatic aneurysms, regardless of diameter. Standard treatment has traditionally been surgery. Elective open therapy of aneurysms is associated with a substantial short-term treatment mortality incidence of 10–20%.

In recent years, endovascular aortic repair (EVAR) of descending aneurysms has shown great promise (Fig. 2.2). Volodos published the first report on endovascular stent grafting for a thoracic aortic lesion in 1991 [20] while the first clinical series was published by the Stanford group in 1994 [21]. Typically short-term mortality for stent grafting of the aorta for aneurysms and type B dissec-

tions are less than for open surgery [22, 23]. New improved stent grafts for thoracic use are available on the market. Since this is an evolving technology even better devices are likely to appear.

The aim of EVAR is to prevent rupture by exclusion of the aneurysm sac, decrease pressure stress on the wall of the aneurysmal sac, or to reduce the pressure in the false lumen with subsequent obliteration. Transluminal endovascular stent-graft deployment is less invasive than standard operative repair and, as a result, patients who were previously not eligible for surgery may now be considered for treatment.

Each year in Europe, an estimated 16,000 patients are diagnosed with descending thoracic aortic lesions. There seems to be a need in the vascular community to confidently treat more challenging thoracic descending thoracic aortic lesions. The thoracic aorta is as described in the context above, vulnerable to the development of aneurysms and dissections, which can be signaled by chest or back pain, but are usually present without symptoms. Associated pain may indicate acute expansion or leakage of the lesion. The thoracic aorta also can be impacted by outside trauma, such as injuries sustained in an automobile accident. If the thoracic aorta becomes dissected or severed during an accident, patients invariably face high mortality rates if normal blood flow is not restored quickly. The

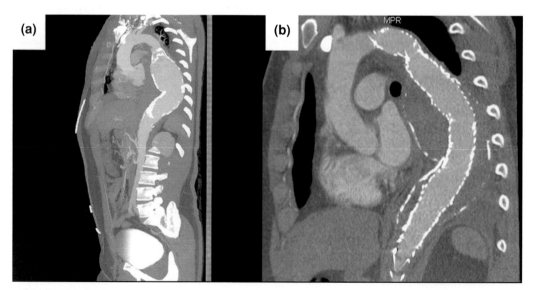

Figure 2.2 (a) Computed tomography of a thoracic aortic aneurysm before treatment (CT, 3D MIP, sagittal projection). (b) Thoracoabdominal aneurysm after EVAR (CT, 3D, MIP, sagittal projection).

thoracic endovascular clinical history now includes thousands of implanted grafts in various anatomical positions. The new generation of devices seems to be more robust, at least in the midterm follow-up. In future there is a demand that the new systems should provide more options with increased control. So in order to be the first line treatment for aortic lesions also in the long run, devices must show improved performance, especially regarding key attributes such as conformability, track ability, and deployment added to long-term durability without migration.

Thoracoabdominal aortic aneurysms

Thoracoabdominal aortic aneurysms (TAA) constitute about 10–15% of all aortic aneurysms. They are among the most difficult to treat and in about 20 to 30% there is an aneurysm in some other part of the aorta. Chronic dissection is the cause of these aneurysms in approximately 20% of the cases [24]. Women seem affected as often as men which is at variance with abdominal aneurysms which predominantly are a male disorder. The TAAs are classified, as originally described by Crawford (Table 2.1), according to their size. Type II aneurysms are the most extensive and difficult to treat. They also have the highest morbidity and mortality.

Modern treatment of TAA was pioneered by Stanley Crawford who introduced the "inlay"-technique [25] which since has been the standard approach to these aneurysms. Results of open surgery have improved considerably with time but even with precautions such as spinal fluid drainage and visceral vessel perfusion with partial by-pass these procedures are associated with significant morbidity and mortality. Complication rate is related to the extent of the aneurysm. While overall

Table 2.1 Crawford classification of thoracoabdominal aortic aneurysm.

Type	Extent
Type I	Descending aorta + part of visceral branches
Type II	Descending aorta + abdominal aorta
Type III	Distal part of descending aorta + abdominal aorta
Type IV	Visceral branches

mortality from a leading center is around 5% and paraplegia 5% [26, 27], the figures for type II repair are slightly higher, 10% and 7.5%, respectively [28]. By using motor evoked potential to monitor motor function of the spinal cord during surgery the risk for paraplegia can be reduced further to around 2% [29]. There are a substantial number of other complications, pulmonary, renal, abdominal and cardiovascular, which contribute to the significant morbidity in these patients.

Indication for intervention in asymptomatic patients is aneurysm size of 6.0 cm and above. In patients with Marfan's syndrome the upper limit is usually 5.0 cm. Symptomatic patients need immediate surgery. Significant comorbidities in most patients make the decision difficult and complicated. Due to the age profile of the patients, atherosclerotically damaged vessels in one or several organs increase the risk for complications. Approximately 1/3 of the patients have clinically significant cerebrovascular, cardiovascular, renal, or peripheral atherosclerotic disease.

Many are smokers with chronic obstructive lung disease. Reduced FEV1, reduced kidney function with elevated serum creatinine, or symptomatic coronary disease will increase the risks significantly. Preventive measures must be instituted preoperatively, such as CABG or PCI, and a proper risk assessment must be performed. Probably due to the risks involved in elective repair, a large proportion of patients, approximately 25%, are treated urgent due to acute symptoms [26]. Of course, the risks are even higher under these emergent circumstances.

Given the risk scenario with open repair, endovascular approaches are attractive. The endovascular development in this area has taken two ways that partly merge. One is the stent-graft technique based on fenestrated or branched grafts, which both share a common goal, i.e. the exclusion of flow to vital aortic branches. The other is hybrid operations, combining a less extensive open repair to secure visceral perfusion with stent-graft exclusion of the aortic aneurysm (Fig. 2.3).

Fenestrated (scalloped) grafts were developed first to enable free flow through vital side branches such as renal arteries, but apposition to the wall is necessary to create a seal as well as providing a secure landing zone for the stent graft [30]. The cutting edge technology today implies multiple fenestrations to

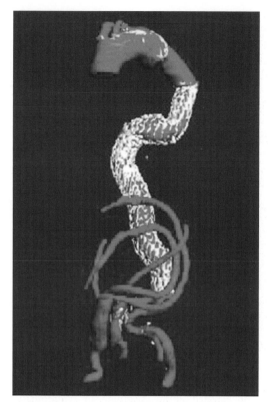

Figure 2.3 Hybrid aortic surgery. Revascularization of the four visceral vessels by grafts from right common iliac artery. Abdominal and thoracic aorta covered with stent grafts. 3D CT reconstruction in work-station (Medical Media Systems, Lebanon, NH).

commercially manufactured branched grafts, now available, are likely to speed up the utilization of this very exciting technique.

In *hybrid operations* both open and endovascular techniques are used. The logics are usually to spare the compromised patient a large open repair by reducing the magnitude of the interventional/surgical trauma. Revascularization of the visceral vessels can be accomplished by several routes. By raising four grafts from one common iliac artery it is possible to achieve this with minimal ischemic time. The aneurysmal segments of the aorta can then be stented as shown in Fig. 2.3.

Abdominal aneurysms (AAA)

Abdominal aorta is the main location for aortic aneurysms (65%, Fig. 2.4). The incidence is 21 per 100,000 person-years [9]. Only about 15% of patients with AAA die from rupture. The majority die from other causes. Women develop their aneurysms about 10 years later than men. There is a high prevalence in male relatives (about 25–30%) [33]. Screening for AAA is debated but male siblings is one focus group. Screening studies have demonstrated that a normal aortic diameter at the age of 65 very seldom leads to aneurysm formation. Screening at that age seems cost-effective [34].

Most AAA grow with time, 5 mm/y as a mean. The risk for rupture is exponentially related to aneurysmal diameter. Unfortunately even small aneurysms can rupture. A recent trial has documented that the operative risks are larger than the risks for rupture in aneurysms below 55 mm diameter [35]. Of particular interest is the high incidence of popliteal aneurysms in AAA patients indicative of a generalized arterial degeneration. The widely accepted indication for elective surgical intervention is a diameter of 55 mm or above, unless the patient has strong contraindications. Open surgery is still the gold standard. It can be performed with a perioperative mortality less than 5%.

The last decade has seen a boost in endovascular treatment. Even if EVAR can be performed with low mortality and morbidity there is hitherto no reason to change the indication for intervention. In the short- and midterm follow-up outcome is satisfactory. Long-term benefit may be obviated by problems of migration or endoleaks necessitating

cover all visceral orifices. The branches are usually stented with a bare or a small covered balloon-expandable stent.

Branched devices have incorporated side branches and their use is for those aneurysms with no neck/proximal landing zone at all. The zone between the side branch and the target vessel can be bridged as described above for fenestrated grafts with a junctional piece of stent graft or a covered stent. These advanced devices can be classified according to target region (abdominal or thoracic or thoracoabdominal) and subdivided into fenestrated or branched stent-graft systems [31]. The first endovascular thoracoabdominal aneurysm operation using *branched grafts* was reported by Chuter in 2001 [32]. Progress in this field has been slow due to the immense technological problems. However, improved and

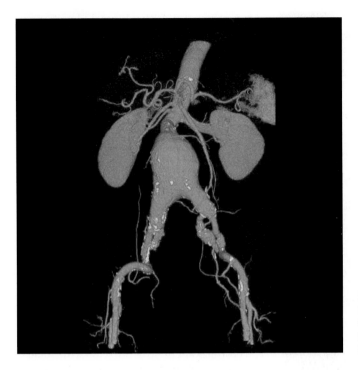

Figure 2.4 Three-dimensional (3D) reconstruction of a computed tomography angiography (CTA) of an infrarenal abdominal aortic aneurysm (AAA).

repeated interventions. Still there is a reduced rate in freedom from rupture with time in these patients. All EVAR patients must be submitted to long-term surveillance.

Rupture is the most dreaded complication to AAA. The majority of patients (70%) never make it to the hospital. Operative mortality is still high, 30–50%. Standard operation in most institutions is an open repair with exclusion of the aneurysm by means of a tube or a bifurcated graft. Urgent EVAR has been introduced at many institutions. Probably about half of patients with rupture will be eligible for the endovascular treatment. Preliminary data demonstrate the feasibility of the concept and that EVAR for ruptured AAA can be performed with low mortality, about 20% or less [36, 37].

Inflammatory aneurysm is a particular form of AAA characterized by an intense inflammation in the vessel wall, periaortitis. It occurs in about 5% of all AAA. The wall is adherent to the intestines and sometimes the urethers are involved in the inflammatory process, leading to hydronephrosis. Steroids are advocated to reduce the inflammatory component and to obviate ureteral obstruction.

The inflammatory aneurysms are not less prone to rupture than ordinary AAA. Elective surgery through a retroperitoneal approach is recommended but EVAR has been used successfully.

Mycotic aneurysms

This infection in these aortic aneurysms is of hematogenous origin (most frequently gram positive agents). Local invasion of the vessel wall can lead to abscess or pseudo aneurysm formation. The risks are septic embolization and rupture. Early diagnosis is essential and the condition should be suspected in patients presenting clinically with signs of sepsis.

Signs on CT of mycotic aneurysm of the aorta include adjacent soft-tissue mass around the aortic wall with eventual rupture, gas-forming inflammation, and fluid in an unusual location. Mycotic (infectious) aortic aneurysms have been described throughout the whole arterial tree. Therefore, whenever a mycotic aneurysm is suspected, the whole vasculature should be investigated in order to localize other mycotic "aneurysmatic siblings."

In the thoracic aorta mycotic aneurysms can occur in conjunction with endocarditis, coarctation, persistent ductus arteriosus, and endovascular manipulations within the aorta. Aortic pseudo- or mycotic aneurysms following aortic vascular surgery occur rarely but with high mortality.

Excision of the aneurysm with insertion of an anatomical graft is the recommended treatment in combination with long-term antibiotics. In contained mycotic ruptures life-saving endovascular stent grafts have been proven effective [22, 38].

Thoracic dissections

Aortic dissection is a unique, complex aortic emergency with an incidence double that of ruptured abdominal aortic aneurysms, i.e. of 10–20 cases/million/y. An intimal focal tear or an intramural hematoma will result in a rapid surge of pulsatile blood to enter and propagate into and through the media layers of the aortic wall (Fig. 2.5). The dissection may propagate both proximally and distally from the point of initial injury. Aortic dissections are classified by location, duration of injury, and presence of ischemic complications. The creation of the false aortic lumen predisposes the patient to a sequence of dangerous events, which also are the indications for intervention and calls for immediate action:

1 rapid aortic aneurysm formation
2 ongoing organ ischemia caused by obstruction of primary aortic branch vessels
3 adverse hemodynamics
4 cardiac tamponade
5 aortic rupture

According to one of the commonly used classifications, The Stanford, type A dissection involves the ascending aorta and type B the descending. With the De Bakey classification type I involves the entire aorta, type II the ascending aorta, and type III the descending aorta. Atherosclerotic degeneration of the wall inherited disorders such as Marfan's and Ehlers–Danlos syndromes and hypertension predispose for dissection.

The intimal tear allows blood to flow into medial part of the wall separating the intima from the rest of the wall. The intimal flap separates the true and false lumens. The separation of the wall can obstruct branches, avulse, or thrombose them. The obstruction can be dynamic or static leading to malperfusion. Reentry into the true lumen unloads the dynamic stress on the wall by causing a spontaneous "fenestration." Multiple reentries are common, and should be thoroughly investigated

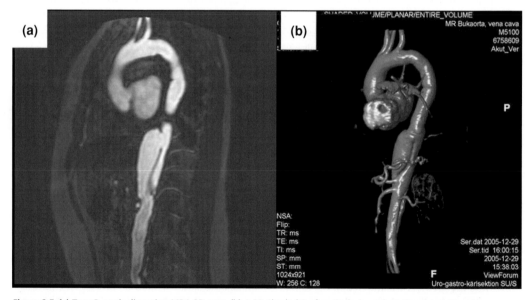

Figure 2.5 (a) Type B aortic dissection MRA 3D scan. (b) A 3D Shaded Surface Technique depicting a type B aortic dissection.

by the "state-of-the-art" imaging technique at the hospital.

The symptoms are usually very abrupt with severe chest pain, irradiating to the neck or arms. Back pain is typically seen in type B dissections. Other symptoms depend on the extent of dissection and organs involved. Abdominal pain, renal failure, paraplegia, or ischemia in the lower extremity can occur.

Type A dissection is particularly hazardous with high mortality if misdiagnosed or left untreated. Occlusion of the coronaries or carotids, aortic insufficiency or pericardial tamponade needs immediate surgery if the patient will have a fair chance of survival. The mortality is 1–2%/h during the early phase [39]. Medical treatment is not an option in type A dissection. The outcome, 40% 1-week mortality, is far inferior to surgical treatment even if open surgery still has an operative mortality of about 10%.

Type B dissections are routinely managed medically by a strict hypotensive regime. The aim is to limit the extent of the dissection, minimize stress on the aortic wall, prevent dilatation, and to create thrombosis of the false lumen. In-hospital mortality of medically treated type B patients is around 10%. In surgically treated patients mortality is over 30% [39].

Treatment strategies for type B dissection are constantly evolving. Endovascular treatment of dissections has been attempted for both types A and B. In both instances this treatment must be considered as experimental. This new treatment modality has been extensively explored in type B dissections. Others and we have reported preliminary results of both elective and emergency endoluminal treatment of type B dissection with a satisfactory outcome [23, 40].

The indication for treatment with endovascular stent grafts is still debatable in patients with acute or chronic aortic dissections [41]. Proximal dissections are not well suited for endovascular therapy because of the severe angulations of the aortic arch and the proximity to the coronary vasculature. Chronic dissections are often difficult to treat due to residual false lumen flow after deployment and ischemic complications from coverage of vessels arising from the false lumen. Uncomplicated dissections are typically managed with antihypertensive

medications. Thus, only acute complicated distal dissections may be appropriate for endovascular therapy, i.e. progressive aortic dilatation, aortic rupture, and in selected cases with end-organ ischemia. A recent large meta-analysis indicates that the endovascular treatment is technically possible in over 98% of the cases and that acute and midterm results are very promising. However, major complications occurred in 11% of the patients including neurological complications in 3% [40]. A proper comparison to medical treatment is needed to establish the future role of endovascular type B treatment.

Paraplegia is a concern in open surgery, but less so with endovascular treatment of thoracic diseases. The risk is higher if a long stent graft is used in the aorta (>20 cm) and when the region of eighth to tenth thoracic intercostal arteries is covered. In our opinion spinal drainage should be considered in these cases. Earlier percutaneous fenestration between true and false lumens with guide wires and balloons could reestablish blood-flow peripherally and may be used with or without concomitant treatment of the intimal tear by endoluminal stent grafting.

Intramural hematoma

The intramural hematoma (IMH) is one variant of dissection (Fig. 2.6). It may be caused by an intimal tear with a localized hematoma formation or by bleeding from a ruptured vasa vasorum. They constitute approximately 5–20% of all acute aortic syndromes. Hypertension is a predisposing factor in about half of the patients, the majority of which are men. A comprehensive meta-analysis of intramural hematomas was published some years ago, based on published reports from 143 cases [42]. Hematoma developed on the basis of an atherosclerotic ulcer had a progressive course as opposed to hematoma without ulcer that were more stable [43].

The symptoms do not differ initially from other acute aortic syndromes such as dissection with chest or back pain. CT, MRI, or transesophageal echocardiography (TEE) have a diagnostic sensitivity for intramural hematoma of 100% [44]. The hematoma is seen as a crescentic thickening of the wall extending for a distance of 5–20 cm. Typically, no entry point can be demonstrated in patients with intramural

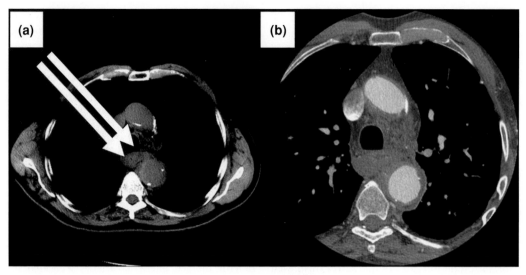

Figure 2.6 (a) Intramural hematoma without intravenous contrast. (b) Same image with intravenous contrast. Note the high density of the aortic wall even without contrast enhancement (arrow).

hematoma as opposed to dissections. Imaging is an essential part of management [45].

Many IMH resolve spontaneously. In one large single center study the majority (about 90%) had resolved after 1 year [6]. There does not seem to be a difference in outcome between type A and B hematoma even if type A may be a more serious event [46]. Medical, conservative treatment, including β-blockers, is inferior to open surgery in type A hematoma [42]. β-blockers seem to be an essential part of conservative management [46]. A more aggressive approach, which includes use of endovascular techniques, seems to be the current strategy [47]. Evangelista and coworkers have shown that the outcome of IMH is still like "flipping the coin." There is no evidence yet to predict which IMH that needs treatment [48].

Trauma in thoracic aorta

Most patients with a traumatic aortic rupture are involved in high velocity motor vehicle accidents, i.e. a blunt force trauma. Blunt aortic injury results in mortality of 70–90%. Of the approximately 20% who survive transport to a hospital, 50% die within 24 h and 90% within 4 months without expedient therapeutic measures. If the initial lesion is left untreated a chronic pseudo aneurysm will develop. Only patients with contained ruptures have

the chance of surviving long enough to get to a hospital. Short-term mortality in patients who survive open surgical repair ranges from 12 to 31%.

Arteriography is by many regarded as the "gold standard" for diagnosis. The classical widening of the aorta on a plain chest X-ray is notoriously unreliable. An enhanced multidetector CT examination with contrast of the whole aorta will diagnose the rupture with high accuracy. A 3D reconstruction can be of great value in characterizing the injury. The technique is rapidly becoming a new "gold standard."

Most lesions are situated just distal to the subclavian artery. A contained rupture will allow time enough for detailed surgical planning. A transesophageal echocardiogram can be very helpful in delineating details of the traumatic lesion but is very operator dependent. Patients with transection of the thoracic aorta usually have multiple traumatic injuries with damage to several other organs. Conventional open surgical repair adds a substantial trauma to these already heavily traumatized patients. Hemodynamically unstable patients have a very high mortality (up to 100%) but stable patients can be managed with very low or zero mortality [49]. Operative strategies and techniques are beyond the scope of this chapter. Access can be achieved through sternotomy or posterolateral thoracotomy, depending on the location of the injury. Repair can in simple cases be by clamp-and-sew technique or by left atrio-femoral bypass using a centrifugal pump. Full cardiopulmonary bypass under heparinization is seldom necessary. The risk for paraplegia seems to be higher after clamp-and-sew than after bypass unless clamping time is below 30 min [50].

In recent years endovascular treatment of hemodynamically stable patients with traumatic thoracic aortic injuries has been reported. The stent graft can be placed with a minimal invasive procedure, even under local anesthesia, if necessary. Few and small, noncontrolled studies on endovascular treatment of traumatic thoracic aortic injuries have been published. The endovascular approach seems at least in the short and midterm perspective at least as good as the open surgical alternative. Low mortality and few neurological complications, such as stroke or paraplegia, have been noticed with the stent-graft technique [49, 51–54].

Aortobronchial and aortoesophageal fistulas, although different in etiology, are similar to aneurysmal rupture in that massive hemorrhage is a common outcome. *Aortoenteric fistulas* are rare but life-threatening emergencies that demand immediate intervention. They are defined as a communication between aorta and the digestive system, the duodenum most commonly engaged. Causes of primary aortoenteric fistulas include aneurysms, pseudoaneurysms, infection, peptic ulcers, trauma, foreign body ingestion, inflammatory bowel disease (Crohn's disease), neoplasms, and radiotherapy. Secondary fistulas are well-documented late complications of open abdominal paraaortic surgeries, aortic aneurysm repair and endovascular aortic aneurysm repair.

Short-term mortality with open surgical repair for aortic fistula is high, up to 40%. Even if there is a substantial risk of continued infection in prosthetic graft, endovascular treatment might be a safe and effective alternative to open repair also in these high-risk patients. Mainly case reports have been published [55, 56].

References

1 Hass WK, Fields WS, North RR, Kircheff II, Chase NE, Bauer RB. Joint study of extracranialarterial occlusions: II. Arteriography, techniques, sites and complications. JAMA 1968; **203**: 961–968.

2 Gosselin C, Walker PM. Subclavian steal syndrome: Existence, clinical features, diagnosis and management. Semin Vasc Surg 1996; **9**: 93–97.

3 Sonesson B, Länne T, Hansen F, Sandgren T. Infrarenal aortic diameter in the healthy person. Eur J Vasc Surg 1994; **8**: 89–95.

4 Åstrand H, Rydén-Ahlgren Å, Sandgren T, Länne T. Age-related increase in wall stress of the human abdominal aorta: An in vivo study. J Vasc Surg 2005; **42**: 926–931.

5 Sonesson B, Länne T, Vernersson E, Hansen F. Sex difference in the mechanical properties of the abdominal aorta in human beings. J Vasc Surg 1994; **20**: 959–969.

6 Cho KR, Stanson AW, Potter DD, Cherry KJ, Schaff HV, Sundt TM. Penetrating atherosclerotic ulcer of the descending thoracic aorta. J Thorac Cardiovasc Surg 2004; **127**: 1393–1401.

7 Absi TS, Sundt TM, Camillo C, Schuessler RB, Gutierrez FR. Penetrating atherosclerotic ulcers of the descending thoracic aorta may be managed expectantly. Vascular 2004; **12**: 307–311.

8 Tittle SL, Lynch RJ, Cole PE, Singh HS, Rizzo JA, Kopf GS *et al.* Midterm follow-up of penetrating ulcer and intramural hematoma of the aorta. J Thorac Cardiovasc Surg 2002; **123**: 1051–1059.

9 Bickerstaff LK, Pairolero PC, Hollier LH, Melton LJ, VanPeenen HJ, Cherry KJ *et al.* Thoracic aortic aneurysms: A population-based study. Surgery 1982; **92**: 1103–1108.

10 McNamara JJ, Pressler VM. Natural history of arteriosclerotic thoracic aortic aneurysms. Ann Thorac Surg 1978; **26**: 468–473.

11 Clouse WD, Hallett JW, Schaff HV, Gayari MM, Ilstrup DM, Melton DM. Improved prognosis of thoracic aortic aneurysms: A population based study. JAMA 1998; **280**: 1926–1929.

12 Johansson G, Markström U, Swedenborg J. Ruptured thoracic aneurysms: A study of incidence and mortality rates. J Vasc Surg 1995; **21**: 985–988.

13 Diethrich EB, Ghazoul M, Wheatley GH, Alpern J, Rodriguez-Lopez J, Ramaiah V *et al.* Surgical correction of ascending type a thoracic aortic dissection: Simultaneous endoluminal exclusion of the arch and distal aorta. J Endovasc Ther 2005; **12**: 6660–6666.

14 Inoue K, Hosokawa H, Iwase T, Sato M, Yoshida Y, Ueno K *et al.* Aortic arch reconstruction by transluminally placed endovascular branched stent graft. Circulation 1999; **100**(Suppl): 316–321.

15 Ischimaru S. Endografting of the aortic arch. J Endovasc Ther 2004; **11**(Suppl 2): 62–71.

16 Greenberg RK, Haddad F, Svensson L, O'Neill S, Walker E, Lyden SP *et al.* Hybrid approaches to thoracic aortic aneurysms: The role of endovascular elephant trunk completion. Circulation 2005; **112**: 2619–2626.

17 Bergeron P, Coulon P, De Chaumaray T, Ruiz M, Mariotti F, Gay J *et al*. Great vessel transposition and aortic arch exclusion. J Cardiovasc Surg (Torino) 2005; **46**: 141–147.

18 Joyce JW, Fairbairn JF, Kincaid OW, Juergens JL. Aneurysms of the thoracic aorta. A clinical study with special reference to prognosis. Circulation 1964; **29**: 176–181.

19 Juvonen T, Ergin A, Galla JD, Lansman SL, Nguyen KH, McCullough JW *et al*. Prospective study of the natural history of thoracic aortic aneurysms. Ann Thorac Surg 1997; **63**: 1533–1545.

20 Volodos ML, Karpovich IP, Troyan VI, Kalashnikova YV, Shekhanin VE, Ternyuk NE *et al*. Clinical experience of the use of self-fixating synthetic prosthesis for remote endoprosthesis of the thoracic and abdominal aorta and iliac arteries through the femoral artery and as intraoperative endoprosthesis for aortic reconstruction. Vasa 1991; **33**(Suppl): 93–95.

21 Dake MD, Miller DC, Semba CP, Mitchell RS, Walker PJ, Liddell RP. Transluminal placement of endovascular stent-grafts for the treatment of of descending thoracic aortic aneurysms. N Engl J Med 1994; **331**: 1729–1734.

22 Lepore V, Lönn L, Delle M, Bugge M, Jeppsson A, Kjellman U *et al*. Endograft therapy for aneurysms and dissections of the thoracic aorta in 43 consecutive patients. J Endovasc Ther 2002; **9**: 829–837.

23 Lönn L, Delle M, Falkenberg M, Lepore V, Klingenstierna H, Rådberg G *et al*. Endovascular treatment of type B thoracic aortic dissections. J Card Surg 2003; **18**: 539–544.

24 Svensson LG, Crawford ES, Hess KR, Coselli JS, Safi HJ. Experience with 1509 patients undergoing thoracoabdominal aortic operations. J Vasc Surg 1993; **17**: 357–370.

25 Crawford ES. Thoracoabdominal and abdominal aortic aneurysm involving renal, superior mesenteric and celiac arteries. Ann Surg 1974; **179**: 763–772.

26 Coselli JS, LeMaire SA, Miller CC, Schmittling ZC, Koksov C, Pagan J *et al*. Mortality and paraplegia after thoracoabdominal aortic aneurysm repair: A risk factor analysis. Ann Thorac Surg 2000; **69**: 409–414.

27 LeMaire SA, Miller CC, Conklin LD, Schmittling ZC, Coselli JS. Estimating group mortality and paraplegia rates after thoracoabdominal aortic aneurysm repair. Ann Thorac Surg 2003; **75**: 508–513.

28 Coselli JS, LeMaire SA, Conklin LD, Koksov C, Schmittling ZC. Morbidity and mortality after extent II thoracoabdominal aortic aneurysm repair. Ann Thorac Surg 2002; **73**: 1107–1115.

29 Jacobs MJ, Mess WH. The role of motor evoked potential monitoring in operative management of type I and type II thoracoabdominal aortic aneurysms. Semin Thorac Cardiovasc Surg 2003; **15**: 353–364.

30 Stanley BM, Semmens JB, Lawrence-Brown MM, Goodman MA, Hartley DE. Fenestration in endovascular grafts for aortic aneurysm repair: New horizons for preserving blood flow in branch vessels. J Endovasc Surg 2001; **8**: 16–24.

31 Verhoeven EL, Zeebregts CJ, Kapma MR, Tielliu IF, Prins TR, van den Dungen JJ. Fenestrated and branched endovascular techniques for thoracoabdominal aneurysm repair. J Cardiovasc Surg (Torino) 2005; **46**: 131–140.

32 Chuter TA, Gordon RL, Reilly LM, Pak LK, Messina LM. Multi-branched stent-graft for type III thoracoabdominal aortic aneurysm. J Vasc Interv Radiol 2001; **12**: 391–392.

33 Bengtsson H, Norrgård Ö, Ängkvist KA, Ekberg O, Öberg L, Bergqvist D. Ultrasonographic screening of the abdominal aorta among siblings of patients with abdominal aortic aneurysms. Br J Surg 1989; **76**: 598–601.

34 Multicentre Aneurysm Screening Study (MASS): Cost effectiveness analysis of screening for abdominal aortic aneurysm based on four year results from a randomised controlled trial. BMJ 2002; **325**: 1135.

35 The UK small aneurysm trial. Mortality results for randomised controlled trial of early elective surgery or ultrasonographic surveillance for small abdominal aortic aneurysms. Lancet 1998; **253**: 1649–1655.

36 Peppelenbosch N, Cuypers PW, Vahl AC, Vermassen F, Buth J. Emergency endovascular treatment for ruptured abdominal aortic aneurysm and the risk for spinal cord ischemia. J Vasc Surg 2005; **42**: 608–614.

37 Resch T, Malina M, Lindblad B, Dias NV, Sonesson B, Ivancev K. Endovascular repari of ruptured abdominal aortic aneurysms: Logistics and short-term results. J Endovasc Ther 2003; **10**: 440–446.

38 Smith JJ, Taylor PR. Endovascular treatment of mycotic aneurysms of the thoracic and abdominal aorta: The need for level I evidence. Eur J Vasc Endovasc Surg 2004; **27**: 569–570.

39 Hagan PG, Nienaber CA, Isselbacher EM, Bruckman D, Karavite DJ, Russman PL *et al*. The international registry of acute aortic dissection (IRAD): New insights into and old disease. JAMA 2000; **283**: 897–903.

40 Eggebrecht H, Nienaber CA, Neuhäuser M, Baumgart D, Kische S, Schmermund A *et al*. Endovascular stent-graft placement in aortic dissection: A meta-analysis. Eur Heart J 2006 Feb; **27**(4): 489–498.

41 Eggebrecht H, Lönn L, Herold U, Breukmann F, Leyh R, Jakob HG *et al*. Endovascular stent-graft placement for complications of acute type B aortic dissections. Curr Opin Cardiol 2005; **20**: 477–483.

42 Maraj R, Rerkpattananpipat P, Jacobs LE, Makornwattana P, Kotler MN. Meta-analysis of 143 reported cases of aortic intramural hematoma. Am J Cardiol 2000; **86**: 664–668.

43 Ganaha F, Miller DC, Sugimoto K, Minamiguchi H, Saito H, Mitchell RS *et al*. The prognosis of aortic intramural

hematoma with and without penetrating atherosclerotic ulcer: A clinical and radiological analysis. Circulation 2002; **106**: 342–348.

44 Nienaber AC, von Kodolitsch Y, Petersen B, Loose R, Helmchen U, Haverich A *et al*. Intramural hemorrhage of the thoracic aorta. Diagnostic and therapeutic implications. Circulation 1995; **92**: 1465–1472.

45 Nienaber CA, Sievers HA. Intramural hematoma in acute aortic syndrome. Circulation 2002; **106**: 284–287.

46 von Kodolitsch Y, Csosz SK, Koschvk DH, Schalwat I, Loose R, Karck M *et al*. Intramural hematoma of the aorta: Predictors of progression to dissection and rupture. Circulation 2003; **107**: 1158–1163.

47 Dake M. Aortic intramural haematoma: Current therapeutic strategy. Heart 2004; **90**: 375–378.

48 Evangelista A, Dominguez R, Sebastia C, Salas A, Permanyer-Miralda G, Avegliano G *et al*. Prognostic value of clinical and morphological findings in short-term evaluation of aortic intramural haematoma. Therapeutic implications. Eur Heart J 2004; **25**: 81–87.

49 Stampfl P, Greitbauer M, Zimpfer D, Fleck T, Schoder M, Lammer J *et al*. Mid-term results of conservative, conventional and endovascular treatment for acute traumatic aortic lesions. Eur J Vasc Endovasc Surg 2006 May; **31**(5): 475–480.

50 Fabian TC, Richardson JD, Croce MD, Smith JS, Rodman G, Kearny PA *et al*. Prospective study of blunt aortic injury: Multicenter trial of the American association for the surgery of trauma. J Trauma 1997; **42**: 374–383.

51 Wellons ED, Milner R, Solis M, Levitt A, Rosenthal D. Stent-graft repair of traumatic thoracic aortic disruptions. J Vasc Surg 2004; **40**: 1095–1100.

52 Amabile P, Collart F, Gariboldi V, Rollet G, Bartoli JM, Piquet P. Surgical versus endovascular treatment of traumatic thoracic aortic rupture. J Vasc Surg 2004; **40**: 873–879.

53 Eggebrecht H, Schmermund A, Herold U, Baumgart D, Martini S, Kuhnt O *et al*. Endovascular stent-graft placement for acute and contained rupture of the descending aorta. Catheter Cardiovasc Interv 2005; **66**: 474–482.

54 Dunham MB, Zygun D, Petrasek P, Kortbeek JB, Karmy-Jones R, Moore RD. Endovascular stent grafts for acute blunt aortic injury. J Trauma 2004; **56**: 1173–1178.

55 Chuter TA, Ivancev K, Lindblad B, Brunkwall J, Ahren C, Risberg B. Endovascular stent-graft exclusion of an aortobronchial fistula. J Vasc Interv Radiol 1996; **7**: 357–359.

56 Bockler D, Schumacher H, Schwartzbach M, Ockert S, Rotert H, Allenberg JR. Endoluminal stent-graft repair of aortobronchial fistulas: Bridging of definitive long-term solution? J Endovasc Ther 2004; **11**: 41–48.

CHAPTER 3

Thoracic aortic aneurysms: classification, incidence, etiology, natural history, and results

Hazim J. Safi

In the mid-1950s, the first thoracoabdominal aortic aneurysm (TAAA) repairs were performed, first with a homograft in 1955 then using a Dacron tube graft in 1956. In the following decades (1960s, 1970s, and early 1980s), results of TAAA and descending thoracic aortic aneurysm (DTAA) repair varied tremendously from center to center. This was probably due to the lack of coherent methods of reporting and an agreed-upon classification of the aneurysms.

With this in mind, we are going to describe our rationale for classifications of the DTAA and TAAA. In the last decade, we began classifying descending thoracic aneurysms based upon whether they affect the upper half, lower half, or entire thoracic aorta, known as types A, B, and C, respectively (Fig. 3.1). Type A involves the upper half, type B involves the 6th intercostal space to T12, and type C comprises the entire thoracic aorta. During the era of the clamp-and-sew technique, some reported cases showed that the maximum incidence of neurological deficit involved types B and C.

TAAA is an extensive aneurysm involving the thoracic aorta and varying degrees of the abdominal aorta. We categorize these using the modified "Crawford classification," which is shown in Fig. 3.2. Extent I is from the left subclavian artery to above the renal arteries. Extent II is from the left subclavian artery to below the renal arteries, and extent III is from the 6th intercostal space to below the renal arteries. Extent IV involves the total abdominal aorta from T12 to below the renal arteries. Extent V, which has been described in the last half decade, is

from the upper extent of the 6th intercostal space to the lower extent above the renal arteries. In the past, we found that the extent of the aneurysm correlated with a high incidence of neurological deficit, the highest being in extent II and then extents I, III, and IV. In the era of the clamp-and-sew technique, the clamp time and the extent of the aneurysm correlated to neurologic deficit. In extent II, the overall incidence of neurological deficit was 31% [1].

Incidence

Ruptured aortic aneurysms remain the 13th leading cause of death in the United States with an increasing prevalence [2]; this may be attributable to improved imaging techniques, increasing mean age of the population, and overall heightened awareness [3]. The incidence of rupture abdominal aortic aneurysms is estimated to be 9.2 cases per 100,000 person-years [4–6]. The incidence of rupture thoracic aortic aneurysms and acute aortic dissection is estimated to be 2.7 and 3.0 cases per 100,000 person-years, respectively [7–10]. The mean age of this population is between 59 and 69 years with a male to female ratio of 3:1 [7].

Etiology

Arteriosclerosis has long been associated with aortic aneurysms, but each affects different layers of the aortic wall. Atherosclerosis mainly affects the intima, causing occlusive disease, while aortic

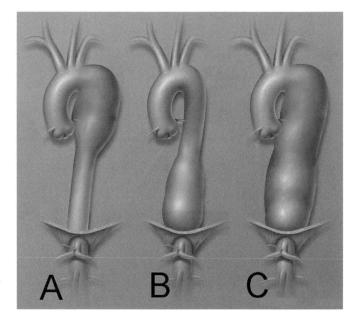

Figure 3.1 Classification of descending thoracic aortic aneurysms (DTAAs): Type A involves the upper half of the DTAA, type B involves the 6th intercostal space to T12 of the DTAA, and type C comprises the entire DTAA.

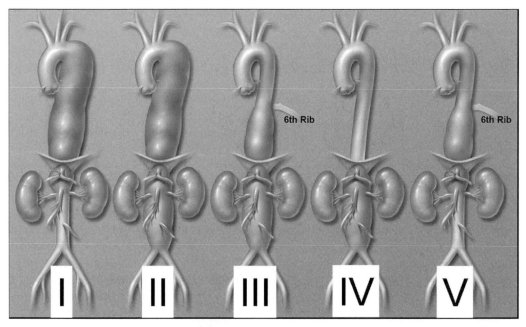

Figure 3.2 The modified Crawford classification of thoracoabdominal aortic aneurysms (TAAAs). Extent I is from the left subclavian artery to above the renal arteries. Extent II is from the left subclavian artery to below the renal arteries. Extent III is from the 6th intercostal space to below the renal arteries. Extent IV involves the total abdominal aorta from T12 to below the renal arteries. Extent V is from the upper extent of the 6th intercostal space to the lower extent above the renal arteries.

aneurysm is a disease of the media and adventitia. They are distinct conditions that nonetheless often occur together. An aortic aneurysm is typically characterized by a thinning of the media and destruction of smooth muscle cells and elastin as well as infiltration of inflammatory cells. The infiltrate consists of macrophages as well as T and B lymphocytes, which excrete proteases and elastases causing wall degradation [11]. The reason for this migration is unclear. In both clinical and experimental studies, metalloproteinases (MMP), a most prominent group of elastases, have emerged as playing a role in the development of aortic aneurysms [11–14].

Familial clustering of aortic aneurysms is evident as up to 20% of patients have one or more first-degree relatives who have also suffered from the disease [15–17]. Genetic mapping studies have recently identified a number of chromosomal loci that are responsible for familial thoracic aneurysms and dissections. A mutation in transforming growth factor-β receptor type II is responsible for approximately 5% of familial aneurysms and dissections [18]. Future studies may further elucidate the role of genetics in this disease process.

Marfan syndrome, a connective tissue disorder causing skeletal, ocular, and cardiovascular abnormalities, is the disorder most commonly associated with TAAA as well as aortic dissection. It occurs in approximately 1 in 5000 people worldwide. Aortic dilation in individuals with Marfan has been linked to a mutation in fibrillin-1. Other such disorders include Ehlers–Danlos syndrome, Turner syndrome, polycystic kidney disease, as well as other not yet identified familial disorders [19]. In the majority of these families, the phenotype for TAAA and dissection are inherited in an autosomal dominant manner with a marked variability in age and decreased penetrance [19].

At times, an aneurysm may be caused by an extrinsic factor, such as infection (mycotic aneurysm) or trauma (pseudoaneurysm). A mycotic aneurysm is caused by bacteria or septic emboli that seed the aortic wall or resulting from a contiguous spread from empyema or adjacent infected lymph node. Though any organism can be the cause of a mycotic aneurysm, the most commonly described are salmonella, hemophilus influenza, staphylococcus, and treponema pallidum spirochetes species [20, 21].

There is also a connection between TAAA and aortic dissection. One quarter of TAAA are associated with aortic dissection, and 24% of patients with an aortic dissection will develop TAAA within 2 to 5 years [15–17]. Persistent patency of the false lumen has been shown to be a significant predictor for aneurysm formation, though neither dissection nor false lumen has been linked to higher risk of rupture [22–25].

Natural history

The survival rate for patients with untreated thoracic aortic aneurysms is dismal, estimated to be between 13 and 39% at 5 years [7, 26–28]. The lifetime probability of rupture in untreated thoracic aneurysms and TAA is between 75 and 80% [7, 26]. The most common cause of death is rupture [29]. Moreover, the few patients who survive to operation sustain significant morbidity, prolonged hospital course, and, ultimately, a poor quality of life.

The time that elapses between aneurysm formation and rupture is influenced by aneurysm size and growth rate, hypertension, smoking, history of chronic obstructive pulmonary disease, presence of pain, etiology, and age. The size of the aortic aneurysm remains the single most important determinant of the likelihood of rupture. Rupture is more likely to occur in TAAs exceeding 5 cm in diameter with the likelihood increasing significantly as the aneurysm enlarges [26, 30–33]. Growth rate is a component in formulating the rate of rupture or indication for surgical intervention [30, 34]. The rate of growth is exponential with larger aneurysms growing at greater rates; at 0.12 cm/y for aneurysms greater than 5.2 cm in diameter [34, 35].

Hypertension and subsequent increased aortic wall tension play a significant role in aneurysm formation. The law of Laplace states that as the diameter of a cylinder increases, the tension applied to the wall also increases. This indicates that the wall tension is directly related to pressure. Though systemic hypertension is widely recognized as a risk factor for aneurysm formation, it is diastolic blood pressure that has been specifically correlated with aneurysm rupture. Multiple reports have noted an association of increased diastolic blood pressure (greater than 100 mmHg) with rupture of both abdominal and thoracic aortic aneurysms [30, 34, 36]. As was demonstrated by Wheat in his work on aortic dissections, decreasing the force of myocardial contraction or *dp/dt* may decrease the progression of disease and the likelihood of rupture [37]. Consequently, it is recommended that beta-adrenergic blocking agents be included in the antihypertensive treatment regimen for patients with known aortic aneurysms.

Although smoking has been implicated as a risk factor for rupture in abdominal aortic aneurysms [38, 39], a stronger association with chronic obstructive pulmonary disease has been identified [30, 34]. In one study, chronic obstructive pulmonary disease was defined as a forced expiratory volume in 1 s (FEV1) of less than 50% of predicted [39]. This correlation may be related to increased collagenase activity as seen in smokers [40]. It is theorized that the proteolytic activity may weaken the aortic wall of those patients that are susceptible [41]. Patients with chronic obstructive pulmonary disease have demonstrated a connective tissue intolerance to smoke-related toxicity, which may be seen as an indicator of susceptibility [42]. In addition, it has been documented that patients with a history of smoking have a more rapid expansion of thoracic aneurysms [34, 43]. This evidence justifies the cessation of smoking in the presence of an aortic aneurysm.

Further implicated in the increased likelihood of aortic rupture are pain, chronic dissection, and age. Vague or uncharacteristic pain in the presence of TAA has been significantly associated with subsequent rupture [30]. Generally, the etiology of TAA has been attributed to a degenerative process. It has also been suggested that rupture is associated with chronic dissection, but the evidence is not compelling [7, 44]. In a prospective study by Juvonen *et al.* aneurysms associated with chronic dissection were observed to be smaller (median diameter of 5.4 cm) than degenerative aneurysms (median diameter of 5.8 cm) [45]. Significant alterations in the structure of the aortic wall occur with aging that are distinct from the formation of aneurysms. However, age in TAA patients has been associated with increased risk of rupture [9]. Furthermore, Juvonen *et al.* demonstrated that the relative risk for rupture increased by a factor of 2.6 for every decade of age [9].

The natural course of the majority of aortic aneurysms is rupture and death. Aneurysm size and growth rate, patient age, medical history, and symptoms must be carefully weighed while considering when to intervene surgically; however, elective surgery for TAA repair has been demonstrated to improve long-term survival [28]. Methods have been devised to attempt to predict the risks of surgical repair for TAAs [30, 34]. Although these formulas may allow one to preoperatively stratify the risks of surgery for a patient, the decision to operate still remains with the surgeon based upon the surgeon's clinical evaluation and the patient's preference.

Results

Between February 1991 and March 2005, we performed 1887 operations for ascending/arch or descending thoracic/TAAAs. Seven hundred eighty one of these cases involved the proximal aorta (ascending and transverse arch). The 30-day mortality in this group of patients was 11.5% (90/781). The stroke rate was 2.1% (16/781).

We performed 1106 operations for repair of the distal aorta (descending thoracic, $n = 305$, and TAAAs, $n = 801$). The 30-day mortality rate was 14.5% with an immediate neurological deficit rate of 3.2%. The mortality rate highly correlates with preoperative renal function as determined by calculated glomerular filtration rate (GFR). Patients with a GFR greater than 90 ml/min/1.73 m^2 had a mortality rate of 5.6% compared to a rate of 27.8% in patient with a GFR less than 49 ml/min/1.73 m^2 [46].

Approximately 80% of patients who underwent surgical repair of the descending thoracic aorta in our series did so with the adjunct (cerebrospinal fluid drainage and distal aortic perfusion). The remaining 20% underwent simple crossclamp with or without the use of a single adjunct [47]. Aortic crossclamp times have increased significantly (34 s/y) since 1991. Despite this increase in crossclamp time, neurologic deficit rates have declined from the first to the fourth quartile. This decrease in neurologic deficit is most pronounced with extent II TAAAs (21.1% to 3.3%). The use of the adjunct (cerebrospinal fluid drainage and distal aortic perfusion) increased the crossclamp time by a mean of 12 min, but was associated with a significant protective effect against neurologic deficit.

Although other previously established risk factors remained significantly associated with neurologic deficit, crossclamp time is no longer significant [48]. The adjunct significantly reduced the risk of neurologic deficit, despite increasing crossclamp time. The use of the adjunct appears to blunt the effect of the crossclamp time and may provide the surgeon the ability to operate without being hurried. Because crossclamp time has been effectively eliminated as a risk factor with the use of the adjunct, using this variable to construct risk models becomes irrelevant in our experience.

In repairs of DTAA, the incidence of neurologic deficit after all repairs was 2.3%. The incidence of neurologic deficit (immediate and delayed) in the adjunct group was 1.3%, and in the nonadjunct group was 6.5%. One case of delayed paraplegia occurred in each group. All neurologic deficits occurred in patients with aneurysmal involvement of the entire descending thoracic aorta. Statistically significant predictors for neurologic deficit were the use of the adjunct, previously repaired abdominal aortic aneurysm, type C aneurysm, and cerebrovascular disease history. Significant multivariate predictors of 30-day mortality were preoperative renal dysfunction and female sex.

Remarkable progress in the treatment of TAAAs has been achieved in the last decade. Morbidity and mortality have declined which we attribute to the adoption of the adjuncts distal aortic perfusion and CSF drainage as well as the evolution of surgical techniques to include sequential aortic crossclamp, intercostal artery reattachment, and moderate hypothermia. Currently, the overall incidence of neurological deficit in DTAA is 0.8% and mortality rate in patients with normal renal function is 5%.

The introduction of endovascular repair has added a new approach to the armamentarium of surgeons treating this disease. Currently available technology is limited by patients' anatomical criteria. Future advances will widen the availability of this approach to a larger group of patients.

For now, aortic surgeons need to maintain expertise in both open and endovascular approaches. Regardless of the technique, complex aortic aneurysms should be treated in centers with the capability and experience necessary to manage this challenging group of patients.

References

1 Svensson LG, Crawford ES, Hess KR *et al.* Experience with 1509 patients undergoing thoracoabdominal aortic operations. J Vasc Surg 1993; **17**: 357–368; discussion 368–370.

2 Coady MA, Rizzo JA, Goldstein LJ, Elefteriades JA. Natural history, pathogenesis, and etiology of thoracic aortic aneurysms and dissections. Cardiol Clin 1999; **17**: 615–635; vii.

3 LaRoy LL, Cormier PJ, Matalon TA *et al.* Imaging of abdominal aortic aneurysms. AJR Am J Roentgenol 1989; **152**: 785–792.

4 Bengtsson H, Bergqvist D. Ruptured abdominal aortic aneurysm: A population-based study. J Vasc Surg 1993; **18**: 74–80.

5 Bickerstaff LK, Hollier LH, Van Peenen HJ *et al.* Abdominal aortic aneurysms: The changing natural history. J Vasc Surg 1984; **1**: 6–12.

6 Choksy SA, Wilmink AB, Quick CR. Ruptured abdominal aortic aneurysm in the Huntingdon district: A 10-year experience. Ann R Coll Surg Engl 1999; **81**: 27–31.

7 Bickerstaff LK, Pairolero PC, Hollier LH *et al.* Thoracic aortic aneurysms: A population-based study. Surgery 1982; **92**: 1103–1108.

8 Clouse WD, Hallett JW, Jr., Schaff HV *et al.* Acute aortic dissection: Population-based incidence compared with degenerative aortic aneurysm rupture. Mayo Clin Proc 2004; **79**: 176–180.

9 Johansson G, Markstrom U, Swedenborg J. Ruptured thoracic aortic aneurysms: A study of incidence and mortality rates. J Vasc Surg 1995; **21**: 985–988.

10 Meszaros I, Morocz J, Szlavi J *et al.* Epidemiology and clinicopathology of aortic dissection. Chest 2000; **117**: 1271–1278.

11 Ailawadi G, Eliason JL, Upchurch GR, Jr. Current concepts in the pathogenesis of abdominal aortic aneurysm. J Vasc Surg 2003; **38**: 584–588.

12 Longo GM, Xiong W, Greiner TC *et al.* Matrix metalloproteinases 2 and 9 work in concert to produce aortic aneurysms. J Clin Invest 2002; **110**: 625–632.

13 Annabi B, Shedid D, Ghosn P *et al.* Differential regulation of matrix metalloproteinase activities in abdominal aortic aneurysms. J Vasc Surg 2002; **35**: 539–546.

14 McMillan WD, Pearce WH. Increased plasma levels of metalloproteinase-9 are associated with abdominal aortic aneurysms. J Vasc Surg 1999; **29**: 122–127; discussion 127–129.

15 Biddinger A, Rocklin M, Coselli J, Milewicz DM. Familial thoracic aortic dilatations and dissections: A case control study. J Vasc Surg 1997; **25**: 506–511.

16 Coady MA, Davies RR, Roberts M *et al.* Familial patterns of thoracic aortic aneurysms. Arch Surg 1999; **134**: 361–367.

17 Hasham SN, Willing MC, Guo DC *et al.* Mapping a locus for familial thoracic aortic aneurysms and dissections (TAAD2) to 3p24-25. Circulation 2003; **107**: 3184–3190.

18 Pannu H, Fadulu VT, Chang J *et al.* Mutations in transforming growth factor-beta receptor type II cause familial thoracic aortic aneurysms and dissections. Circulation 2005; **112**: 513–520.

19 Milewicz DM, Chen H, Park ES *et al.* Reduced penetrance and variable expressivity of familial thoracic aortic aneurysms/dissections. Am J Cardiol 1998; **82**: 474–479.

20 Jarrett F, Darling RC, Mundth ED, Austen WG. Experience with infected aneurysms of the abdominal aorta. Arch Surg 1975; **110**: 1281–1286.

21 Bakker-de Wekker P, Alfieri O, Vermeulen F *et al.* Surgical treatment of infected pseudoaneurysms after replacement of the ascending aorta. J Thorac Cardiovasc Surg 1984; **88**: 447–451.

22 Bernard Y, Zimmermann H, Chocron S *et al.* False lumen patency as a predictor of late outcome in aortic dissection. Am J Cardiol 2001; **87**: 1378–1382.

23 Marui A, Mochizuki T, Mitsui N *et al.* Toward the best treatment for uncomplicated patients with type B acute aortic dissection: A consideration for sound surgical indication. Circulation 1999; **100**: II275– II280.

24 Juvonen T, Ergin MA, Galla JD *et al.* Risk factors for rupture of chronic type B dissections [In Process Citation]. J Thorac Cardiovasc Surg 1999; **117**: 776–786.

25 Sueyoshi E, Sakamoto I, Hayashi K *et al.* Growth rate of aortic diameter in patients with type B aortic dissection during the chronic phase. Circulation 2004; **110**: II256– II261.

26 Perko MJ, Norgaard M, Herzog TM *et al.* Unoperated aortic aneurysm: A survey of 170 patients. Ann Thorac Surg 1995; **59**: 1204–1209.

27 Pressler V, McNamara JJ. Thoracic aortic aneurysm: Natural history and treatment. J Thorac Cardiovasc Surg 1980; **79**: 489–498.

28 Crawford ES, DeNatale RW. Thoracoabdominal aortic aneurysm: Observations regarding the natural course of the disease. J Vasc Surg 1986; **3**: 578–582.

29 Bonser RS, Pagano D, Lewis ME *et al.* Clinical and pathoanatomical factors affecting expansion of thoracic aortic aneurysms. Heart 2000; **84**: 277–283.

30 Juvonen T, Ergin MA, Galla JD *et al.* Prospective study of the natural history of thoracic aortic aneurysms. Ann Thorac Surg 1997; **63**: 1533–1545.

31 Lobato AC, Puech-Leao P. Predictive factors for rupture of thoracoabdominal aortic aneurysm. J Vasc Surg 1998; **27**: 446–453.

32 Elefteriades JA, Hartleroad J, Gusberg RJ *et al.* Long-term experience with descending aortic dissection: The complication-specific approach. Ann Thorac Surg 1992; **53**: 11–20; discussion 20–21.

33 Cambria RA, Gloviczki P, Stanson AW *et al.* Outcome and expansion rate of 57 thoracoabdominal aortic aneurysms managed nonoperatively. Am J Surg 1995; **170**: 213–217.

34 Dapunt OE, Galla JD, Sadeghi AM *et al.* The natural history of thoracic aortic aneurysms. J Thorac Cardiovasc Surg 1994; **107**: 1323–1332; discussion 1332–1333.

35 Rizzo JA, Coady MA, Elefteriades JA. Procedures for estimating growth rates in thoracic aortic aneurysms. J Clin Epidemiol 1998; **51**: 747–754.

36 Szilagyi DE, Smith RF, DeRusso FJ *et al.* Contribution of abdominal aortic aneurysmectomy to prolongation of life. Ann Surg 1966; **164**: 678–699.

37 Palmer RF, Wheat MW. Management of impending rupture of the aorta with dissection. Adv Intern Med 1971; **17**: 409–423.

38 Strachan DP. Predictors of death from aortic aneurysm among middle-aged men: The Whitehall study. Br J Surg 1991; **78**: 401–414.

39 Cronenwett JL, Murphy TF, Zelenock GB *et al.* Actuarial analysis of variables associated with rupture of small abdominal aortic aneurysms. Surgery 1985; **98**: 472–483.

40 Cannon DJ, Read RC. Blood elastolytic activity in patients with aortic aneurysm. Ann Thorac Surg 1982; **34**: 10–15.

41 Busuttil RW, Abou-Zamzam AM, Machleder HI. Collagenase activity of the human aorta: A comparison of patients with and without abdominal aortic aneurysm. Arch Surg 1980; **115**: 1373–1378.

42 Ergin MA, Spielvogel D, Apaydin A *et al.* Surgical treatment of the dilated ascending aorta: When and how? Ann Thorac Surg 1999; **67**: 1834–1839; discussion 1853–1856.

43 Lindholt JS, Jorgensen B, Fasting H, Henneberg EW. Plasma levels of plasmin–antiplasmin-complexes are predictive for small abdominal aortic aneurysms expanding to operation-recommendable sizes. J Vasc Surg 2001; **34**: 611–615.

44 Pitt MP, Bonser RS. The natural history of thoracic aortic aneurysm disease: An overview. J Card Surg 1997; **12**: 270–278.

45 Juvonen T, Ergin MA, Galla JD *et al.* Risk factors for rupture of chronic type B dissections. J Thorac Cardiovasc Surg 1999; **117**: 776–786.

46 Huynh TT, van Eps RG, Miller CC, 3rd *et al.* Glomerular filtration rate is superior to serum creatinine for prediction of mortality after thoracoabdominal aortic surgery. J Vasc Surg 2005; **42**: 206–212.

47 Estrera AL, Miller CC, 3rd, Chen EP *et al.* Descending thoracic aortic aneurysm repair: 12-year experience using distal aortic perfusion and cerebrospinal fluid drainage. Ann Thorac Surg 2005; **80**: 1290–1296; discussion 1296.

48 Safi HJ, Estrera AL, Miller CC *et al.* Evolution of risk for neurologic deficit after descending and thoracoabdominal aortic repair. Ann Thorac Surg 2005; **80**: 2173–2179; discussion 2179.

CHAPTER 4

Angiographic aortic anatomy and variants

Louis G. Martin

From day 29 to week 7 of human cardiovascular development a common arterial trunk, the truncus arteriosis, emerges from the bulbus cordis. Two primitive ventral (ascending) aortae continue via symmetrical aortic arches into primitive dorsal (descending) aortae [1]. The proximal portions of the ventral aortae fuse to form a single midline trunk (the aortic sac). The paired dorsal aortae fuse to form a midline descending aorta. Between the ventral and dorsal aortae, the first two pairs of symmetrical branchial aortic arches develop. Six paired branchial arches eventually develop between the dorsal and ventral aortas. Although there are six primitive pairs of arches, they are not all present at the same time [1, 2]. As the branchial arches are developing and regressing the aortic sac divides into what will become the pulmonary trunk and ascending aorta. The third arches and dorsal aorta cephalad to these arches become the internal carotid arteries. The ventral aorta cephalad to the third arches forms the external carotid arteries. The fourth branchial arches form paired (double) aortic arches. The fifth branchial arches regress completely. The sixth branchial arches form the ductus arteriosis and the pulmonary arteries. The seventh branchial arteries migrate cephalad to a position between the ductus arteriosis and the common carotid arteries and become the subclavian arteries [1]. At this point in development a double arch is formed (Fig. 4.1). The hypothetical "Edwards double arch" [2] can now be used to explain the further development of the aortic arch and its variations [3].

The normal *left aortic arch* results from interruption of the dorsal segment of the embryonic right arch between the right subclavian artery and the descending aorta with regression of the right

ductus arteriosis (Figs. 4.2 & 4.3). The midline dorsal aorta shifts to the left of the spine to become the descending aorta (Fig. 4.4) [2]. Not infrequently, a small diverticulum arises from the medial (inner) aspect of the left arch just distal to the origin of the left subclavian artery. Although this structure is in anatomic proximity to the left ductus arteriosis it is not caused by traction of the ductus but rather it represents persistence of the most distal portion of the embryonic right arch [4]. It is important not to confuse this normal structure with a traumatic dissection when performing catheter based or computerized tomographic aortography following chest trauma.

The *left aortic arch* with an aberrant (anomalous) right subclavian artery is the most common variation of the thoracic aortic arch affecting 0.5% of the normal population. Its incidence is somewhat higher, reported in up to 2.9%, in patients with congenital heart disease. The aberrant right subclavian artery results from interruption of the dorsal segment of the embryonic right arch between the right common carotid artery and the right subclavian artery (Figs. 4.5 & 4.6). It may cause an oblique left posterior indentation of the esophagus on a barium swallow, but it does not cause respiratory or swallowing difficulties [3, 5]. Their relative positions are important when aberrant right subclavian artery coexists with aortic coarctation. The aberrant right subclavian artery will be a low pressure vessel if it arises distal to the coarctation in which case there may be large retrograde flow to the descending aorta through this artery and rib notching will occur on the left side only. This abnormality results from interruption of the right arch between the common carotid and right subclavian arteries. The right

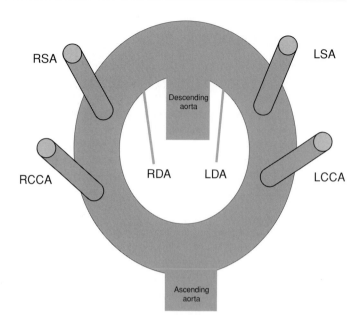

Figure 4.1 Edwards hypothetical double arch.

subclavian artery origin from the aorta may have an aneurismal or bulbous appearance. This is called the diverticulum of Kommerell; it represents persistence of the most distal portion of the embryonic right arch [6].

The *right aortic arch* is a very rare variation. It courses to the right of the trachea and esophagus and continues as the upper thoracic aorta to descend either to the right or to the left of the spine. The most common type of right aortic arch is right aortic arch with an aberrant left subclavian artery. Its frequency is about 0.1% and it is 2–3 times more common than right arch with mirror image branching of the brachiocephalic vessels (Figs. 4.7 & 4.8) [7]. Right arch and aberrant left subclavian artery has a 5–12% incidence of associated congenital heart disease while right arch with mirror branching of the brachiocephalic vessels has a 98% incidence of

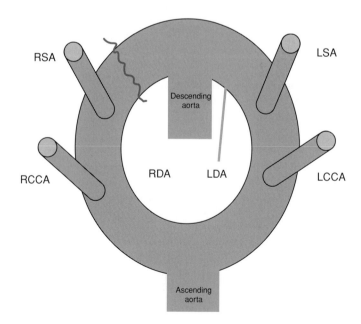

Figure 4.2 Interruption of the dorsal segment of the embryonic right arch between the right subclavian artery and the descending aorta.

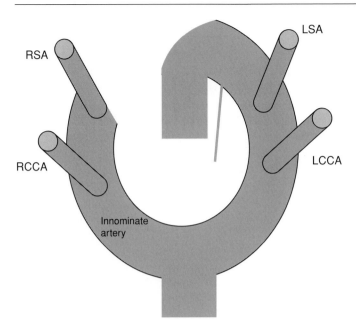

Figure 4.3 Regression of the arch between the right subclavian artery and the descending aorta and regression of the right ductus arteriosis.

associated congenital heart disease [8]. The right aortic arch has been classified into types depending on where interruption of the hypothetical Edwards double arch occurs (Fig. 4.9). The first two types result in mirror image branching of the arch vessels. In type 1, the most common form of the interruption

occurs between the left ductus arteriosis and the descending aorta. The interruption occurs between the left ductus and the left subclavian artery in the extremely rare type 2 right aortic arch. A vascular ring is possible with type 1, but not with type 2. The interruption is between the left subclavian artery

The arch rotates anteriorly and to the right

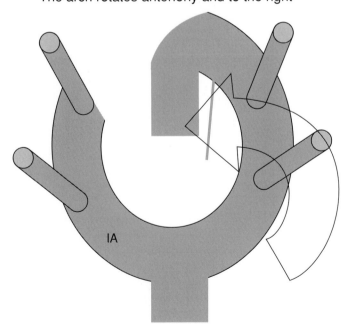

Figure 4.4 The right side of the "Edwards double arch" persists as the innominate artery. The left side of the "Edwards double arch" rotates anteriorly and to the right resulting in the innominate artery being the first branch of the "left arch" followed by the left common carotid artery and the left subclavian artery in turn.

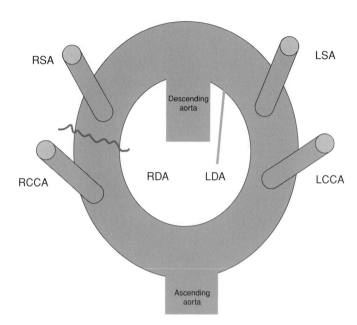

Figure 4.5 Interruption of the dorsal segment of the embryonic right arch between the right common carotid artery and the right subclavian artery.

and the left common carotid artery in type 3 right aortic arch. This results in an aberrant origin of the left subclavian artery which becomes the last artery arising from the aortic arch. There is interruption of the anterior portion of the embryonic left arch proximal to the left common carotid artery in type 4 right aortic arch resulting in a left innominate artery that becomes the last artery arising from the aortic arch and gives rise to the left common carotid and the left subclavian arteries. In type 5 right aortic

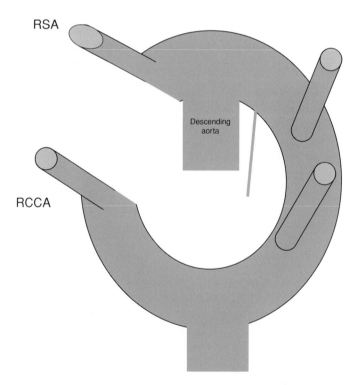

Figure 4.6 Regression of the arch between the common carotid artery and the right subclavian artery and regression of the right ductus arteriosis.

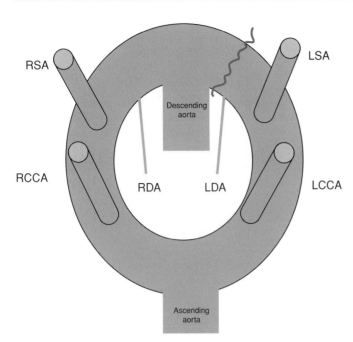

Figure 4.7 Interruption of the dorsal segment of the embryonic left arch between the left subclavian artery and the descending aorta.

arch, interruption of the left arch occurs on both sides of the left subclavian artery which, now isolated from the aorta receives its blood supply from the left ductus arteriosis. This anomaly is frequently associated with cyanotic congenital heart disease, especially the tetralogy of Fallot [3].

The *double aortic arch* is characterized by the presence of two aortic arches. The ascending aorta arises anterior to the trachea and divides into two arches which pass on either side of the trachea and esophagus. The right common carotid and subclavian arteries and the left common carotid and subclavian arteries arise independently from their ipsilateral arches. It is not possible for an innominate artery to be present with a double arch. The two arches join posteriorly to form the descending

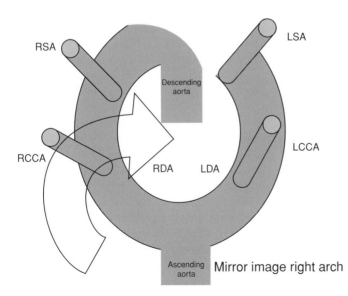

Mirror image right arch

Figure 4.8 Regression of the arch between the left subclavian artery and the descending aorta and regression of the right ductus arteriosis. The left ductus usually persists. The left side of the "Edwards double arch" persists as a left innominate artery. The right side of the "Edwards double arch" rotates anteriorly and to the left resulting in the innominate artery being the first branch of the "mirror image right arch" followed by the right common carotid artery and the right subclavian artery in turn.

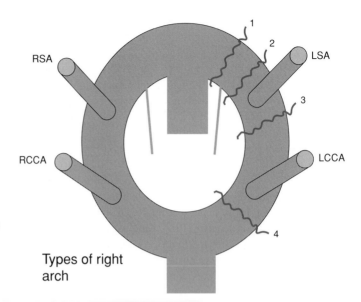

RSA

LSA

RCCA

LCCA

1

2

3

4

Types of right arch

Figure 4.9 Interruptions in the numbered locations explain the formation of four variations of the anomalous right arch. "*Type 5*" right arch is explained by interruption of the "Edwards double arch" at locations 1 and 3 resulting in isolation of the left subclavian artery, which remains connected to the pulmonary artery by way of the left ductus arteriosis.

aorta, which descends on the left more often than the right. The right arch is usually larger. There are two variations of the double arch. In type 1, the most common, both arches are patent and functioning and in type 2 both arches are intact, but one arch is atretic. Theoretically in type 2 the atresia can occur in either the right or the left arch; however in all reported cases the atresia has only occurred in the left arch. Double arches are rarely associated with congenital cardiac anomalies but is the most important arch anomaly resulting in vascular rings [8, 9].

There are two forms of *interruption of the aortic arch*; both are rare. In one form, there is complete anatomic interruption of the arch; in the other, an atretic fibrous remnant connects the arch with the descending aorta. The latter is referred to as "atresia of the aortic arch." This anomaly is one of the causes of the hypoplastic left heart syndrome. Interruption of the aortic arch can occur in almost any location and can be multiple [3].

Hypoplasia of the aorta refers to a state of arrested development in which the lumen of the aorta is narrowed but patent and the vessel is small in size. The term is used here to refer to a segment of aorta with a narrowed lumen in which the media is histologically normal. Although hypoplasia may be a focal lesion as in coarctation, frequently a longer segment of the aorta may be involved such as cases in the ascending

aorta in aortic valve atresia and supravalvular aortic stenosis.

The essential feature of *coarctation* is a "localized deformity of the aortic media resulting in a curtain-like infolding of the wall which causes an eccentric narrowing of the aortic lumen. Although a normal lumen may be present distal to the coarctation, more often a zone of hypoplasia is present [10]." Coarctation most often involves the isthmus of the aorta, the portion of the aorta between the left subclavian artery and the ductus arteriosis, but on rare occasions may be proximal to the left subclavian artery. The appearance of the aorta is related to the relationship of the ductus arteriosis to the coarctation during fetal development. When the coarctation is proximal to the ductus, fetal blood flow is through the ductus to the distal descending aorta which may result in hypoplastic development of the portion of the aortic arch between the left subclavian artery and the coarctation. When the coarctation is distal to the ductus fetal flow is directed into the normally developed proximal arch and left subclavian artery [10, 11]. Coarctation is twice as common in males. Approximately 50% of patients with coarctation will present in the first year with symptoms of severe congestive heart failure, the majority of which will have other cardiac defects [12]. Rib notching secondary to collateral blood supply to the hypotensive descending aorta via the intercostal arteries can provide information on the relationship between the coarctation and the origin of the subclavian arteries. Bilateral rib notching is present when the coarctation is below the origins of the right and left subclavian arteries, but may be on the left only, if it occurs between the left subclavian artery and an aberrant right subclavian artery or is absent on the rare occasion that the coarctation is above the origin of the left subclavian artery [3, 13, 14].

The *Midaortic Syndrome* also known as *Abdominal Coarctation* may be located in the descending thoracic aorta, abdominal aorta, or both. It accounts for 0.5 to 2% of all coarctations. The midaortic syndrome is characterized by severe narrowing of the abdominal aorta with progressive involvement of the renal arteries in 90% of the cases and superior mesenteric and celiac axis in 20–40% of cases; it almost never involves the inferior mesenteric artery. Several congenital or acquired etiologies have been suggested. Hypoplasia may occur during development of the aorta and the vitelline and metanephric vasculature. The association of Midaortic Syndrome with fibromuscular dysplasia, neurofibromatosis, mucopolysaccharidosis, Alagille syndrome, and William's syndrome would suggest a genetic etiology. The Midaortic Syndrome has also been associated with fetal alcohol syndrome, rubella, Takayasu's arteritis and several autoimmune diseases which suggest an acquired etiology. The natural history of untreated symptomatic midaortic syndrome is death before the 4th decade frequently associated with the complications of hypertension and renal failure. Therapeutic options are usually surgical and percutaneous angioplasty and stenting [15, 16].

The abdominal aorta

Compared to the aortic arch, little has been written about the development and variations of the abdominal aorta. Because of interest in the construction of abdominal aortic endografts which can accommodate side branches of juxtarenal and suprarenal abdominal aortic aneurysms, there has been recent interest in anatomic variations of the mesenteric and renal artery origins. Of significance to the development of the visceral circulation,

both dorsal aortas provide ventral segmental (omphalomesenteric) arteries to the viscera which give rise to the vitelline arteries. The ventral roots fuse at about the fourth week and there is reduction of the primitive ventral segmental arteries. As the embryo continues to develop, most of the segmental arteries regress, except for the precursors of segmental arteries to the three major mesenteric *vessels*. The 10th segmental artery gives rise to the celiac artery, which supplies the foregut, which in turn includes the region extending between the esophagus and the distal duodenum. The 13th segmental artery becomes the SMA that supplies the midgut, which corresponds to the intestinal segment between the proximal jejunum and the midtransverse colon. Lastly, the 22nd segmental artery develops into the IMA to supply the hindgut from the midtransverse colon to the rectum [17, 18].

The more common variations the *origin and positions* of visceral and renal *abdominal aortic branches* are listed in Table 4.1. The greatest variation occurs in the blood supply to the liver, which normally is supplied by right and left hepatic arterial branches of the common hepatic artery which originates from the celiac axis. The right hepatic artery completely originates from the SMA in approximately 16% and from both the celiac and SMA in 5%. Rarely the common hepatic artery or the splenic artery can originate from the SMA or the splenic artery can originate as a separate branch from the aorta. At least one kidney is supplied by more than one renal artery originating from the aorta in approximately 30%; neither kidney is more commonly affected [17]. The right renal artery originates ventral to a

Table 4.1 Variations of major abdominal aortic branches [17]. Incidence (%)

Hepatic branches for the SMA (overall)	18–20
Totally replaced right hepatic artery from SMA	14–18
Accessory right hepatic artery from SMA	4–6
Common hepatic artery from SMA	2.5
Celiacomesenteric trunk from the aorta	<1
Splenic artery off the SMA	<1
Splenic artery from the aorta	<0.1
Multiple renal arteries (2–4)	30*
Multiple renal arteries – unilateral	32
Multiple renal arteries – bilateral	12

*No more common on the right or left

Table 4.2 Normal diameter of the adult thoracic aorta* [23].

	Male	Female
Ascending aorta at the level of the right pulmonary artery	34.1 ± 5.8	28.2 ± 3.7
Ascending segment of the aortic arch	30.4 ± 5.6	25.6 ± 3.4
Distal segment of the aortic arch	26.1 ± 4.3	21.1 ± 3.2
Descending aorta at the level of the right pulmonary artery	25.4 ± 4.0	20.7 ± 4.0
Descending aorta at the level of the left ventricle	24.2 ± 4.3	18.0 ± 3.4

*Measured in millimeters on magnetic resonance images of 15 females and 51 males

horizontal plane through the axis of the abdominal aorta and the left renal artery originates dorsal to this plane in 93% and 80% respectively [19].

The aortic diameter varies with body size, sex, and ageing. Dilatation and loss of compliance are accelerated by factors such as atherosclerosis and hypertension. Several series have produced tables of normal ranges in adults and these are useful for reference. There is quite a wide range of normality. The diameter of the mid ascending aorta in young men is approximately 33 mm ± 3 and the descending aorta 22 mm ± 3. The ratio of ascending to descending aorta should normally be about 3:2 but the descending aorta becomes relatively larger with age, particularly over 60 years. Women have slightly smaller aortas than men, even at the same body surface area. When measuring the progress of aortic dilatation by serial CT or MRI, it is convenient to choose a readily recognizable level such as the right pulmonary artery. It is also important to measure the shortest diameter if the image plane is not absolutely perpendicular to the axis of the aorta. Normal diameters in the thoracic and abdominal aortas are presented in Tables 4.2, 4.3 and 4.4.

Fleischmann *et al.* (Table 4.3) found a significant effect of **sex**, with men having 1.9 mm larger aortic

diameters. They also found a significant stepwise decrease of diameter from the supraceliac abdominal aorta to the aortic bifurcation. Segmental diameters increased significantly with *age*, with the slopes of these linear relations being steeper proximally (0.14 mm/y above the celiac axis, $P < 0.0001$) than distally (0.03 mm/y between the IMA and aortic bifurcation, $P = 0.013$) [20]. They conclude that "in healthy, 19- to 67-year-old individuals, the age-related increase of aortic diameter is strongly associated with the relative anatomic position along the abdominal aorta. The "growth rate" was highest (0.14 mm/y) in the most proximal (supraceliac) segment of the abdominal aorta, diminished gradually when moving down the aorta, and was minimal (0.03 mm/y) near the bifurcation. Consequently, the aortic geometry also changes gradually and systematically in healthy subjects. In general, this causes an increase of tapering of the entire abdominal aorta from proximal to distal with time [20]." Fleischmann *et al.* found no tapering or observed a mild proximal-to-distal increase of diameter in the infrarenal aorta in young individuals. It must be noted that only 9 of the patients that were studied were 55 years or older. In an older, more diverse population-based study from the Netherlands [21]

Table 4.3 Normal diameter of the adult abdominal aorta* [20].

	Male	Female
Supraceliac abdominal aorta	19.3 ± 2.2	17.6 ± 2.3
Aorta between the celiac and SMA	18.6 ± 1.8	16.5 ± 2.2
Aorta between the SMA and the renal arteries	17.5 ± 1.6	15.5 ± 2.2
Aorta between the renal arteries and the IMA	17.1 ± 1.7	14.6 ± 2.0
Aorta between the IMA and aortic bifurcation	15.0 ± 1.3	13.1 ± 1.7

*Measured on CT angiographic images of 33 males and 44 females

Table 4.4 Autopsy study of 30 men without aneurysm [24].

Aortic dimensions (mm)	Thoracic (n = 30)*	Abdominal (n = 30)**
Luminal diameter	17.00 ± 0.43	14.88 ± 0.70
External diameter	20.30 ± 0.50	17.80 ± 0.70
Media thickness	1.01 ± 0.03	0.48 ± 0.03
Wall thickness	1.63 ± 0.05	1.50 ± 0.06
Plaque thickness	0.65 ± 0.06	1.01 ± 0.09
Plaque area (mm^2)	44.30 ± 5.40	59.20 ± 5.70

*Midway between the left subclavian artery and the celiac artery
**Midway between the renal arteries and the aortic bifurcation

in 5419 subjects aged 55 years and older revealed slower growth rates of the abdominal aorta proximally (0.03 mm/y, measured with ultrasound scan) than distally (0.07 mm/y). These findings were confirmed in a subsequent study based on the same patient population ($n = 5419$) combined with data from another large population-based study from the United Kingdom conducted in 6053 men older than 50 years [22].

Acknowledgments

I would like to acknowledge my debt and gratitude to my mentors Wade H. Shuford, MD, and Robert G. Sybers, MD, PhD, who are responsible for whatever knowledge that I might have regarding aortic arch and great vessel development. Most of my discussion of the aortic arch and its development were taken directly from their book "The Aortic Arch and its Malformations." Readers are encouraged to refer to this text for information that I was not able to include.

References

1 Barry A. Aortic arch derivatives in the human adult. Anatomic Records 1951; **111**: 221.

2 Edwards JE. Anomalies of the derivatives of the aortic arch system. Med Clin North Am 1948; **32**: 925.

3 Shuford WH, Sybers RG. The Aortic Arch And Its Malformations. Thomas, Springfield, IL, 1974.

4 Grollman JH. The aortic diverticulum: a remnant of the partially involuted dorsal aortic root. Cardiovasc Intervent Radiol 1989; **12**(1): 14–17.

5 Felson B, Cohen S et al. Anomalous right subclavian artery. Radiology 1950; **54**(3): 340–349.

6 van Son JAM, Konstantinov IE. Burckhard F. Kommerell and Kommerell's diverticulum. Tex Heart Inst J 2002; **29**(2): 109–112.

7 Hastreiter AR, D'Cruz IA, Cantez T, Namin EP, Licata R. Right-sided aorta. I. Occurrence of right aortic arch in various types of congenital heart disease. II. Right aortic arch, right descending aorta, and associated anomalies. Br Heart J 1966; **28**(6): 722–739.

8 Stewart JR, Kincaid OW. An Atlas of Vascular Rings and Related Malformations of the Aortic Arch System. Thomas, Springfield, IL, 1964.

9 Shuford WH, Sybers RG, Weens HS. The angiographic features of double aortic arch. Am J Roentgenol Radium Ther Nucl Med 1972; **116**(1): 125–140.

10 Edwards JE, Carey LS, Henfield HN, Lester RG. Congenital Heart Disease. Saunders, Philadelphia, 1965.

11 Perloff JK. The Clinical Recognition of Congenital Heart Disease. Saunders, Philadelphia, 1970.

12 Fuster V, Alexander RW, O'Rourke RA. Hurst's The Heart. McGraw-Hill, New York, 2004.

13 Drexler CJ, Stewart JR, Kincaid OW. Diagnostic implications of rib notching. Am J Roentgenol Radium Ther Nucl Med 1964; **91**: 1064–1074.

14 Grollman JH, Jr., Horns JW. The collateral circulation in coarctation of the aorta with a distal subclavian artery. Radiology 1964; **83**: 622–625.

15 Zeltser I, Parness IA, Ko H, Holzman IR, Kamenir SA. Midaortic syndrome in the fetus and premature newborn: A new etiology of nonimmune hydrops fetalis and reversible fetal cardiomyopathy. Pediatrics 2003; **111** (6 Pt 1): 1437–1442.

16 Stadlmaier E, Spary A, Tillich M, Pilger E. Midaortic syndrome and celiac disease: A case of local vasculitis. Clin Rheumatol 2005; **24**(3): 301–304.

17 Kadir S. Atlas of Normal and Varient Angiographic Anatomy. Saunders, Philadelphia, 1991.

18 Lin PH, Chaikof EL. Embryology, anatomy, and surgical exposure of the great abdominal vessels. Surg Clin North Am 2000; **80**(1): 417–433.

19 Verschuyl EJ, Kaatee R, Beek FJ, *et al.* Renal artery origins: Location and distribution in the transverse plane at CT. Radiology 1997; **203**(1): 71–75.

20 Fleischmann D, Hastie TJ, Dannegger FC *et al.* Quantitative determination of age-related geometric changes in the normal abdominal aorta. J Vasc Surg 2001; **33**(1): 97–105.

21 Pleumeekers HJ, Hoes AW, van der Does E *et al.* Aneurysms of the abdominal aorta in older adults. The Rotterdam study. Am J Epidemiol 1995; **142**(12): 1291–1299.

22 Wilmink AB, Pleumeekers HJ, Hoes AW, Hubbard CS, Grobbee DE, Quick CR. The infrarenal aortic diameter in relation to age: Only part of the population in older age groups shows an increase. Eur J Vasc Endovasc Surg 1998; **16**(5): 431–437.

23 Garcier JM, Petitcolin V, Filaire M *et al.* Normal diameter of the thoracic aorta in adults: A magnetic resonance imaging study. Surg Radiol Anat 2003; **25**(3–4): 322–329.

24 Zarins CK, Xu C, Glagov S. Atherosclerotic enlargement of the human abdominal aorta. Atherosclerosis 2001; **155**(1): 157–164.

CHAPTER 5

Patient selection for thoracic endografts: today and tomorrow

Mark A. Farber

It has been over a decade since the first implantation of a thoracic stent graft was reported and only recently has the first device been approved by the FDA [1, 2]. Even though this technology has been approved by the FDA for more than 6 years for infrarenal aneurysmal repair, devices for use in the thoracic aorta are considered first generation and are limited by constraints similar to those for infrarenal devices. Additionally, complicated devices that allow for fenestrated or branched designs are lacking, or are only in the initial phases of development [3].

In the beginning, hand-made devices were used to treat "ideal" isolated descending thoracic aortic aneurysms in straight regions of the aorta. These initial results were met with great enthusiasm and interest [1, 4, 5]. More extensive lesions were avoided secondary to fear of inducing paraplegia from sacrificing critical intercostals arteries. This myth was dispelled however after more extensive lesions were treated in high risk, nonoperative patients with a surprisingly low incidence of ischemic spinal cord complications. Additionally, advancements in both device technology and techniques allowed for better navigation and treatment of more challenging pathologies. While this broadened the scope of thoracic endovascular procedures, it also increased the number and incidence of associated complications. This learning curve and the desire to "push the envelope" is nothing new to device technology and was previously experienced by many individuals during the early phases of infrarenal EVAR development. One must keep this in mind and realize that successful thoracic endovascular repairs are governed by many of the same principles as infrarenal EVAR repair; mainly that patient selection plays a vital role in obtaining excellent results with limited complications. Thoracic aortic anatomy can be very complicated and challenging to assess. It should be evaluated and sized on a workstation with multiplanar reformatting and never be based upon axial imaging alone. This allows for more precise measurements and compensates for the inherent tortuosity present in the thoracic aorta. Most imaging protocols involve 2–3 mm axial imaging with reconstructions; however, the specific details vary among institutions.

Device sizes

In the United States there have been four different devices trialed for the treatment of thoracic disease to date. Each manufacturer has different diameter ranges and lengths for their devices. Both of these device characteristics play an important role in selecting the best device for the patient. Appropriate device oversizing and limiting the number of component junctions may help to improve patient outcomes and reduce complication rates.

Neck anatomy

Neck anatomy still remains the "Achilles heel" of all EVAR procedures. When diseased implantation sites are selected for device fixation, increased complications occur. Providing adequate proximal and distal fixation and accomplishing aneurysm exclusion with an appropriate sealing region is the most challenging task in many patients [6]. Almost all infrarenal devices require 1.5 cm of aortic neck length to provide adequate fixation and seal for aneurysmal exclusion. Additional length is needed in the thoracic aorta, however given its larger size; 2.0–3.0 cm is generally thought to be sufficient. Some experts rely upon a ratio calculation and target a fixation length of 0.75 times the aortic diameter as a minimal acceptable length. During patient selection if inadequate neck length exists, the patient should be evaluated for proximal and/or distal debranching techniques to accomplish aneurysm exclusion or traditional open repair. Some devices provide additional fixation without sacrificing branched arteries with bare stent regions.

It is also crucial that the aortic walls be fairly parallel and free of significant calcification and thrombus. Implantation into funnel shaped necks is not advised and alternative options including hybrid procedures or open repair should be considered in these patients. While isolated thoracic aortic lesions can still meet these requirements, many thoracic aortic processes involve the entire descending thoracic aorta and end at, or near, the crus of the diaphragm or in the visceral section. In these cases, obtaining adequate distal fixation can be problematic. The angle of the descending thoracic aorta also plays a major role in the migration of thoracic stent grafts, possibly causing a cephalad migration of the caudal aspect of the device. It can also make precise deployment rather difficult; many times it is necessary to deploy an additional distal extension [7]. Implanting the device in a region where significant angulation exists can jeopardize the durability of the endovascular repair. Finally, most stent-graft deployment mechanisms are designed for precise proximal placement with minimal or no control over the distal attachment site or landing zone. Therefore accurate deployment near the celiac artery becomes more challenging. Given the aforementioned issues, it is advisable to lengthen the distal neck by performing aortic debranching techniques in a small but not insignificant number of patients.

While additional fixation can be obtained on the proximal aspect of the aneurysm by either carotid subclavian bypass or coverage of the left subclavian artery, the visceral section of the aorta is less forgiving. While there are reports of celiac artery coverage without incident, severe complications may arise from either hepatic or splenic ischemia, resulting in potential demise of the patient [8, 9]. It has been our approach to routinely revascularize all celiac arteries if coverage is planned unless certain contraindications exist [10]. These include prohibitive abdominal surgical risks, diminutive hepatic or inflow vessels potentially jeopardizing collateral flow or patients with documented celiac occlusion.

Neck angulation can also impose significant restrictions on proximal thoracic pathologies. Since the arch of the aorta is fixed by the great vessels, proximal aneurysms often induce an acute angle change at or just distal to the left SCA. Passage of some devices can be difficult in these situations and are often associated with an increased risk of stroke during endovascular exclusion. It is advisable in these patients to evaluate the extent of arch atherosclerotic disease and council the patient about potential stroke risks.

Aortic morphology

Tortuosity in other regions of the aorta can also cause intent to treat failures. The thoracic aorta is a complex three-dimensional (3D) structure, which when dilated from aneurysmal disease can pose many challenges for the interventionalist. One should be familiar with the available devices and their relative ability to traverse various thoracic anatomies (flexibility). This becomes especially important when treating extensive regions of the thoracic aorta. Each component implanted into the thoracic aorta results in a relative compliance change and potentially limits the insertion of the next component. There have been instances when exclusion of the aneurysm cannot be completed after the deployment of the initial device because secondary devices are not able to traverse the thoracic aorta. One approach is to evaluate the radius of curvature. In the cases where the aortic arch radius is less than 25–35 mm endovascular repair may be problematic. In addition, when the aortic angles exceed 75°, the deliverability of the device often becomes extremely difficult or impossible.

Device position

During patient selection, the location of the proximal implantation region of the device should be determined. Adjustments to the ideal position of the proximal seal are not only governed by the neck location, but also the orientation and conformation of the device and the sealing stents to the thoracic aorta. In angled regions, especially in the arch, this can alter the intended implantation site and result in unanticipated coverage of branched vessels. When preoperative evaluation predicts that this may occur, cerebral evaluation should be completed prior to implantation [11]. This generally includes carotid and subclavian artery duplex ultrasonography, as well as CT and/or MRA of the great vessels, vertebral arteries and the Circle of Willis. As previously described the left subclavian artery can be managed expectantly without preprocedural revascularization with few exceptions [11, 12]. These include patients with aberrant or dominant left vertebral arteries and LIMA bypass grafts. When more proximal implantation is desired, aortic arch debranching can be performed. This can be accomplished with numerous procedures that include carotid–subclavian bypass or transposition, carotid–carotid bypass and ascending arch to innominate and carotid bypass.

Paraplegia risks

While it has been shown with open thoracoabdominal aneurysm repair that the length of aorta replaced is associated with an increased risk of paraplegia, this has not been the experience with thoracic endovascular procedures. Therefore, generous sealing regions (3–5 cm) that exceed the IFU recommendations are usually chosen for the patient to maximize the potential for long-term success. An association with paraplegia has been identified however in those patients who have had prior abdominal aortic aneurysm repairs. It appears that the risk is increased approximately two-fold, from 4% to 8% [6, 13]. In this cohort care should be taken when planning the procedure. Preservation of left SCA flow should be stressed because it provides an excellent collateral pathway in potentially preventing spinal cord ischemia. Additionally, many surgeons will insert a prophylactic spinal drainage catheter. This practice has arisen from several anecdotal case reports of resolution of spinal cord ischemic complications after placement of a lumbar drain in patients.

Access issues

Access complications are often due to a combination of iliofemoral arterial calcification, tortuosity, and stenosis that can be identified with preoperative imaging. While the presence of any one of these aspects can easily be overcome, their combination

can lead to access failure or vascular complications during the procedure. Critical assessment of the iliac vessels should be undertaken with axial imaging characterizing the caliber of access vessels (common iliac, external iliac, and common femoral) and the degree, location, extent, and circumferential nature of calcium; and 3D reconstructions can map out vessel tortuosity. Delivery catheter sizes are still relatively large and have a size range of 22–25 Fr. Approximately 15–20% of patients will require an iliac or aortic conduit for successful device implantation. While this can be tolerated in most patients in the elective situation, it does add additional morbidity to the procedure. When emergent conversion from iliac rupture occurs, it imparts significant risks to the patient. If any potential access issues are identified preoperatively, an elective conduit placement should be planned.

Conclusion

Despite advancements in devices and technology over the past decade, patient selection criteria have remained relatively the same and are mainly governed by aortic neck characteristics both proximally and distally. When compromises are made in either of these two regions, patient outcomes are negatively impacted. Detailed axial imaging with multiplanar reconstruction capabilities is crucial for proper evaluation, planning and sizing for thoracic endovascular procedures. In the future, branched and fenestrated devices will allow for the treatment of lesions involving either the great vessels or the visceral section with less invasive methods compared to hybrid procedures performed today.

References

1 Dake MD, Miller DC, Semba CP, Mitchell RS, Walker PJ, Liddell RP. Transluminal placement of endovascular stent-grafts for the treatment of descending thoracic aortic aneurysms. N Engl J Med 1994; 331(26): 1729–1734.

2 Volodos NL, Karpovich IP, Shekhanin VE, Troian VI, Iakovenko LF. A case of distant transfemoral endoprosthesis of the thoracic artery using a self-fixing synthetic prosthesis in traumatic aneurysm. Grudn Khir 1988; 2(6): 84–86.

3 Saito N, Kimura T, Odashiro K et al. Feasibility of the Inoue single-branched stent-graft implantation for thoracic

aortic aneurysm or dissection involving the left subclavian artery: Short- to medium-term results in 17 patients. J Vasc Surg 2005; **41**(2): 206–212; discussion 12.

4 Htay T, Fujiwara H, Sato M, Tanaka M, Sasayama S, Inoue K. Transcatheter Inoue endovascular graft for treatment of canine aortic dissection. Heart Vessels 1996; **11**(2): 80–85.

5 Semba CP, Mitchell RS, Miller DC *et al.* Thoracic aortic aneurysm repair with endovascular stent-grafts. Vasc Med 1997; **2**(2): 98–103.

6 Criado FJ, Clark NS, Barnatan MF. Stent graft repair in the aortic arch and descending thoracic aorta: A 4-year experience. J Vasc Surg 2002; **36**(6): 1121–1128.

7 Ellozy SH, Carroccio A, Minor M *et al.* Challenges of endovascular tube graft repair of thoracic aortic aneurysm: Midterm follow-up and lessons learned. J Vasc Surg 2003; **38**(4): 676–683.

8 Sunder-Plassmann L, Orend KH. Stentgrafting of the thoracic aorta-complications. J Cardiovasc Surg (Torino) 2005; **46**(2): 121–130.

9 Greenberg RK, O'Neill S, Walker E *et al.* Endovascular repair of thoracic aortic lesions with the Zenith TX1 and TX2 thoracic grafts: Intermediate-term results. J Vasc Surg 2005; **41**(4): 589–596.

10 Fulton JJ, Farber MA, Marston WA, Mendes R, Mauro MA, Keagy BA. Endovascular stent-graft repair of pararenal and type IV thoracoabdominal aortic aneurysms with adjunctive visceral reconstruction. J Vasc Surg 2005; **41**(2): 191–198.

11 Gorich J, Asquan Y, Seifarth H *et al.* Initial experience with intentional stent-graft coverage of the subclavian artery during endovascular thoracic aortic repairs. J Endovasc Ther 2002; **9**(Suppl) 2: II39–II43.

12 Tiesenhausen K, Hausegger KA, Oberwalder P *et al.* Left subclavian artery management in endovascular repair of thoracic aortic aneurysms and aortic dissections. J Card Surg 2003; **18**(5): 429–435.

13 Fattori R, Napoli G, Lovato L *et al.* Descending thoracic aortic diseases: Stent-graft repair. Radiology 2003; **229**(1): 176–183.

CHAPTER 6

Noninvasive aortic imaging modalities: CT, MRI, intravascular ultrasound (IVUS), and transesophageal echocardiography (TEE)

Tae K. Song, & Rodney A. White

Noninvasive imaging modalities are the principal methods used to determine which patients are candidates for thoracic aortic endovascular intervention and allow for surveillance monitoring following aortic endovascular procedures. Current modalities being utilized include computed tomography (CT), magnetic resonance imaging (MRI), transesophageal echocardiography (TEE), and intravascular ultrasound (IVUS). Each modality provides information that is useful for preinterventional selection of patients, deployment of endografts, and assessment of long-term outcomes.

Preintervention CT and MRI are replacing contrast angiography as the primary imaging studies for thoracoabdominal pathology in determining patient candidacy for endovascular therapy. Angiography can be particularly misleading regarding adequacy of landing zone length and the distribution of thrombus at the fixation sites. In fact, many interventionalists feel that contrast enhanced CT scans (preferably centerline images with three-dimensional (3D) reconstructions) are the most accurate method to determine aneurysm morphology, aortic dissection characteristics, and adequacy of fixation sites for endograft deployment in aortoiliac procedures. MRI provides similar information as CT scans if high quality software is available.

IVUS and TEE are ultrasound-based imaging modalities that are enhancing the 3D, real-time imaging of aortic segments prior to, during, and following endovascular therapy. These nonionizing radiation imaging technologies supplement conventional angiography and cinefluoroscopy. Appropriately employed in conjunction with preintervention CT images, IVUS interrogation can expedite preprocedural planning and reduce fluoroscopic and contrast requirements.

IVUS can also be used to determine aortic morphology such as the presence of thrombus or calcification. IVUS provides real-time observation of endograft stent expansion and assessment of apposition of endograft stents to the aortic wall before the procedures are completed. In comparison, TEE offers some of the same advantages as IVUS but also produces a unique perspective of cardiac function, ascending and descending aortic anatomy.

Computed tomogaphy

3D spiral CT imaging methods are dramatically improving the utility of CT for interpreting the distribution of thoracoabdominal disease and for assessing appropriate endovascular therapy. Images can be reconstructed using maximum intensity projection (MIP), producing two-dimensional (2D) images that can differentiate mural calcification from intraluminal contrast. Alternatively, a shaded surface display (SSD)-rendering technique may be used, producing 3D images depicting the surface of the contrast-enhanced structures. CT angiography (CTA) then allows an infinite number of viewing angles of the 3D reconstructed image.

CT has become the gold standard in preinterventional planning of thoracoabdominal aortic aneurysms, thoracic aortic dissections, grafts, and stents for endovascular therapy. CT offers precise anatomic information needed for preplanning of endovascular therapy. Thin cut CT slices of 2 to 3 mm can be converted into 3D reconstructions using specialized computer software (Medical MetRx Solutions, West Lebanon, NH). Thus, CT allows assessment of the cross-sectional morphology of vascular structures with clear delineation of luminal and wall components (i.e. thrombus or calcifications), aortic dimensions (i.e. stent selection), size of femoral access vessels, and involvement of branch vessels [1]. With thoracic aortic dissections, CT accurately determines the extent of dissection flaps and which visceral vessels are supplied by the true or false lumen (Fig. 6.1). This information may be important when planning interventions such as

fenestration to alleviate the ischemic sequelae of a thoracic dissection. CT is also sensitive (92%) and specific (83%) for the detection of hemodynamically significant renal artery stenosis [2]. CT accurately delineates the splanchnic vessel anatomy, including identifying accessory renal arteries, stenoses involving mesenteric vessels, and collateral vessels [3].

CT is helpful in monitoring the long-term function of devices and is the primary modality for establishment of long-term surveillance. Patients selected for endovascular treatment are often enrolled in follow-up surveillance programs with serial CT scans obtained preoperatively and postoperatively at 1 month, 6 month, and yearly thereafter (Fig. 6.2). Serial CT scans can then help delineate the effects of endovascular therapy on the natural history of thoracoabdominal pathology. CT will also detect complications of endograft treatment such as stent fracture, stent migration, thrombosis, and endoleaks. Compared to digital subtraction angiography, CTA is sensitive (86%) in detecting the presence of endoleaks, but demonstrates less specificity in differentiating the type of endoleak [4].

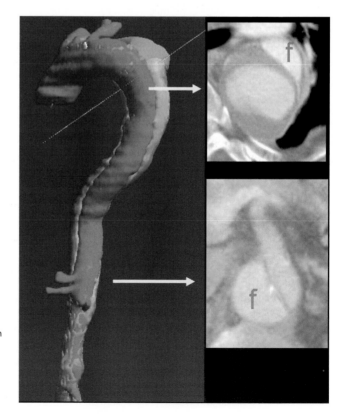

Figure 6.1 Interactive 3D CT image of a chronic descending aortic dissection depicting a true and false lumen (f) with an entry point distal to the left subclavian artery and extending below the celiac axis (celiac origin is derived from true lumen). Corresponding axial images depict the 2D findings found on conventional CT.

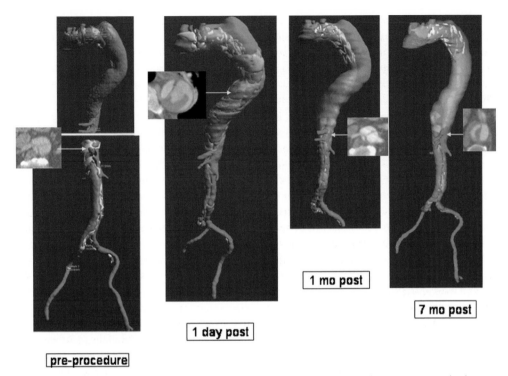

Figure 6.2 Composite interactive 3D CT images of complete regression over 7 months of a 7 cm aneurysmal enlargement of a chronic proximal descending aortic dissection following coverage of the proximal entry site with a single 130-mm-long Talent thoracic endograft.

Magnetic resonance imaging

The principle of "flow void," where rapidly moving protons fail to elicit a perceptible signal, forms the basis for imaging blood vessels using MRI methods (magnetic resonance angiography) essentially producing a "luminogram" of the thoracic aorta [5]. More sophisticated techniques based on gradient-echo (GRE) pulse sequences produce bright blood images from 2D or 3D data sets that can be processed for optimal viewing angles.

MRI is an important and noninvasive diagnostic tool to screen patients for endovascular therapy. MRI can also be used as an alternative method for monitoring long-term outcomes following endograft placement. A comparison of MRI to CT as the sole preoperative imaging modality for endovascular therapy showed no differences in aborted procedures, conversions to open procedures, or inability to access vessels for deployment [6, 7].

MRI provides information regarding luminal dimensions, vessel wall, and the relation of pathology to the arch vessels and paraaortic structures. Like CT, MRI is effective for diagnosing aortic dissec-tions, but MRI is more sensitive for demonstrating the dissection entry site and endpoint. On MRI scans, intimal flaps are seen as linear structures of intermediate signal density, with blood flowing in the adjacent lumens appearing as flow void or anomalous intraluminal flow signal. MRI is also well suited to the evaluation of aortic aneurysmal disease detecting the presence of a mural thrombus, outer dimensions of the aorta, size of the residual lumen, and the relation of the aneurysm to major branch vessels. Dynamic MR is developing as a powerful method for evaluating intravascular 3D hemodynamics and flow and is enhancing the assessment of complicated aortic pathologies such as dissections.

Increasingly, MRI is commonly used as an adjunct to ultrasound imaging for the assessment of patients who are not suitable for radiologic contrast infusion due to renal insufficiency or contrast allergy. The incidence of anaphylactic reaction to gadolinium is extremely low. MRI can also be used to establish long-term surveillance outcomes as the nitinol stent material is compatible with magnets; however MRI does not allow assessment of the stent lumen. Artifacts created by the presence of intravascular steel coils [5] from previous embolization vessel occlusion reduce image resolution. In contrast, the use of platinum intravascular coils would allow for MRI compatibility.

More recently, application of MRI using faster magnetic resonance gradients to allow for time-resolved magnetic resonance angiography (TR-MRA) has been employed not only to detect the presence of endoleak, but also to characterize the type of endoleak with much greater sensitivity than CTA [8, 9]. The ability to characterize the type of endoleak is important in directing the need for future intervention for type I and type III endoleaks. Currently, the gold standard for detecting the type of endoleak is digital subtraction angiography. Haulon *et al.* [9] suggest the failure of the aneurysm to shrink based on 6 month CTA surveillance should be followed by a MRI with gadolinium to detect an endoleak with a high degree of sensitivity. Cine MRA has also been used to correlate aneurysm pulsatility to differentiate between type I and type II endoleaks [10]. Type II endoleaks have not been associated with continued endotension [11] and are often monitored with serial imaging.

MRI, however, is not suitable for all patients. Exclusion from MRI scanning includes metal implants, inability to hold one's breath (i.e. ventilator-dependent patients), and claustrophobia. MRI shows a limited ability to determine the degree and distribution of calcification within a vessel lumen making assessment of the suitability of femoral access vessels difficult. MRI does not accurately detect the presence of accessory renal vessels or the degree of renal artery stenosis well.

Ultrasound imaging

Transesophageal echocardiography

The role of TEE during endovascular therapy is evolving and is probably the least utilized noninvasive imaging modality. Primarily employed for the assessment and treatment of thoracic aortic dissections, TEE provides a unique perspective of cardiac function and ascending and descending thoracic aortic anatomy. TEE allows precise localization of entry sites and relationship to the brachiocephalic artery, depicts the anatomical relationship of the true and false lumens, and can detect endoleaks [12]. Similar to IVUS, TEE can verify placement

of the guide wire within the true lumen prior to endograft deployment and assess for stent apposition following endograft deployment with color flow Doppler. Because TEE does not interfere with deployment, TEE can be used in real time to assess successful exclusion of the false lumen (i.e. "smoke phenomenon") as well as to detect the presence of endoleaks including a higher sensitivity in detecting Type IV endoleaks [12, 13].

In contrast to IVUS, TEE requires general anesthesia and allows limited visualization of the transverse aortic arch and abdominal aorta and its branches. Similar to IVUS, the assessment of PTFE stents with TEE will be less useful. With its higher degree of sensitivity in detecting thoracic dissections and its utility in endograft deployment, the role of TEE may continue to expand in the treatment of aortic dissections.

Intravascular ultrasound

IVUS is particularly useful in the treatment of thoracoabdominal pathology [14]. For instance, IVUS can establish aortic wall morphology, locate the origins of branch vessels, size vessel lumen dimensions, and select proximal and distal landing zones for endograft deployment [15]. In conjunction with cinefluoroscopy, IVUS can be used to assess the accuracy of endograft deployment, degree of device expansion, and stent apposition of the prosthesis to the vascular wall (Fig. 6.3). An advantage of IVUS is the ability to map additional segments of the aorta either proximal or distal to the endograft in preparation for additional endograft stent placement. IVUS is particularly useful when combined with fluoroscopy to identify the origin of the visceral vessels, thus enhancing precise deployment. Through the use of IVUS and pulsed fluoroscopy, the amount of radiation exposure and potentially nephrotoxic contrast use can be minimized significantly. This reduced exposure and limited contrast use may benefit those with contrast allergies or renal insufficiency.

As an appealing alternative to contrast angiography, IVUS can be used independently to investigate pathologic lesions. Its ability to identify branch vessels relative to a calibrated ruler placed beneath the patient and anatomic landmarks has been used to deploy endografts without the need for fluoroscopy (Fig. 6.4).

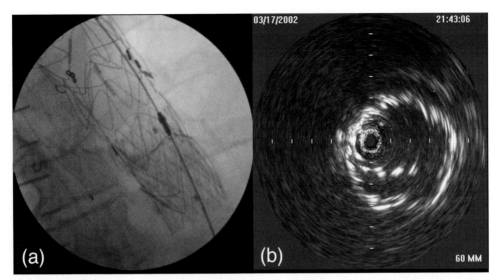

Figure 6.3 Postendograft deployment (a) image on fluoroscopy and corresponding IVUS image (b) demonstrating poor apposition of the endograft to the aortic wall. The endograft underwent balloon dilatation with subsequent improved apposition.

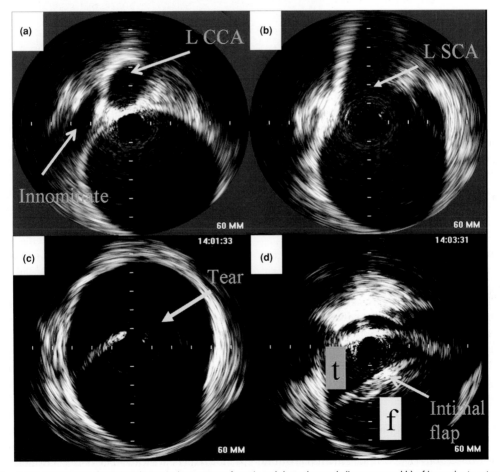

Figure 6.4 IVUS image depicting the typical sequence of aortic arch branch vessels (images a and b) of innominate artery, left common carotid artery (CCA) and left subclavian artery (SCA). An entry site (tear) is demonstrated (image c) distal to the left subclavian artery. An intimal flap separating the true (t) and false (f) lumen is shown by IVUS (image d).

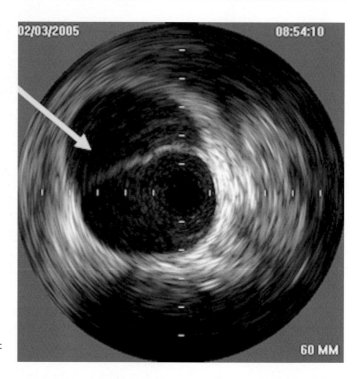

Figure 6.5 Entry site (arrow) of an aortic dissection is depicted by IVUS.

IVUS utilization requires an understanding of the principals of ultrasound interpretation in vascular anatomy. The ultrasound signal may be attenuated by calcification in the vessel wall, and may show enhancement by prosthetic graft material. Analysis of aortic wall morphology may show the presence of thrombus, dissection flaps, and pulsatile flow within the true and false arterial lumens in a dissected artery.

Artifacts can be produced by wires and catheters in the arterial lumen. Catheter designs that enable delivery of the ultrasound elements without a monorail delivery wire eliminate wire artifact and enhance 360° views of the arterial anatomy. For this reason, coaxial phased array systems that produce images utilizing electronically rotating signals rather than mechanically rotating systems over eccentric wire delivery provide enhanced optimal resolution.

In our practice, IVUS is particularly useful in the endograft treatment of aortic dissections [16]. IVUS can help identify entry and reentry tears in aortic dissections (Fig. 6.5), identify the origin of aortic and visceral branch vessels, and determine the proximal fixation point relative to the brachiocephalic vessels. Selective endograft exclusion of the false lumen can be aided by use of IVUS to carefully navigate a guide wire pathway within the true lumen and assess for successful reperfusion of the true lumen following endograft deployment. IVUS may also help determine adequacy of stent length coverage for false lumen exclusion by demonstrating the return of systolic pulsatile flow to the true lumen as well as concomitant stagnation of flow and thrombus development within the false lumen (Fig. 6.6) [16]. The major drawback to the use of IVUS is the need for invasive arterial access for catheter placement.

Conclusion

There exist a number of noninvasive imaging modalities that are currently available for use in the treatment of thoracoabdominal pathology with endovascular therapy. Each modality has particular advantages and will likely continue to evolve as more experience with endografts is accumulated and long-term outcomes are better understood.

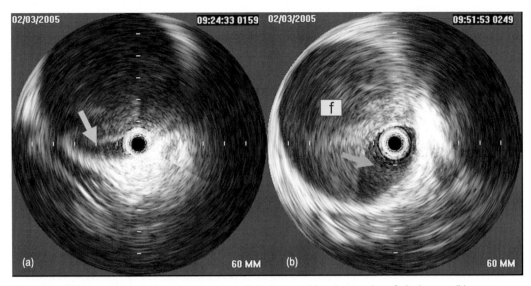

Figure 6.6 IVUS images of aortic dissection preendograft deployment (a) and postendograft deployment (b) demonstrating the dimensions of the true lumen (arrows) at the same aortic level. Real-time predeployment images show pulsatile flow in the false lumen with severe compromised flow in the true lumen. The postprocedure IVUS image (b) demonstrates enlargement of the true lumen with pulsatile flow in the true lumen and stagnation of flow in the false lumen (f) following coverage of the proximal entry site.

Spiral CT remains the gold standard for preoperative assessment for patient selection and postoperative surveillance. For instance, spiral CT is particularly useful for choosing appropriate candidates for complex reconstructive procedures such as endoluminal vascular prosthesis placement, where preintervention assessment of the lesions, sizing of proximal and distal vessels, and identification of collateral beds is indispensable. Moreover, TEE and IVUS are under-utilized modalities that may play an expanding role in endovascular therapy given its applicability within the operating room.

References

1 Rubin GD, Walker PJ, Dake MD, Napel S, Jeffrey RB, McDonnell CH et al. Three-dimensional spiral computed tomographic angiography: An alternative imaging modality for the abdominal aorta and its branches. J Vasc Surg 1993; **18**: 656–665.

2 Rubin GD, Dake MD, Napel S, Jeffrey RB, McDonnell CH, Sommer FG, Wexler L et al. Spiral CT of renal artery stenoses: Comparison of three-dimensional rendering techniques. Radiology 1994; **190**: 181–189.

3 Rubin GD et al. Three-dimensional CT angiography of the splanchnic vasculature. Radiology 1993; **189**(Suppl): 229.

4 Stavropoulos SW, Clark TW, Carpenter JP, Fairman RM, Litt H, Velazquez OC et al. Use of CT angiography to classify endoleaks after endovascular repair of abdominal aortic aneurysms. J Vasc Interv Radiol 2005; **16**: 663–667.

5 Neschis DG, Velazquez OC, Baum RA, Roberts D, Carpenter JP, Golden MA et al. The role of magnetic resonance angiography for endoprosthetic design. J Vasc Surg 2001; **33**: 488–494.

6 Glazer HS, Gutierrez FR, Levitt RG, Lee JK, Murphy WA. The thoracic aorta studied by MR imaging. Radiology 1985; **157**: 149–155.

7 Ludman CN, Yusuf SW, Whitaker SC, Gregson RH, Walker S, and Hopkins BR. Feasibility of using dynamic contrast-enhanced magnetic resonance angiography as the sole imaging modality prior to endovascular repair of abdominal aortic aneurysm. Eur J Vasc Endovasc Surg 2000; **19**: 524–530.

8 Lookstein RA, Goldman J, Pukin L, Marin ML. Time-resolved magnetic resonance angiography as a noninvasive method to characterize endoleaks: Initial results compared with conventional angiography. J Vasc Surg 2004; **39**: 27–33.

9 Haulon S, Lions C, McFadden EP, Koussa M, Gaxotte V, Halna P et al. Prospective evaluation of magnetic

resonance imaging after endovascular treatment of infrarenal aortic aneurysms. Eur J Vasc Endovasc Surg 2001; **22**: 62–69.

10 Faries PL, Agarwal G, Lookstein R, Berhneim JW, Cayne NS, Cadot H *et al.* Use of cine magnetic resonance angiography in quantifying aneurysm pulsatility associated with endoleak. J Vasc Surg 2003; **38**: 652–656.

11 Veith FJ, Baum RA, Ohki T, Amor M, Adiseshiah M, Blankensteijn JD *et al.* Nature and significance of endoleaks and endotension: summary of opinions expressed at an international conference. J Vasc Surg 2002; **35**: 1029–1035.

12 Rocchi G, Lofiego C, Biagini E, Piva T, Brachetti G, Lovato L *et al.* Transesophageal echocardiography-guided algorithm for stent-graft implantation in aortic dissection. J Vasc Surg 2004; **40**: 880–885.

13 Gonzalez-Fajardo JA, Guiterrez V, Roman J, Serrador A, Arreba E, del Rio *et al.* Utility of intraoperative transesophageal echocardiology during endovascular stent-graft repair of acute thoracic aortic dissection. Ann Vasc Surg 2002; **16**; 297–313.

14 White RA, Donayre D, Kopchock G, Walot I, Wilson E, de Virgilio C. Intravascular ultrasound: The ultimate tool for abdominal aortic aneurysm assessment and endovascular graft delivery. J Endovasc Surg 1997; **4**: 45–55.

15 White RA. (2001) Intravascular ultrasound imaging. Current Surgical Therapy, 7th edn. Mosby, Saint Louis, MO, 2001: 800–806.

16 Song TK, Donayre CE, Walot I, Kopchok GE, Litwinski RA, Lippmann M *et al.* Endograft exclusion of acute and chronic descending thoracic aortic dissections. J Vasc Surg 2006; **43**: 247–258.

CHAPTER 7

Preoperative imaging and device sizing in endovascular management of thoracic aortic aneurysms

Panagiotis Kougias, Hosam El Sayed, & Wei Zhou

Thoracic aortic pathology in a variety of forms continues to represent a significant health challenge. The incidence of thoracic aortic aneurysms (TAAs) is estimated to be as high as 10 cases per 100,000 population per year [1, 2], whereas acute aortic dissection occurs in 10 to 20 individuals per million population [3] and traumatic aortic tears occur in up to 18% of motor vehicle accidents [4]. Until recently, the only effective treatment method was surgical graft replacement, involving high morbidity and at times technically complex operations. Endovascular stent-graft repair recently emerged as a viable alternative and has now gained acceptance as an innovative, safe treatment method associated with substantially less morbidity and reduced hospital stay.

Unlike open TAA repair, where the surgeon can make decisions on graft size at the time of surgery, endoluminal repair requires meticulous preoperative imaging to precisely define the aneurysm morphology and choose the appropriate size graft. This quickly became evident in the early era of endovascular abdominal aortic aneurysm (AAA) repair, when failure to correctly measure the aneurysm led to endoleaks, graft thrombosis, graft misalignment, and failure to exclude the aneurysm [5]; and is particularly true for aneurysms of the thoracic aorta, where high flow velocities and acute arch angles pose a formidable challenge in accurate graft placement and aneurysm exclusion. Evaluation must include measurements of various diameters and lengths of the aortic arch and proximal and distal thoracic aorta. In addition, iliac artery size,

tortuosity, angulation, and calcification may impact graft delivery and need to be taken into account. This chapter summarizes the most important aspects and highlights commonly made pitfalls in endograft sizing prior to endovascular repair of TAA.

Preoperative imaging

An ideal preoperative imaging modality to evaluate a patient for endovascular TAA repair would be accurate in depicting aneurysm morphology, minimize radiation and contrast exposure, and be noninvasive, inexpensive, and easily tolerated by the patient. Such a modality is not available. Techniques that are available and currently in use, sometimes in combination, include computed tomography (CT) scans, aortography, intravascular ultrasound scanning, and magnetic resonance angiography. The most commonly used diagnostic modalities are CT scan and marking aortography [6].

CT angiography with intravenous administration of contrast and 3-mm-thick slices, widely used in the assessment of TAAs, may be the only study required prior to an open repair. Traditional axial CT images over a tortuous portion of the aorta will overestimate the true diameter of the vessel and should thus be interpreted cautiously when sizing a thoracic endograft. Digital modification of CT-acquired images has been used with success for both abdominal and TAAs. Reconstruction of the image with curved linear reformats allows visualization of the vascular lumen in a plane perpendicular to the central arterial axis. To achieve this, central lumen lines are created by placing markers in the center of the vessel of interest (Fig. 7.1). The reconstruction obtained using this method may provide more accurate information on aortic length than traditional arteriography with marking catheter, since the position of the central lumen line can be adjusted to the anticipated position of the endograft. If the aorta is elliptical at the level of the measurement, then the mean diameter can be used to select the appropriate graft [7]. In addition, three-dimensional (3D), interactive digital reconstruction is possible using proprietary software (Preview Software, Medical Media Systems [MMS], West

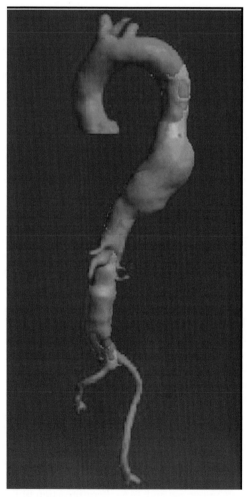

Figure 7.1 Three-dimensional reconstruction of CT scans is invaluable in permitting accurate measurements of thoracic aorta aneurysms. Length measurements are optimized; however, lumen diameters are best measured directly from transverse slices.

Lebanon, NH). Encouraging results with this technology indicate that 3D reconstruction might be the only diagnostic modality necessary for preoperative planning in patients with AAAs, eliminating the need for preoperative angiography [8]; however, others take a more conservative approach, suggesting that for the straightforward aneurysm, 3D reconstruction does not really alter or improve decision making compared to traditional CT angiography [6]. Studies comparing 3D CT reconstruction with traditional CT angiography and other imaging modalities in terms of preoperative thoracic endograft planning are not currently available. The complex structure of the aortic arch and the tortuosity present in the distal descending aorta – the two common landing zones of thoracic endografts – lend themselves to a more sophisticated level of imaging, and most authors use 3D reconstruction routinely [1].

Aortography provides important information on arterial tortuosity, length of the various segments, and the presence of concomitant occlusive disease. Distinct disadvantages include complications associated with the invasive nature of the procedure; and inability to reliably measure diameter, because of the presence of mural thrombus, or detect calcification that can be a major cause of fixation and delivery problems. When performed as a separate procedure prior to endograft placement, arteriography also adds to the overall cost of the procedure. In our experience, sizing the endograft with CT angiography and performing the arteriogram with a marking catheter just prior to the deployment of the stent graft is preferable, except for the most complicated aneurysms or those associated with chronic dissection.

Intravascular ultrasound (IVUS) has become an invaluable intraoperative imaging tool, particularly in difficult cases and those associated with aortic dissection. IVUS gives information on aortic diameter without the confounding magnification effect of arteriography; measures the length of proximal and distal landing zones; confirms aortic branch anatomy; verifies the optimal stent-graft placement after deployment; confirms wire passage in the true lumen and adequate coverage of the entry site in the cases of dissection; and offers information on adequate graft apposition and relation to adjacent branches [9, 10].

Device sizing

Selection of appropriate length and diameter of the endoprosthesis used in endovascular TAA repair is closely linked to the sophistication and accuracy of the preoperative imaging modalities. The importance of accurate sizing cannot be overemphasized. Some of the major postoperative complications, including type I endoleak, kinking and collapse, and obstruction at branch orifice points, are directly related to poor sizing.

Diameter considerations (Fig. 7.2)

CT scan imaging with or without 3D reconstruction indicates the aneurysmal portion of the aorta and the adjacent segments of normal caliber that can serve as landing zones. Diameter measurements of the true lumen from inner wall to inner wall at 1 and 2 cm from the proximal and distal implantation sites are recommended to assess for a conically shaped neck, which may increase the risk of graft migration. A graft diameter 6–19% larger than the aortic diameter is desirable to allow for good wall apposition. For the Gore thoracic aortic graft (TAG) device, this means that aortic diameters from 23 to 37 mm can be treated using six different prosthesis diameters from 26 to 40 mm (Fig. 7.3). Further oversizing the graft does not add anything to the procedure and can in fact be dangerous if the end point of the graft protrudes into the aortic lumen, especially if the proximal landing zone is just distal to an acutely angled aortic arch. This has the potential for graft collapse, which can lead to continuous pressurization of the aneurysmal sac. In an even worse case scenario, high blood flows within the aortic arch can make the graft fold into itself, causing obstruction of the aorta and death. This is of particular concern in young patients with relatively small aortas who present with aortic trauma and for whom appropriately small endoprostheses are not available.

The size of the introducer sheath utilized to deliver the endoprosthesis is closely linked to the diameter of the endograft and may vary from 20 Fr (7.6 mm) to 24 Fr (9.2 mm). This is an important consideration when planning the operation and mandates careful evaluation of the diameter of the access vessels. Small, calcified, and tortuous iliac and femoral vessels will not accommodate the large

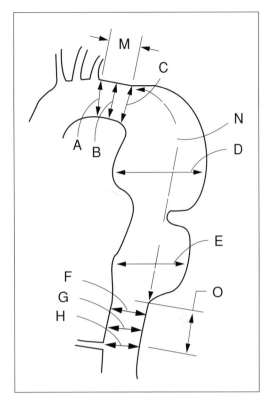

Figure 7.2 This is a typical sizing diagram for sizing of the descending thoracic aorta. A minimum of six diameters are used to characterize the proximal and distal landing zones. For the Gore TAG device, these are lumen-to-lumen measurements, not adventitial-to-adventitial measurements. Consequently appropriate sizing requires a contrast-enhanced CT scan, angiogram, or IVUS. A: Proximal implantation site. B: 1 cm from proximal implantation site. C: 2 cm from proximal implantation site. D: Aneurysm. E: 2 cm from distal implantation site. F: 1 cm from proximal implantation site. G: Distal implantation site. H: Right common iliac artery. M: Aneurysm length. N: Distal neck, distance from aneurysm to celiac axis. O: Total treatment length.

delivery devices. Placement of a temporary prosthetic conduit in the common iliac artery is recommended in these situations to avoid vascular injuries in the iliac and femoral territory. If using a conduit, select a graft with a large enough inner diameter for the sheath, such as a 10-mm Dacron graft.

Length considerations (Figs. 7.4–7.6)

At least 2 cm neck length proximally and distally is recommended by most authors to allow adequate stent-graft seal and minimize the risk of type I

Device diameter	Vessel diameter	Oversizing (%)
26	23—24	8—14
28	24—26	8—17
31	26—29	7—19
tt	29—32	6—17
37	32—34	9—16
40	34—37	9—18

Figure 7.3 A TAG (W.L. Gore) sizing chart.

endoleaks. In the cases where this was not possible, continuous sac pressurization with deleterious consequences has been described [11]. When the aneurysm starts at least 2 cm distal to the left subclavian artery, the endograft deployment is rather straightforward. Aneurysms with more proximal extent may necessitate complex debranching procedures that will allow coverage of one or more of the arch branches in order to achieve the desirable 2 cm sealing zone. Distal neck length, measured as the distance of the aneurysm from the celiac axis, also needs to be adequate, although debranching procedures have been described [12] and can optimize the neck to appropriate length.

Lengths of thoracic stent grafts are limited; the TAG endoprosthesis, for instance, is available in lengths of 10, 15, and 20 cm. Therefore, more than one piece of stent graft is often required to completely exclude the aneurysm. Several factors should be considered in the decision making process: (1) A minimum of 3 cm of overlap should be used for devices of different sizes. (2) Five centimeter overlap should be used for same size devices. (3) Many physicians use 5 cm overlap in most situations. (4) Implant the smallest device, which may be the distal device, first. (5) If the diameters of the proximal and distal landing zones are different enough to require endografts of different

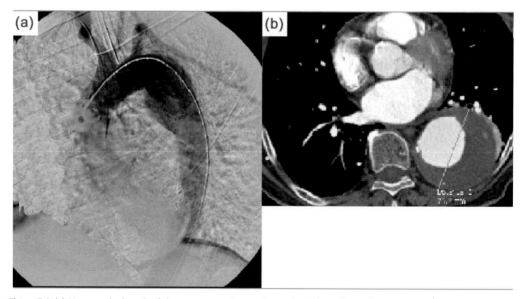

Figure 7.4 (a) Measure the length of the aneurysm using angiography with marker catheter present. (b) Measure the maximum lumen-to-lumen diameter using CT.

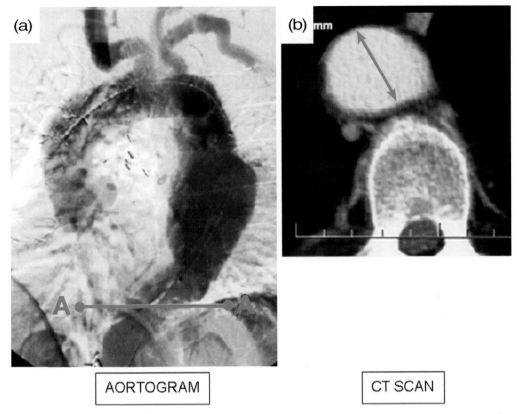

Figure 7.5 Diameter measured in angled necks seen on an aortogram (a). For device sizing purpose, measure the smaller width of the ellipse on the CT scan (b).

diameters, which is often the case, a bridging device may be necessary between the devices.

Difficult scenarios

Small iliac arteries

Vascular trauma or thrombosis occurred in 14% of patients in the Gore TAG pivotal trial, most of them access-related iliac artery injuries. Iliac artery rupture is the most commonly reported complication since US Food and Drug Administration (FDA) approval of the device. Judging iliac artery ability to accommodate a sheath is very difficult. Size requirements vary depending on the diameter of the graft to be utilized, which in turn determines diameter of the sheath to be inserted:

20 Fr sheath: OD = 7.6 mm
22 Fr sheath: OD = 8.3 mm
24 Fr sheath: OD = 9.2 mm.

Typically a rupture will not be identified until the sheath is being removed. If sheath insertion has been difficult, have an occlusion balloon prepped and on the table or insert one into the distal aorta while slowly withdrawing the sheath and injecting dye. Although some ruptures can be salvaged by insertion of a stent graft, usually the external is avulsed and back bleeding can occur from the internal iliac artery. In our experience, open surgical repair is usually required. As a result, we have adopted a very liberal policy for insertion of a retroperitoneal conduit: If in doubt, place a conduit.

Significant aortic tortuosity

Numerous curves can develop within the aorta. When there is angulation and tortuosity at the arch, coupled with tortuosity immediately prior to penetrating the diaphragmatic hiatus, these double curves can lead to difficulty in advancing the

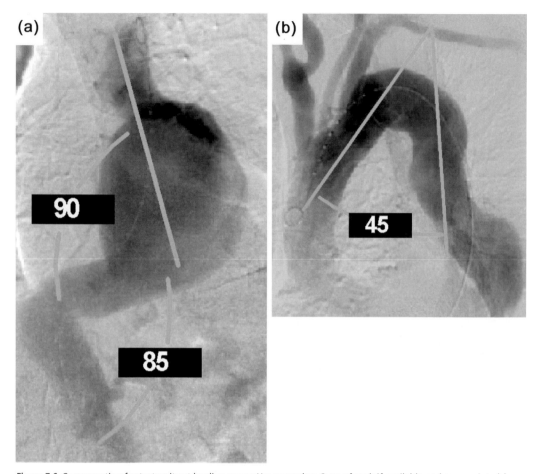

Figure 7.6 Compensating for tortuosity at landing zones: Use more than 2 cm of neck if available and appropriate (a). Greater than 2 cm of neck is recommended when a severe angle exists (<60° angle) (b).

device over the arch. The device tends to buckle into the curve above the diaphragm and fails to advance in the arch. Ensuring that the wire is advanced as much as possible, advancing the wire and catheter together, or placing a second wire to straighten the aorta as much as possible are adjunctive techniques for this problem.

Debranching techniques to extend the application of thoracic endografts

Selective carotid–subclavian bypass was the first technique used to extend the proximal landing zone to permit endograft deployment up to the origin of the left common carotid artery. Since device approval, clinicians have developed techniques to further debranch the aorta. Carotid-to-carotid bypass with selective carotid–subclavian

bypass permits device deployment up to the innominate. In patients with a normal ascending aorta or a prior ascending graft, aorto–innominate bypass with carotid-to-carotid and carotid–subclavian bypass permits total debranching of the aortic arch. Debranching of the abdominal aorta can also be performed from either an infrarenal graft, infrarenal aorta, or iliac arteries. Retrograde bypass to the celiac, superior mesenteric artery, and renal arteries allows a sequential increase in the length of the distal landing zone.

Conclusion

Careful preoperative planning is essential for the success of endovascular treatment of thoracic aortic pathology (ETAP). CT scans with or without 3D reconstruction in conjunction with arteriography provides the information needed for graft selection. Careful diameter oversizing and adequate coverage of the proximal and distal landing zones will allow for aneurysm exclusion. Debranching procedures enable treatment of aneurysms adjacent to or involving the aortic arch branches, providing flexibility on landing zone selection. Characteristics of the iliofemoral vessels need to be taken into account, in conjunction with the delivery sheath size, in order to avoid serious injury to the access vessels.

References

1 Lee JT, White RA. Current status of thoracic aortic endograft repair. Surg Clin North Am 2004; **84**: 1295–1318; vi–vii.

2 Johansson G, Markstrom U, Swedenborg J. Ruptured thoracic aortic aneurysms: A study of incidence and mortality rates. J Vasc Surg 1995; **21**: 985–988.

3 Pate JW, Richardson RL, Eastridge CE. Acute aortic dissections. Am Surg 1976; **42**: 395–404.

4 Cardarelli MG, McLaughlin JS, Downing SW, Brown JM, Attar S, Griffith BP. Management of traumatic aortic rupture: A 30-year experience. Ann Surg 2002; **236**: 465–469; discussion 469–470.

5 Broeders IA, Blankensteijn JD. Preoperative imaging of the aortoiliac anatomy in endovascular aneurysm surgery. Semin Vasc Surg 1999; **12**: 306–314.

6 Parker MV, O'Donnell SD, Chang AS, Johnson CA, Gillespie DL, Goff JM, Rasmussen TE, Rich NM. What imaging studies are necessary for abdominal aortic endograft sizing? A prospective blinded study using conventional computed tomography, aortography, and three-dimensional computed tomography. J Vasc Surg 2005; **41**: 199–205.

7 Broeders IA, Blankensteijn JD, Olree M, Mali W, Eikelboom BC. Preoperative sizing of grafts for transfemoral endovascular aneurysm management: A prospective comparative study of spiral CT angiography, arteriography, and conventional CT imaging. J Endovasc Surg 1997; **4**: 252–261.

8 Wyers MC, Fillinger MF, Schermerhorn ML, Powell RJ, Rzucidlo EM, Walsh DB, Zwolak RM, Cronenwett JL. Endovascular repair of abdominal aortic aneurysm without preoperative arteriography. J Vasc Surg 2003; **38**: 730–738.

9 Lee JT, White RA. Basics of intravascular ultrasound: An essential tool for the endovascular surgeon. Semin Vasc Surg. 2004; **17**: 110–118.

10 Dake MD, Kato N, Mitchell RS, Semba CP, Razavi MK, Shimono T, Hirano T, Takeda K, Yada I, Miller DC. Endovascular stent-graft placement for the treatment of acute aortic dissection. N Engl J Med 1999; **340**: 1546–1552.

11 Criado FJ, Clark NS, Barnatan MF. Stent graft repair in the aortic arch and descending thoracic aorta: A 4-year experience. J Vasc Surg 2002; **36**: 1121–1128.

12 Fulton JJ, Farber MA, Marston WA, Mendes R, Mauro MA, Keagy BA. Endovascular stent-graft repair of pararenal and type IV thoracoabdominal aortic aneurysms with adjunctive visceral reconstruction. J Vasc Surg 2005; **41**: 191–198.

CHAPTER 8

Intramural hematoma and penetrating ulcer

Michael D. Dake

Over the past decade, advances in vascular imaging technology have led to increasing recognition of aortic intramural hematomas (IMHs) in patients with acute aortic syndromes. Considered by many to be a variant of aortic dissection, the pathogenesis of IMH still remains unclear. Two different pathophysiological processes can lead to intramural hematoma formation. One is IMH without intimal disruption; in this entity, it is believed that spontaneous rupture of aortic vasa vasorum is responsible for hematoma formation within the aortic wall [1]. The other type of IMH is associated with an atherosclerotic ulcer that penetrates into the internal elastic lamina and allows hematoma formation within the media of the aortic wall [2–4]. In previous reports, these two types of IMH are rarely distinguished in discussing prognoses and optimal treatment methods [3, 5, 6]. The concept of the Stanford classification scheme for aortic dissection has been applied to IMH because the prognostic impact of the location of IMH and its standard treatment have been considered similar to those for classic aortic dissection [5]. It is generally accepted that patients with type B (exclusive involvement of the descending aorta) IMH can be managed conservatively in the absence of disease progression, whereas early surgical interventions are recommended for type A (involvement of the ascending aorta) IMH [5,6]. On the other hand, Coady *et al.* [7] recently reported that the prognoses of acutely symptomatic hospitalized patients with penetrating atherosclerotic ulcers (PAUs) were worse than those with classic aortic dissection due to a higher incidence of aortic rupture.

In general, the treatment paradigm for IMH parallels the approach in classical aortic dissection

[8, 9]. A meta-analysis review of 11 IMH studies found cumulative mortality for type A IMH to be 24% for those treated surgically, 47% for those treated medically, and 34% overall; mortality for type B IMH was 14% overall with little difference between surgical (15%) and medical (13%) treatment groups [10]. At present, no consensus therapeutic strategy for PAU exists although a more aggressive surgical approach, independent of location, is being increasingly considered especially in symptomatic patients [7, 11, 12]. The Yale Thoracic Aortic Diseases Group has identified a 40% rupture rate among PAU patients managed medically [7, 11]. At a minimum, PAU patients with complications should undergo surgical treatment [13].

Management strategies

As the profile of clinical factors, imaging findings, acute outcomes, and long-term results of various management strategies comes into sharper focus, some patterns are emerging and serve as a basis for establishing the initial standard treatment algorithms for IMH. One of the aspects of IMH, however, that confounds attempts to set indications for intervention, much less precise management techniques, is the wide variety of morphologic appearances of aortic IMH observed with common diagnostic imaging modalities, including transesophageal echo (TEE) or magnetic resonance imaging/computed tomographic (MRI/CT) scans. Traditionally, IMH refers to hemorrhage contained within the medial layer of the aortic wall, and is distinguished from typical aortic dissection and penetrating atherosclerotic aortic ulcer by the absence of an associated tear in the intima or direct communication between the media and the aortic lumen.

Unfortunately, this seemingly straightforward differentiation is not always possible because of the rapid tempo of morphologic evolution noted frequently on sequential imaging exams of patients with IMH. Thus, depending on the exact time after the onset of symptoms when an imaging "snapshot" is performed, the appearance may be interpreted differently than an impression made from images obtained only hours before or after. In practical terms, because there are limitations in our ability to repeat imaging at frequent intervals, assignment of precise diagnostic labels in a dogmatic manner is not always possible. Indeed, in many patients with acute aortic symptoms, a healthy bit of confusion between the related diagnoses of aortic dissection without intimal rupture, IMH, and penetrating atherosclerotic aortic ulcer with associated IMH is expected, and reflects the natural history of IMH.

In addition to the potential for diagnostic confusion that exists when imaging "samples" one point in the rapid tempo of morphological evolution characteristic of some IMH patients, other factors limit the facile development of criteria that would permit the blanket application of a general therapeutic strategy to manage patients with IMH. Some of the critical features identified in the medical literature that appear to influence the outcome of IMH, in terms of whether it has a complicated, progressive course or follows an uncomplicated, benign disease pattern include: the presence of acute symptoms at the time of imaging diagnosis; involvement of the ascending aorta, and presence of an associated penetrating ulcer or ulcer-like projection in the involved aortic segment [14–19].

Born out of these initial clinical observations and despite the recognized limitations to formulating prognostic criteria for IMH, recent attention focused on this entity over the last five years led to the identification of numerous new features of disease involvement that may allow a more reliable determination of the relative risk for an individual patient. It is hoped that these disease characteristics will be further refined in the future to better define those patients with an increased relative risk of progression to aortic dissection, rupture, aneurysm formation, IMH expansion, and those in which partial regression or complete resorption is likely.

Predictors of disease progression

Some of the current predictive factors of disease progression proposed for patients with IMH exclusively, without an associated ulcer or intimal erosion, include: involvement of the ascending aorta; maximum aortic diameter of 50 mm or greater on initial CT scan; persistent pain; progressive maximal aortic wall thickness; and enlarging aortic diameter [15, 18–20]. Other predictors of disease progression in patients with IMH and an associated aortic ulcer or intimal erosion include: interval increase of associated pleural effusion; recurrent pain; ulcer located in the ascending aorta or arch; initial maximum ulcer diameter of 20 mm or more; and initial maximum ulcer depth of 10 mm or greater [14, 15].

Given this background and with the recognition that roughly half the cases of IMH progress despite medical treatment while the others show spontaneous resolution of the process without clinical sequelae, a loosely held consensus regarding IMH management has coalesced around the traditional treatment algorithms applied to classic aortic dissection [15, 21]. Thus, one of the pivotal criteria used to direct treatment is based around the location of aortic involvement with the Stanford classification of aortic dissection commonly used to categorize IMH. In this regard, in many institutions, the standard treatment over the past decade for patients with type A IMH with or without an ulcer has been early surgical graft replacement.

Published 30 day mortality after surgery is reported to range from 10 to 50% [15, 20–23]. Despite the uncertain risk of operative repair, it is a firmly held belief that for acute IMH presenting within a few hours of symptom onset and involving the ascending aorta, observation and medical treatment are far more dangerous than surgery [15, 20–23]. Alternatively, other investigators have advocated conservative treatment for type A IMH and report favorable results without progression to classic dissection, rupture, tamponade, or compression of coronary ostia [16, 24–26]. Song and colleagues suggest that medical treatment initially with frequent imaging follow-up and elective surgery in cases that develop complications is a prudent strategy [27]. These conservative approaches currently, however, remain minority opinions for dealing with acutely symptomatic patients.

Asymptomatic patients

Conversely, in asymptomatic patients or those beyond 48 h from the onset of symptoms with IMH located in the arch or descending aorta, watchful waiting and aggressive antihypertensive treatment appear a safe strategy; however, frequent follow-up imaging evaluations for evidence of intimal erosion or disease progression are required and a low threshold for intervention should be maintained if symptoms recur [14, 15]. This conservative approach to type B IMH is supported by studies that document similar survival statistics for medical treatment and surgical repair in the setting of descending thoracic IMH [17, 18, 22]. In a series of 53 cases of type B IMH, Harris and colleagues reported similar survival results for 33 patients managed medically and 20 who underwent surgery (91% and 80%, respectively) [22]. Thus, although the cumulative risk of a conservative management policy is not defined precisely for type B IMH, there exists no clear advantage to an operative strategy.

There are clinical scenarios, however, that are considered exceptions to this approach. Most notably, the presence of a penetrating aortic ulcer in an acutely symptomatic patient or an unstable or enlarging distal ulcer associated with type B IMH should undergo more aggressive treatment [14]. Expeditious surgical intervention is recommended in this setting; however, conventional open repair requiring graft interposition is associated with high morbidity and mortality rates, especially in this complicated setting in patients that typically are not ideal operative candidates because of advanced age and/or coexisting medical diseases. Consequently, less invasive strategies that rely on the endovascular placement of stent grafts to cover the ulcer and some extent of the IMH have been recently investigated with promising initial results, including a lack of early pseudoaneurysm formation in the treated aortic segment. Indeed the endovascular approach may have considerable advantages in this disease compared with conventional open surgical repair [14, 28]. Application of this minimally invasive technology to cases of type B IMH without associated intimal disruption or ulcer has not been reported. As additional correlative studies from larger clinical series than previously published and the results of new therapies are reported in the literature, there is an opportunity to refine management approaches to IMH and establish treatment guidelines that will improve outcomes and benefit patients beyond what is achieved currently.

References

1 Gore I. Pathogenesis of dissecting aneurysm of the aorta. Arch Pathol Lab Med 1952; **53**: 142–153.

2 Stanson AW, Kazmier FJ, Hollier LH *et al.* Penetrating atherosclerotic ulcers of the thoracic aorta: Natural history and clinicopathologic correlations. Ann Vasc Surg 1986; **1**: 15–23.

3 Harris KM, Braverman AC, Gutierrez FR *et al.* Transesophageal echocardiographic and clinical features of aortic intramural hematoma. J Thorac Cardiovasc Surg 1997; **114**: 619–626.

4 Mohr-Kahaly S, Erbel R, Kearney FP *et al.* Aortic intramural hemorrhage visualized by transesophageal echocardiography: findings and prognostic implications. J Am Coll Cardiol 1994; **23**: 658–664.

5 Nienaber CA, von Kodolitsch Y, Petersen B *et al.* Intramural hemorrhage of the thoracic aorta: Diagnostic and therapeutic implications. Circulation 1995; **92**: 1465–1472.

6 Muluk SC, Kaufman JA, Torchiana DF *et al.* Diagnosis and treatment of thoracic aortic intramural hematoma. J Vas Surg 1996; **24**: 1022–1029.

7 Coady MA, Rizzo JA, Hammond GL *et al.* Penetrating ulcer of the thoracic aorta: What is it? How do we recognize it? How do we manage it? J Vasc Surg 1998; **27**: 1006–1016.

8 Nienaber CA, von Kodolitsch Y, Petersen B, Loose R, Helmchen U, Haverich A, Spielman RP. Intramural hemorrhage of the thoracic aorta. Diagnostic and therapeutic implications. Circulation 1995; **92**: 1465–1472.

9 Robbins RC, McManus RP, Mitchell RS, Latter DR, Moon MR, Olinger GN, Miller DC. Management of patients with intramural hematoma of the thoracic aorta. Circulation 1993; **88**: II1-10.

10 Sawhney NS, DeMaria AN, Blanchard DG. Aortic intramural hematoma: An increasingly recognized and potentially fatal entity. Chest 2001; **120**: 1340–1346.

11 Tittle SL, Lynch RJ, Cole PE, Singh HS, Rizzo JA, Kopf GS, Elefteriades JA. Midterm follow-up of penetrating ulcer and intramural hematoma of the aorta. J Thorac Cardiovasc Surg 2002; **123**: 1051–1059.

12 Eggebrecht H, Baumgart D, Herold U, Jakob H, Erbel R. Multiple penetrating atherosclerotic ulcers of the abdominal aorta: treatment by endovascular stent graft placement. Heart 2001; **85**: 526.

13 Braverman AC. Penetrating atherosclerotic ulcers of the aorta. Curr Opin Cardiol 1994; **9**: 591–597.

14 Ganaha F, Miller DC, Sugimoto K *et al*. The prognosis of aortic intramural hematoma with and without penetrating atherosclerose ulcer: A clinical and radiological analysis. Circulation 2002; **106**: 342–348.

15 Nienaber CA, von Kodolitsch Y, Petersen B *et al*. Intramural hemorrhage of the thoracic aorta: Diagnostic and therapeutic implications. Circulation 1995; **92**: 1465–1472.

16 Nienaber CA, Sievers HH. Intramural hematoma in acute aortic syndrome: More than one variant of dissection? Circulation 2002; **106**: 284–285.

17 Shimizu H, Yohino H, Udagawa H *et al*. Prognosis of intramural hemorrhage compared with classic aortic dissection. Am J Cardiol 2000; **85**: 792–795.

18 von Kodolitsch Y, Cso sz S, Koschyk DH *et al*. Intramural hematoma of the aorta: Predictors of progression to dissection and rupture. Circulation 2003; **107**: 1158–1163.

19 Murray JG, Manisali M, Flamm SD *et al*. Intramural hematoma of the thoracic aorta: MR image findings and their prognostic implications. Radiol 1997; **204**: 349–355.

20 Muluk SC, Kaufman JA, Torchiana DF *et al*. Fate of intramural hematoma of thoracic aortic intramural hematoma. J Vasc Surg 1996; **24**: 1022–1029.

21 Robbins RC, McManus RP, Mitchell RS *et al*. Management of patients with intramural hematoma of the thoracic aorta. Circulation 1993; **88**: II1–II10.

22 Harris KM, Braverman AC, Gutierrez FR *et al*. Transesophageal echocardiographic and clinical features of aortic intramural hematoma. J Thorac Cardiovasc Surg 1997; **114**: 619–626.

23 Moriyama Y, Yotsumoto G, Kuriwaki K *et al*. Intramural hematoma of the thoracic aorta. Eur J Cardiothorac Surg 1998; **13**: 230–239.

24 Sueyoshi E, Matsuoka Y, Sakamoto I, *et al*. Fate of intramural hematoma of the aorta: CT evaluation. J Comput Assist Tomogr 1997; **21**: 931–938.

25 Oliver TB, Murchison JT, Reid JH. Serial MRI in the management of intramural hemorrhage of the thoracic aorta. BR J Radiol 1997; **70**: 1288–1290.

26 Kaji S, Nishigami K, Akasaka T *et al*. Prediction of progression or regression of type A aortic intramural hematoma by computed tomography. Circulation 1999; **100** (Suppl II): II-281–6.

27 Song JK, Kim HS, Kang DH *et al*. Different clinical features of aortic intramural hematoma versus dissection involving the ascending aorta. J Am Coll Cardiol 2001; **37**: 1604–1610.

28 Schoder M, Grabenwoger M, Holzenbein T, Domanovits H, Fleischmann D, Wolf F *et al*. Endovascular stent-graft repair of complicated penetrating atherosclerotic ulcers of the descending thoracic aorta. J Vasc Surg 2002 Oct; **36**(4): 720–726.

CHAPTER 9

Patient follow-up and evaluation of abdominal and thoracic stent grafts

Jan D. Blankensteijn

Introduction

Currently, almost 15 years after the introduction of endovascular aortic aneurysm repair, durability of stent grafts is still an issue. Endovascular aneurysm repair has been demonstrated to be safe and effective, and in two randomized studies it was shown to be superior to open repair, at least for the first postoperative month [1, 2]. Despite this, many surgeons are hesitant to make endovascular aneurysm repair the method of first choice in all eligible patients. This attitude probably finds its origin in the first decade of endovascular aneurysm repair in which many durability issues of stent grafts have been encountered including metal fatigue, fabric tears, disconnecting modules, and graft porosity. While 2- to 4-year results of randomized trials comparing open and endovascular repair have been reported [3, 4], longer term results are required before endovascular aneurysm repair can be labeled a durable alternative for open repair.

Although the new generation endografts have already outperformed their predecessors, the disasters of the recent past are not easily forgotten. As a consequence, endovascular aneurysm repair patients are usually submitted to intensive and frequent follow-up schedules. Recent reports have reiterated the need for a continued, intensive, and accurate surveillance [5].

With the development of endovascular aneurysm repair, imaging modalities have also greatly improved. Initially, plain abdominal films (to detect structural defects), Duplex ultrasound (to detect endoleak and evaluate limb patency), and (helical) CT-angiography (to detect endoleak and size

changes) were predominantly used. More recent modalities such as magnetic resonance imaging, MR-angiography (MRA), and multidetector CT-angiography (MDCT) have dramatically improved image quality in endovascular aneurysm repair follow-up. These novel techniques have allowed for dynamic imaging of aortic wall and endograft movement and of endoleak hemodynamics. In addition, remote pressure sensors (RPS) have made noninvasive, continuous sac-pressure measurement possible.

Simultaneously, the focus of follow-up after endovascular aneurysm repair has shifted from incomplete exclusion (endoleak) and structural defects, to aneurysm sac size changes (diameter and volume), and subsequently to sac-pressure and aortic wall and stent-graft motion.

In this chapter, the following issues will be addressed. What is the best indicator of effectiveness of endovascular aneurysm repair, i.e. prevention of death from aneurysm rupture? Are current endografts reliable as to allow us to relax on the follow-up protocols or will newly developed (potentially less durable) endografts continue to require vigilance? Can a single new modality (MDCT, MRA, or RPS) reliably replace multiple older modalities of follow-up? Is follow-up of thoracic stent grafts different from abdominal endovascular aneurysm repair? What impact do the elaborate follow-up examinations have on the economics of endovascular aneurysm repair, and on patient safety (radiation and dye exposure)? Is the same endovascular aneurysm repair follow-up required for all patients or can tailor-made protocols safely minimize the negative effects of follow-up?

Determinants of success

The primary goal of aneurysm repair is to prevent death from rupture. Conventional open repair has long been established to accomplish this for both abdominal and thoracic aortic aneurysms. Imaging plays a key role in determining the postoperative success of endovascular repair. After stent-graft placement, complete and continued exclusion of the aneurysm sac can be confirmed by the absence of flow outside the endograft (endoleak) using contrast-enhanced imaging (CTA/MRA) or Duplex ultrasound, or by shrinkage or arrest of growth of the aneurysm as determined by diameter or volume measurements.

All endoleaks can lead to aneurysms expansion, which in turn is thought to be associated with elevated extra-luminal sac pressure (ESP). Therefore, aneurysm size is an important marker of persistent pressurization of the aneurysm sac, independent of the presence or absence of endoleak [6]. If the aneurysm is growing after endovascular aneurysm repair, even in the absence of an obvious endoleak, it should be considered at risk for rupture.

It is important to realize that sac shrinkage is a slow process and depending on the method used it may take long before changes can be demonstrated. Using diameter measurements it typically takes over 12 months before 50% of sacs can be demonstrated to shrink. Consequently, in the most optimistic scenario, over 40% of patients cannot be assured that the risk of rupture is removed in the first year. We have shown that serial, standardized, nonluminal aneurysm sac volume measurement (thrombus volume) is the most sensitive tool of following size change after endovascular aneurysm repair [7]. Of all size parameters, volume measurements are the first to identify effectively excluded AAA and the first to identify AAAs that are not excluded from the systemic blood pressure and intervention might be indicated. Using thrombus volume, in over 60% of aneurysms a significant change can be detected after 6 months. Maximum aneurysm sac area and circumference measurements are less sensitive to size changes than volume measurements but more sensitive than diameter measurements [8]. Maximum aortic circumference measurements can be used as an alternative if volume measurements are not available or too time-consuming.

In addition to these imaging techniques, complete exclusion can be tested by direct measurement of ESP using pressure gauges [9], or wireless pressure sensors implanted in the excluded aneurysm sac [10]. Pressure measurements do not rely on slow secondary effects of pressure changes (aneurysm growth) to occur and therefore seem to be the most direct and straightforward determinant of successful endovascular exclusion. However, even a small percentage of false negative pressure readings may cast doubt on pressure sensing as a single follow-up tool. Further studies to determine sensitivity and specificity of these techniques are due.

Imaging modalities

Several modalities are available for postoperative imaging. Plain antero-posterior, lateral, and oblique abdominal X-rays are used for their high spatial resolution. They will show dislocation or failures of the attachment systems and kinking of the graft. This method is inexpensive, fast, and patient friendly. Of course no information is obtained on the arterial wall, lumen, and changes in aneurysm diameters.

Color Duplex ultrasound is also relatively inexpensive and may be used for an early, noninvasive first impression of aneurysm exclusion. It is however operator dependent and size measurements have a low reproducibility. A recent systemic review has suggested Duplex ultrasound to be inadequate for endoleak detection [11].

Computer tomography angiography (CTA) is able to show very small endoleaks, communications with patent aortic branches, changes in aortic diameters and volumes, and malplacement of grafts or attachment systems.

In helical or spiral CTA tomography, the X-ray tube and detector (gantry) rotate continuously as the patient moves through the scanner. The result is a raw dataset, representing the helical path of the X-ray beam through the scanned volume. From this primary raw data, images can be reconstructed (postprocessed) in several planes and even into three-dimensional (3D) models. The diagnostic performance of spiral CTA however depends on the appropriate choice of acquisition parameters [12].

In an attempt to limit scanning time, subsequent tube heating, and motion artifacts, the patient has to be moved through the scanner at high table speeds, leading to an increase in slice collimation and sub-optimal spatial resolution. This inverse relation between scan range and slice collimation has been overcome by the introduction of multidetector spiral computed tomography (MDCT) [13].

MDCT allows the simultaneous acquisition of multiple slices during one gantry rotation. The effect of the number of slices on scanning time and resolution is explained by the following example. The scan range from the celiac artery to the femoral bifurcation is approximately 35 cm. Scanning this range using a single slice spiral CT, with a gantry rotation time of 1 s, a collimation of 5 mm, and a pitch of 1 (table speed/collimation) takes 70 s. Scanning the same area with a 16-slice CT, using the same pitch and twice the table speed, results in a slice collimation of 0.625 mm, increasing both resolution and scanning time.

At our institution, we use a 64-slice CT for the pre- and postoperative evaluation of abdominal aortic aneurysms. Although this scanner produces 64 slices during one gantry rotation "only" 32 slices can be generated for abdominal studies due to the orientation of the detectors. This results in maximal spatial resolution of 0.6 mm (SC) during a total data acquisition time of only 15 s (TF = 23 mm/s).

Besides an improvement in acquisition parameters, MDCT also allows an improvement in reconstruction parameters [13]. MDCT produces large amounts of data. A special interpolation scheme (z-filtering) uses all data for final reconstruction. Due to z-filtering the final reconstructed, effective slice thickness is independent of preset collimation as long as effective slice thickness does not exceed SC. Besides effective slice thickness, spatial resolution is determined by the reconstruction increment (RI). RI determines the degree of overlap between subsequent slices. At our institution we use an effective slice thickness of 1 mm with an RI of 0.7 (30% overlap). This final stack of overlapping reconstructed images is used for further image postprocessing. The most useful postprocessing tools for the assessment of aortic morphology include multiplanar reconstruction (MPR), maximum intensity projections (MIP), volume rendering (VR), and shaded surface display (SSD). Evaluation consists of a comparison of the noncontrast-enhanced scan to the subsequent scans. This is best done on a separate image-processing workstation as described earlier. The use of delayed series has been shown to be an effective tool to trace small type II endoleaks.

Cardiac gated or cardiac triggered MDCT techniques can eliminate pulsatile motion artifacts almost completely and allow for dynamic imaging. In dynamic imaging, the CT gantry is maintained in one position at the level of a certain aortic region and the position of all 64 detectors is therefore fixed during data acquisition. The rotation of the detector row is synchronized with the patient's EKG and by referencing the acquired slices to the EKG position a dynamic reconstruction can be created. This generates a movie-like representation of the motions of aorta, its branches, and the endograft in the interrogated segment. Although the moving images derived by this technique are astonishing, the value of this imaging modality will depend on the prospects of quantifying motion and forces.

As described above, an essential part of our follow-up protocol is tracking size changes using measurements of the nonluminal aneurysm sac volume. Unfortunately, nonluminal aneurysm sac volume measurements cannot be obtained from automated postprocessing tools. Manual segmentation is required and this is a time-consuming and labor-intensive procedure in which the aneurysm is outlined in every single reconstructed CT-slice and processed by an experienced technician. Several commercially available systems can be used. Our segmentations were all done on a separate image postprocessing system, EasyVision™ (Philips Medical Systems, Best, The Netherlands). We have also gained experience with the semiautomated PC-based system, Vitrea™ (Vital Images, Plymouth, MN, USA), which can provide volume data in a less time-consuming way [14]. Scans can also be processed by remote service providers, such as MMS (Preview™, Medical Metrx Solutions, West Lebanon, NH, USA). The raw CT-dataset is forwarded to this company and a fully analyzed CD-ROM with over 50 pre- and postoperative patient-specific measurements is returned or communicated through a secure internet database: PEMS™ (Patient Evaluation & Measurement System).

Endoleak detection with CTA can be difficult because of the relative insensitivity of this technique to iodinated contrast agent. Even with the use of the most dedicated CTA protocols, endoleaks may be missed [15, 16]. There is a significant number of patients with a growing aneurysm sac after endovascular aneurysm repair without a detectable endoleak on CTA or on conventional angiography [6, 17]. In some of these patients, this might be due to a hygroma-like process [18]. In others, it is possible that CTA is not sensitive enough. The superselective digital subtraction angiography technique is mainly reserved for specific cases and cannot be used routinely for surveillance because of its invasive nature [19].

In addition, the evaluation of sac size change, by using diameter or volume measurements, can be difficult using CTA. The moderate amount of soft tissue contrast involved does not always allow an accurate demarcation of the aneurysm wall, especially in inflammatory aneurysms. Another limitation of CTA is the difficulty in detecting stenosis in the endograft. Maximum intensity projections (MIP) not only depict the endograft lumen but also calcium, bone, metal, and other signal intense tissues, making appreciation of the lumen difficult.

Magnetic resonance imaging (MRI) might be more appropriate for follow-up after endovascular aneurysm repair than CTA due to its excellent soft tissue contrast, its inherent three-dimensionality, and its extreme sensitivity to gadolinium contrast agent. Moreover, the signal losses resulting from the metallic stent and calcium cannot be confused with contrast agent and are therefore less disturbing in low artifact metals, such as nitinol or tantalum. The absence of ionizing radiation and the ability to use a nonnephrotoxic contrast agent give MRI an additional advantage over CTA in endovascular aneurysm repair follow-up [20]. Furthermore, recent developments in MR hardware, such as SENSE (parallel imaging) and ultrafast gradient systems, together with cardiac gating have made fast dynamic scanning possible. These techniques have the potential to depict the contrast dynamics in and around the aneurysm sac and might therefore be of use for determining the origin of an endoleak and assessment of endograft patency [21].

The excellent soft tissue contrast of MRI can be used to detect local variations in thrombus consistency on T1- and T2-weighted images as described by Castrucci *et al.* [22]. Hygroma-like processes could also be revealed in this way. The clear liquid-like material from the hygroma will have high signal intensity on T2-weighted image in contrast to older organized thrombus.

The processing of the acquired images of patients after endovascular repair is similar to the preprocedural image postprocessing. CTA or MRI/MRA data are loaded onto a separate graphical workstation. Cine-mode, multiplanar reformats, segmentations of the lumen, and the nonluminal aneurysm sac are useful image postprocessing options in the assessment of an aneurysm after endovascular repair. For a more detailed analysis and for accurate diameter and length measurements, the central lumen line is drawn in the MPR. Curved linear reformats allow accurate measurement of the aneurysm diameter in a plane perpendicular to the vessel axis and accurate length measurements which is used for the evaluation of graft migration and aneurysm deformation.

There is one important disadvantage of MR follow-up of endovascular aneurysm repair. The metal components of one new-generation, abdominal and thoracic, aortic endograft are composed of stainless steel: Zenith^{TM} (Cook Inc., Bloomington, IN, USA). We have evaluated the potential of MR imaging with a large set of endografts [23]. For most endografts, the lumen and structures surrounding the endograft were well visualized. However, the ferromagnetic properties of the Zenith^{TM} device resulted in large susceptibly artifacts that obliterated the endograft lumen as well as adjacent structures. All fully supported grafts showed some amount of signal loss from the graft lumen caused by radiofrequency caging.

Recommended guidelines for follow-up

The failures of the past have guided newer endograft designs. With stronger fabric and metal components, the new-generation endografts have reported better durability than older designs. It must be realized, however, that newer endografts have a shorter duration of follow-up than older designs by definition. Longer term data are due before the commonly recommended guidelines can be relaxed.

In addition, new generation endografts are not always designed to be stronger and more durable than the existing models. Smaller profiles of the delivery systems, unconventional attachment systems, and percutaneous introduction techniques are common objectives and means for the next generation devices. Clearly, lower profiles are associated with thinner fabric and supporting materials. Consequently, "new" does not always imply "more durable" and a relaxation of the current follow-up recommendations seems ill-advised at this moment. The Imaging Guidelines Society for Interventional Radiology, published in 2003 by Geller [5], are similar to those suggested by Eurostar [24, 25]: Imaging studies (CT or MR) at baseline, every 6 months in the first 2 years and yearly thereafter.

Our initial endovascular abdominal aneurysm repair protocol consisted of a three full spiral CTA runs (plain, early-arterial, and late-venous) with 1 mm slices from celiac trunk to the level of the common femoral artery. Between 1993 and 2003, we have used this protocol in over 100 patients. In a retrospective study, we have shown that this was an enormous effort for patients and physicians while the yield was rather limited [26]. For all patients, our protocol required almost 600 CTA-scans, 20 gallons of contrast, and 500 h of radiology technician post-processing time. Individual patients were exposed to 500–1000 mSv which is equivalent to 500–1000 plain X-ray films and a cumulative contrast load of about 1 l after 5 years of follow-up. On the other hand, the yield of this intensive protocol was only a few (maybe too early) conversions for sac size increase and some (in the end unsuccessful) reinterventions for endoleaks.

While the risks of this extremely high radiation dose are obvious, the risks of nephrotoxic contrast administration in this patient population are sometimes not fully appreciated. In the patient cohort of our own DREAM-trial (elective nonhigh-risk AAA repair population) we have noted a prevalence of NHANES stage-3 chronic renal failure (glomerular filtration rate < 60) of around 20% (17–25%, $N =$ 348). In stage-3 CRF, the risk of a more than 25% increase in serum creatinine after a single dose of 150–200 ml of contrast is 20%. This increase may be temporary, but permanent loss of GFR is likely, especially after repeated episodes.

We have therefore modified our protocol. Currently, we use a minimized scan protocol single non-contrast run from a level immediately above the stent graft to immediately below the distal end of the stent graft (120 Kv, collimation 1.2, pitch 1.8, 3 mm reconstructions) which yields a fivefold reduction in radiation exposure (100 mSv at 5 years) and in over 80% of patients no contrast is used at all.

The costs associated with the above-mentioned surveillance protocols are significant [27, 28]. In addition, endoleaks and inadequate sac size changes detected by these rigorous follow-up protocols may lead to a further increase of costs by additional reinterventions [29]. These continued postoperative expenses may cancel out the already marginal cost benefit initially realized by the minimally invasive approach [30].

Finally, the cumulative case load of CT-scans is obviously directly related to the volume of patients entering the surveillance protocol. This case load can be shown to quickly amount to incredible numbers congesting CT-schedules. A simple rule-of-thumb to estimate this case load is the following. Assume we want to calculate the case load (L) of CT-scans required per month for surveillance of an endovascular program at time point t (years after the initiation of the endovascular program). Let N be the number of new patients entering the protocol per month, P the sum of scans in the surveillance protocol through t years (in current guidelines P equals 8 at 5 years), and S the typical yearly survival rate of this patient population. Then the case load at time point t can be calculated by this formula: $L(t) = N \times P \times S^{(t/2)}$. Assume you are running an endovascular program since the year 2000 with a relatively stable new patient entry rate of 4 cases per month ($N = 4$) and you want to know the case load (L) in the first month of 2006 ($t = 6$). With $P = 9$ at 6 years and using a typical 4-year survival rate of 70% in this patient population ($S = 92\%$) [4], $L(t) = 4 \times 9 \times 0.92^{(6/2)} = 28$. In other words, this endovascular program will require 28 CT-scans in the first month of 2006. Using a formula not displayed here, it can be calculated that 227 patients are incorporated in the follow-up program. Likewise, with a caseload of 10 new stent grafts per month since 1996, the same formula yields a staggering 93 CT-scans (acquisition, postprocessing, evaluation, and discussions with the patient!) on a monthly basis with 814 patients in follow-up.

Specifics for thoracic stent-graft follow-up

While aneurysmal disease is almost the exclusive indication for endografts in the abdominal aorta, reasons for placing stent grafts in the thoracic aorta are more diverse. The question arises whether a single generic follow-up protocol is appropriate for traumatic aortic ruptures, thoracic aneurysms, and dissections. Size changes and endoleak are most relevant for aneurysms, but less important after treating dissections and irrelevant after traumatic aortic rupture repair. In the case of dissections, specific aspects such as branch patency (away from the stentgraft), entry/reentry of false channels, and the interaction of endografts with the dissected aortic wall should be addressed. After traumatic aortic repair (typically in young healthy aorta), device integrity is the most important issue. Consequently, the follow-up intervals, the modalities used, and the problems to look for need to be defined for each indication specifically.

In our institution, we use MDCT as the mainstay of endografts follow-up for both thoracic aneurysm repair and aortic dissection. In the case of dissections, repeat scans of the entire aorta down to the groins are made frequently in the first few days after stent-graft placement in order to monitor the highly variable and rather unpredictable progression of the true and false lumens even after stent-graft placement. After discharge, CT-scans are used every 3 months until a regression of the false lumen is noted. Once the outer diameter of the dissected aorta can be demonstrated to shrink and in the absence of endoleak, the CT-follow-up intervals are increased to 6 months and 12 months.

Our follow-up protocol of thoracic aneurysm repair is similar to that of abdominal endovascular aneurysm repair. Contrast-enhanced CT is only performed in the cases where aneurysms cannot be demonstrated to shrink using maximum aneurysm circumference or thrombus volume measurements.

Although MDCT has far better resolution than single slice CT and 3D-reconstructions can produce impressive images of the stent-graft structure, we still prefer plain 4-view X-ray films for monitoring modular stability and stent-graft integrity for all indications. Plain X-rays are fast, inexpensive, and have even better resolution than MDCT.

As endoleaks tend not to be a major issue in thoracic aneurysm repair, the importance of follow-up of thoracic stent grafts is sometimes not fully appreciated. The extreme forces working the stent grafts in the thoracic aorta and the larger sizes of aorta and stent grafts amplify each other in challenging endovascular device integrity. Together with the indications other than aneurysmal disease for which thoracic stent grafts are used (aortic dissection and traumatic arch ruptures), these factors render thoracic endograft follow-up protocols largely unsettled at this moment.

Conclusions

In the absence of durability data of current endografts and with newer endograft continuing to emerge, life-long and frequent follow-up remains the cornerstone of endovascular aneurysm repair for both abdominal and thoracic stent grafts. CTA (MDCTA) is currently the imaging modality of choice for endovascular aneurysm repair follow-up. A dedicated CTA protocol will be able to detect most problems, provided it is combined with an adequate image postprocessing evaluation. All necessary assets of the postoperative follow-up can be evaluated.

Although there is only limited evidence of the value of MRI and MRA techniques for surveillance of endovascular aneurysm repair, this modality seems to be more sensitive to endoleak detection than CTA. Furthermore, the combination of the high soft tissue contrast in the T2-weighted images, the comparison of the T1-weighted scans before and after contract enhancement, and the possibility of performing dynamic contrast-enhanced MRA might very well make MRI the imaging modality of choice after endovascular repair in the future.

These elaborate imaging protocols will continue to have a significant impact on the already marginal cost-effectiveness of endovascular aneurysm repair.

References

1 Greenhalgh RM, Brown LC, Kwong GP *et al.* Comparison of endovascular aneurysm repair with open repair in patients with abdominal aortic aneurysm (EVAR trial 1), 30-day operative mortality results: Randomised controlled trial. Lancet 2004; **364**: 843–848.

2 Prinssen M, Verhoeven EL, Buth J *et al.* A randomized trial comparing conventional and endovascular repair of

abdominal aortic aneurysms. N Engl J Med 2004; **351**: 1607–1618.

3 Blankensteijn JD, De Jong SECA, Prinssen M *et al.* Two-year outcomes after conventional or endovascular repair of abdominal aortic aneurysms. New Engl J Med 2005; **352**: 2398–2405.

4 EVAR trial participants. Endovascular aneurysm repair versus open repair in patients with abdominal aortic aneurysm (EVAR trial 1): randomised controlled trial. Lancet 2005; **365**: 2179–2186.

5 Geller SC. Imaging guidelines for abdominal aortic aneurysm repair with endovascular stent grafts. J Vasc Interv Radiol 2003; **14**: S263–S264.

6 Veith FJ, Baum RA, Ohki T *et al.* Nature and significance of endoleaks and endotension: Summary of opinions expressed at an international conference. J Vasc Surg 2002; **35**: 1029–1035.

7 Prinssen M, Verhoeven ELG, Verhagen HJM, Blankensteijn JD. Decision-making in follow-up after endovascular aneurysm repair based on diameter and volume measurements: A blinded comparison. Eur J Vasc Endovasc Surg 2003; **26**: 184–187.

8 Wever JJ, Blankensteijn JD, Mali WPThM, Eikelboom BC. Maximal aneurysm diameter follow-up is inadequate after endovascular abdominal aortic aneurysm repair. Eur J Vasc Endovasc Surg 2000; **20**: 177–182.

9 Dias NV, Ivancev K, Malina M *et al.* Direct intra-aneurysm sac pressure measurement using tip-pressure sensors: *In vivo* and *in vitro* evaluation. J Vasc Surg 2004; **40**: 711–716.

10 Ellozy SH, Carroccio A, Lookstein RA *et al.* First experience in human beings with a permanently implantable intrasac pressure transducer for monitoring endovascular repair of abdominal aortic aneurysms. J Vasc Surg 2004; **40**: 405–412.

11 Ashoke R, Brown LC, Rodway A *et al.* Color duplex ultrasonography is insensitive for the detection of endoleak after aortic endografting: A systematic review. J Endovasc Ther 2005; **12**: 297–305.

12 Prokop M, Schaefer-Prokop C, Galanski M. Spiral CT angiography of the abdomen. Abdom Imaging 1997; **22**: 143–153.

13 Prokop M. General principles of MDCT. Eur J Radiol 2003; **45**(Suppl) 1: S4–S10.

14 Yeung KK, van der Laan MJ, Wever JJ *et al.* New post-imaging software provides fast and accurate volume data from CTA surveillance after endovascular aneurysm repair. J Endovasc Ther 2003; **10**: 887–893.

15 Gilling-Smith GL, Martin J, Sudhindran S *et al.* Freedom from endoleak after endovascular aneurysm repair does not equal treatment success. Eur J Vasc Endovasc Surg 2000; **19**: 421–425.

16 Gilling-Smith G, Brennan J, Harris P *et al.* Endotension after endovascular aneurysm repair: Definition, classifi-

cation, and strategies for surveillance and intervention. J Endovasc Surg 1999; **6**: 305–307.

17 Wever JJ, Blankensteijn JD, Eikelboom BC. Secondary endoleak or missed endoleak? Eur J Vasc Endovasc Surg 1999; **18**: 458–460.

18 Risberg B, Delle M, Eriksson E *et al.* Aneurysm sac hygroma: A cause of endotension. J Endovasc Ther 2001; **8**: 447–453.

19 Mita T, Arita T, Matsunaga N *et al.* Complications of endovascular repair for thoracic and abdominal aortic aneurysm: An imaging spectrum. Radiographics 2000; **20**: 1263–1278.

20 Haulon S, Lions C, McFadden EP *et al.* Prospective evaluation of magnetic resonance imaging after endovascular treatment of infrarenal aortic aneurysms. Eur J Vasc Endovasc Surg 2001; **22**: 62–69.

21 van der Laan MJ, Bakker CJ, Blankensteijn JD, Bartels LW. Dynamic CE-MRA for endoleak classification after endovascular aneurysm repair. Eur J Vasc Endovasc Surg 2005; **31**: 130–135.

22 Castrucci M, Mellone R, Vanzulli A *et al.* Mural thrombi in abdominal aortic aneurysms: MR imaging characterization – useful before endovascular treatment? Radiology 1995; **197**: 135–139.

23 van der Laan MJ, Bartels LW, Bakker CJ *et al.* Suitability of 7 aortic stent-graft models for MRI-based surveillance. J Endovasc Ther 2004; **11**: 366–371.

24 Harris PL, Buth J, Mialhe C *et al.* The need for clinical trials of endovascular abdominal aortic aneurysm stent-graft repair: The EUROSTAR project. J Endovasc Surg 1997; **4**: 72–77.

25 Leurs LJ, Laheij RJ, Buth J. What determines and are the consequences of surveillance intensity after endovascular abdominal aortic aneurysm repair? Ann Vasc Surg 2005; **19**: 868–875.

26 Blankensteijn JD. Is 3D CTA really necessary for follow-up after EVAR? J Endovasc Ther 2004; **11**(SupplI): I-9.

27 Prinssen M, Wixon CL, Buskens E, Blankensteijn JD. Surveillance after endovascular aneurysm repair: Diagnostics, complications, and associated costs. Ann Vasc Surg 2004; **18**: 421–427.

28 Hayter CL, Bradshaw SR, Allen RJ *et al.* Follow-up costs increase the cost disparity between endovascular and open abdominal aortic aneurysm repair. J Vasc Surg 2005; **42**: 912–918.

29 Steinmetz E, Rubin BG, Sanchez LA *et al.* Type II endoleak after endovascular abdominal aortic aneurysm repair: A conservative approach with selective intervention is safe and cost-effective. J Vasc Surg 2004; **39**: 306–313.

30 Michaels JA, Drury D, Thomas SM. Cost-effectiveness of endovascular abdominal aortic aneurysm repair. Br J Surg 2005; **92**: 960–967.

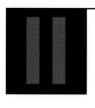

PART II

Thoracic aortic aneurysm

CHAPTER 10

Endovascular therapy of thoracic aneurysms: Gore TAG trial results

Jae-Sung Cho, Shan-e-ali Haider, & Michel S. Makaroun

Device description

The TAG endoprosthesis is a symmetrical expanded polytetrafluoroethylene (ePTFE) tube (Fig. 10.1) externally reinforced with ePTFE/FEP (fluorinated ethylene propylene). A nitinol exoskeleton is attached to the entire external surface of the graft with ePTFE/FEP bonding tape. The ends of the graft have scalloped flares designed to help the graft conform to the tortuous aorta. A PTFE sealing cuff is affixed to the base of the flares. Each cuff is attached on one end with FEP while allowing the other end to remain free. This enhances sealing of the device to the aortic wall and is intended to help prevent type I endoleaks. Two radiopaque gold bands at the base of the flares serve as a guide during deployment and in graft surveillance.

The 100-cm-long delivery catheter is flexible and has tapered oval beads or "olives" at both ends of the device that allow a smooth transition from the delivery catheter to the endograft. Unlike most other endografts that are deployed by a mechanism of unsheathing, deployment of the TAG endoprosthesis is unique (Fig. 10.2). The device is constrained by an ePTFE/FEP sleeve connected to a deployment knob located at the control end of the delivery catheter. The deployment line initiates a rapid release of the TAG device from the middle of the endograft with bidirectional progression. A specially designed trilobed balloon, which allows continuous blood flow during inflation, is used to expand the device after deployment (Fig. 10.3).

Pivotal (phase II) trial

Objectives and hypotheses

The pivotal trial was conducted to determine the safety and efficacy of the device for the treatment of DTAA as compared to an open surgical repair [1]. The primary safety endpoint was the percentage of patients with more than one major adverse event (MAE) through 1-year posttreatment. The primary efficacy endpoint was the percentage of patients free from major device-related events through 1-year follow-up for the TAG group. A predefined estimate of 80% was considered to be a reasonable efficacy outcome since the device was expected to show a significant improvement in safety profile over time; the efficacy for the open repair was assumed to be 100%. The secondary hypotheses were that the operative blood loss, intensive care unit (ICU) and hospital stay and convalescence to normal activities will be lower in the TAG group vs. the surgical control arm.

Study design

The construct of this study was a prospective, non-randomized, controlled multicenter trial. One hundred and forty study patients and ninety four control subjects were recruited through 17 clinical sites in the United States between September 1999 and May 2001. Of the 94 control group patients, 44 were prospectively acquired during the study and 50 were acquired by selecting the most recent surgical patients in a reverse chronological order. All patients

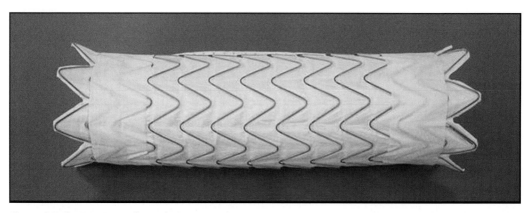

Figure 10.1 The Gore TAG endoprosthesis.

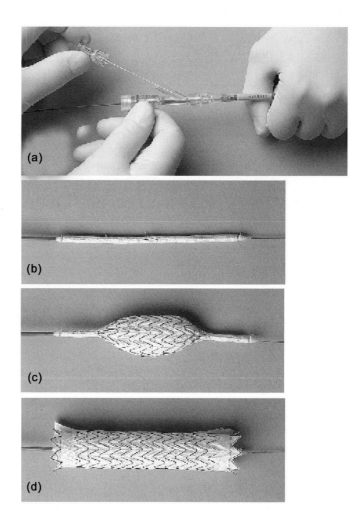

Figure 10.2 Deployment of Gore TAG device in stages. The endoprosthesis is fully constrained on delivery catheter (b). By turning and pulling the deployment knob (a), the deployment begins from the middle (c) and progresses rapidly to both ends (d).

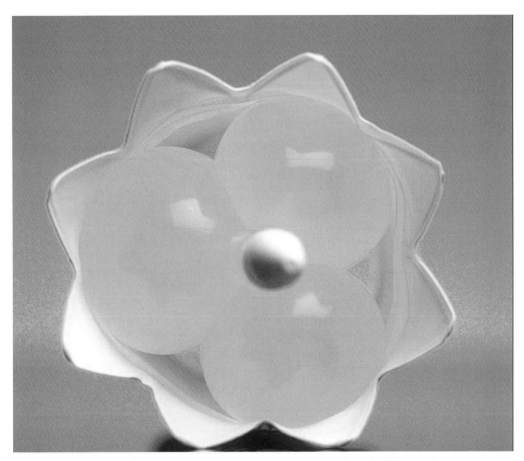

Figure 10.3 Trilobed balloons that allow aortic blood flow during inflation are shown in difference sizes.

were surgical candidates with a life expectancy of at least 2 years. Notable exclusions were ruptured aneurysms, dissections, connective tissue disorders, and mycotic aneurysms. Anatomic requirements for the device included a 2-cm healthy proximal and distal necks.

Follow-up

Physical examinations, plain radiographs, and computed tomography (CT) scans were obtained at 1-, 6- and 12-month intervals and yearly thereafter. For those with early endoleaks, a CT was obtained at a 3-month visit. A core laboratory reviewed all imaging studies. Individual sites reported clinical data which were monitored by sponsor representatives. Major adverse events, defined as those clinical events that required therapy or that resulted in an unintended increase in the level of care, prolonged hospitaliza-

tion, permanent adversity or death, were adjudicated by the Clinical Events Committee [2]. Minor adverse events were those that did not require any therapeutic intervention or those without clinical sequelae. All patients are to be followed for 5 years.

Results

Clinical materials

All major demographic and clinical variables were similar between the two groups (Table 10.1). The mean age of the patients was 71 years and males accounted for 58% of the patients in the TAG group; the corresponding figures were 68 years and 51% in the control group, respectively. Aortic morphology was also comparable between the two groups. The mean aneurysm size was 64 mm in the TAG group and 63 mm in the open control group. Baseline

Table 10.1 Baseline demographics.

	TAG device	Surgical control	P
Age (years)	71	68	NS
Male (%)	57	51	NS
Height (cm)	170	170	NS
Weight (kg)	76	78	NS
Ethnicity (%)			
Caucasian	87	86	
Black	8	10	
Other	5	4	

comorbidities were well-matched between the two groups (Table 10.2). The prevalence of symptomatic aneurysms, however, was significantly higher in the control group although most symptoms were mostly compressive in nature. The higher prevalence of coronary artery disease in the TAG group was of no statistical significance. The risk classification according to the standard ASA classification and the SVS risk score showed no significant difference.

Operative data

Technical success with TAG implantation was achieved in 137 of 140 patients (98%). All three failures resulted from poor vascular access. A conduit was placed to facilitate access in 21 patients (15%). Multiple devices were used in 77 patients (55%). Left carotid-subclavian bypass grafting or subclavian to carotid transposition was utilized in 28 patients (20%) before the left subclavian artery was intentionally covered with the device to assure proper sealing. Unplanned coverage of the left subclavian artery and visceral artery occurred in one patient each. The latter underwent an open abdominal explantation of the device and redeployment of another stent graft without sequelae.

Early outcome

Mortality

Operative mortality, defined as death within 30 days of the procedure or during the same hospitalization, occurred in 3 (2.1%) patients after a TAG repair (Table 10.3). A postoperative stroke, a cardiac event on postoperative day 11, and a late in-hospital death accounted for all three mortalities. This was significantly lower than the 11.7% mortality associated with open repair [3].

Spinal cord ischemia

Spinal cord ischemia (SCI) developed in four patients in the TAG group. One was noted immediately after the procedure without recovery of neurological function despite all supportive measures. Three cases of SCI were delayed in onset and transient. Recovery of motor function was complete in

Table 10.2 Baseline comorbidities.

	Proportion (%)		
	TAG device	Surgical control	P
Smoking	84	82	0.86
Coronary artery disease	49	36	0.06
Prior vascular intervention	45	55	0.14
COPD	40	38	0.89
Other concomitant aneurysms	28	28	1.0
Cardiac arrhythmia	24	31	0.23
Symptomatic aneurysm	21	38	<0.01
Cancer	19	13	0.21
PVD	16	11	0.33
Stroke	10	10	1.0
Hepatic dysfunction	2	1	0.65
Renal dialysis	1	0	0.52
Paraplegia	1	0	1.00

Table 10.3 Comparison of early complications between TAG and open surgical controls in the Gore pivotal trial.

	Patients (%)	
Operative complications	*TAG*	*Open surgical*
Death	2	12
Paraplegia/paraparesis	3	14
Stroke	4	4

one and partial in two, and all were ambulatory at last follow-up. The incidence rate of SCI in the control group was significantly higher at 13.8% (13/94). Of the 13 control patients with SCI, eight suffered paraplegia, resulting in six deaths. One case of paraplegia resolved completely. Spinal drainage was not routinely used in either group.

Cerebrovascular accidents
Perioperative stroke was noted in 4% of patients in both groups and was clustered in the patients with proximal aneurysms involving the arch. Five TAG patients (3.5%) had a stroke resulting in one death. Three occurred in the right hemisphere.

Endoleaks
Early endoleaks were seen in five patients. One patient had a type Ia endoleak and was treated with endovascular revision and additional stent grafting. The remaining endoleaks were thought to be type II.

Other major adverse events
Cardiopulmonary events, bleeding and intraoperative vascular injury accounted for the other most common complications. A higher percentage of postprocedural bleeding and respiratory failure was witnessed in the control group [3]. Only vascular complications were noted to occur more frequently in the TAG group (14%) as compared to the control arm (4%). This is due to introduction of a large sheath through the iliac arteries, causing vascular trauma in 11% of the patients.

Hospital length of stay
The average ICU stay was significantly shorter in the TAG group as compared to the control group (2.6 ± 14.6 days vs. 5.2 ± 7.2 days, $P < 0.001$). This was also true when evaluating the total length of stay (7.4 ± 17.7 days vs. 14.4 ± 12.8 days, $P < 0.001$) [3].

Late outcome

Late survival
Two-year all cause mortality was comparable in both groups at 24% in the TAG group and 26% in the surgical control group (Fig. 10.4). The causes of death were in accordance with associated comorbidities in this elderly population. Aneurysm-related mortality however was significantly better in the TAG group. At 2-year follow-up, the freedom from aneurysm-related mortality was 97% for the TAG group and 90% for the surgical control group ($P = 0.024$). No deaths occurred after the first year (Fig. 10.5).

Major adverse events
The incidence of MAEs at 1-year follow-up was significantly lower in the TAG group as compared to surgical controls, 42% vs. 77%, respectively. The majority (70%) of MAEs were noted to have occurred within 30 days of the original procedure. This advantage to the TAG group persisted through 3-year follow-up. Kaplan–Meier estimates of the probability of freedom from MAEs at 3 years were 48% after TAG repair and 20% after open repair (Fig. 10.6).

Device-related events
During a 3-year follow-up, five patients underwent endovascular revisions and one patient underwent surgical conversion. Three of the revisions took place 24 months after the initial procedure. Three proximal and four component device migrations were noted without clinical adversity at a 2-year follow-up. Sac expansion (>5 mm) was noted in 17% (11/64) of patients, whereas sac shrinkage (>5 mm) was observed in 38% (24/64) of subjects. Out of the 11 patients with sac enlargement 3 had endoleaks at some point in follow-up. A total of 20 fractures were noted in 19 patients, 18 of which were in the longitudinal spine and 2 in the apical nitinol support rings. Clinical sequelae developed in only one patient who manifested a type III endoleak successfully treated with an additional endograft. Freedom from device-related events over 2 years was 94% for the TAG device, which is significantly higher than the predefined limit of 80%. No device-related deaths were noted through 3 years.

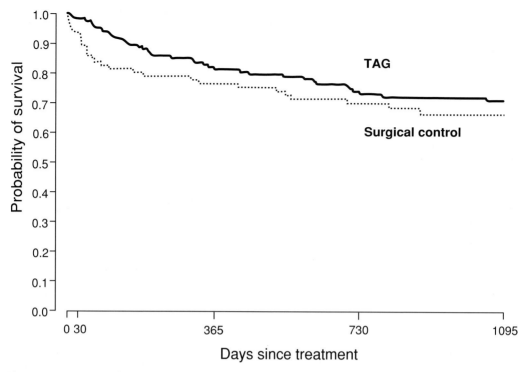

Figure 10.4 Comparison of Kaplan–Meier estimates for all cause mortality through 3-year follow-up between Gore TAG and surgical control groups.

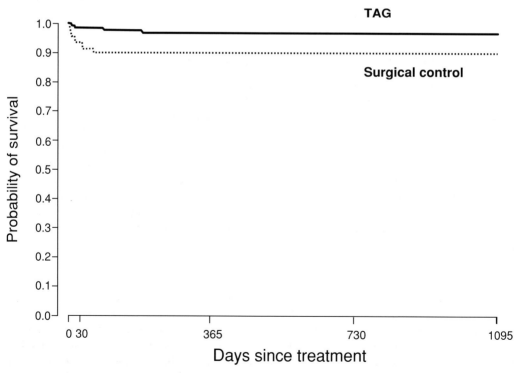

Figure 10.5 Comparison of Kaplan–Meier estimates for aneurysm-related mortality through 3-year follow-up between Gore TAG and surgical control groups.

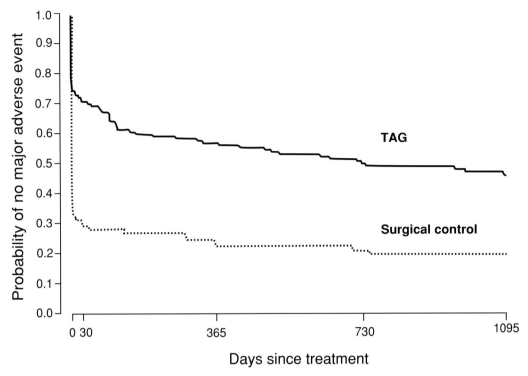

Figure 10.6 Comparison of Kaplan–Meier estimates for freedom from major adverse events through 3-year follow-up between Gore TAG and surgical control.

Confirmatory trial

Objectives and hypotheses

To compare the safety and early results of the modified device with the original device, a confirmatory study was undertaken. A 30-day safety endpoint was chosen as an appropriate measure based on the results of the pivotal study in which the majority of MAEs occurred within the 30-day period. Nevertheless, all patients are to be followed up to 5 years. Inclusion and exclusion criteria and the safety and efficacy endpoints were identical with those of the pivotal study.

Design

The study was a prospective nonrandomized trial. All test subjects were treated with the modified TAG device and compared to the control data from the pivotal study. Fifty-one patients were enrolled and their results compared with the same 94 control subjects used in the pivotal study.

Results

Clinical materials

Baseline demographics, comorbidities, and aortic morphology were similar between the two groups. Although the pivotal study database had a statistically significant prevalence of symptomatic aneurysms in the control group no such difference was noted in this trial. Risk classification according to the ASA was very well-matched between the TAG group and the surgical control group. The SVS risk score was slightly higher in the TAG group, a statistical significance.

Early outcome

Major adverse events
The incidence of MAEs was noted to be 12% in the TAG group and 70% in the control group at a 30-day follow-up. This was a statistically significant difference corresponding to an 83% risk reduction for those with TAG repair. Vascular complication rates

were similar between the two groups in this study. There were no deaths in this TAG cohort. Kaplan–Meier estimates of the probability of freedom from MAEs through 30 days were significantly lower following TAG repair when compared to the surgical controls ($P < 0.001$).

Device-related events
No major device-related events were noted at the 30-day follow-up. This is in comparison to a 4% major device-related complication rate reported in the pivotal study.

Hospital length of stay
The length of hospital stay was shorter in the TAG group (3 days) compared to the control group (10 days). The time to return to normal activities was also significantly shorter following TAG repair (15 days) vs. 78 days for the control group.

Discussion

Due to the high inherent risks of open thoracic aortic repair, greater benefits are anticipated with endovascular therapy of thoracic aneurysmal disease than its abdominal counterpart. The results of the Gore TAG trials have proven that, indeed, endovascular treatment of DTAA is not only safe and effective, but also superior to conventional open surgical repair. Perioperative mortality and morbidity were lower, particularly with respect to spinal cord ischemia, than those with open repairs. This led to the FDA approval of commercial use of the TAG device in March of 2005.

There are, however, several limitations to the Gore TAG device similar to other thoracic endografts. Access with a large profile device continues to present a major challenge. Access issues required a conduit proximal to femoral artery in 15% of patients, and accounted for all three failures and vascular trauma in 11% of patients in the pivotal trial. The increased prevalence of DTAA in women compared to abdominal aneurysms contributes to this problem. Vascular injury was the only category of complications with higher frequency following TAG repair than after open repair. These findings have been reported by others [4] and underline the importance of prophylactic use of conduits to avoid potentially disastrous vascular complications.

It is worth noting that the incidence of vascular complications in the confirmatory trial was only 6% and did not differ significantly from the control group, probably reflecting the increased awareness of iliac access and its potential for complications.

Aneurysm sac shrinkage occurred in 38% and sac expansion in 17% of patients at 2 years. No ruptures were noted. When compared with other thoracic endografts [5, 6] the sac shrinkage rate is lower and the sac enlargement rate higher, much like the phenomenon observed with the Excluder abdominal endograft associated with transudation of fluid [7]. The commercial modified TAG device, however, is composed of a low porosity ePTFE that should eliminate this issue. The results from the confirmatory study may shed light on this subject in the near future.

Despite the low incidence of spinal cord ischemia in the TAG trials compared to open repair and other series in the literature [1, 4, 6, 8, 9], it is still a source of major morbidity when it happens. Prior aortic surgery and long coverage of the thoracic aorta increase the risk of spinal cord ischemia in a cumulative fashion [9–11].

That four of the five strokes occurred in those with planned coverage of the left Subclavian artery warns of the danger of manipulating the aortic arch, particularly when the disease extends proximally. The nature of the strokes was most likely embolic as three were multicentric and three were right-hemispheric. The need to cover the left subclavian artery for proper sealing serves as a marker for the increased risk of stroke, although others have reported coverage of the left subclavian artery without significant problems [12].

Conclusion

In summary, the Gore TAG U.S. trials have demonstrated the safety and efficacy of the TAG device in the endovascular repair of descending thoracic aortic aneurysms and its superiority over open surgical repair. With follow-up extending to 3 years, sustained benefits have been shown with TAG repair. A high-risk trial that is currently underway is expected to broaden the application of this technology for the treatment of other thoracic aortic pathologies.

References

1 Makaroun MS, Dillavou ED, Kee ST, Sicard G, Chaikof E, Bavaria J *et al*. Endovascular treatment of thoracic aortic aneurysms: Results of the phase II multicenter trial of the GORE TAG thoracic endoprosthesis. J Vasc Surg 2005; **41**: 1–9.

2 Sacks D, Marinelli DL, Martin LG, Spies JB. Reporting standards for clinical evaluation of new peripheral arterial revascularization devices. Technology Assessment Committee. J Vasc Interven Radiol 1997; **8**: 137–149.

3 Bavaria JE, Appoo, JJ, Makaroun MS, Verter J, Yu A-F, Mitchell, RS. For the Gore TAG investigators. Endovascular stent grafting versus open surgical repair of descending thoracic aortic aneurysms in low risk patients: A multicenter comparative trial. J Theorac Cardiovasc Surg in press 2006.

4 White RA, Donayre CE, Walot I, Lippmann M, Woody J, Lee J *et al*. Endovascular exclusion of descending thoracic aortic aneurysms and chronic dissections: Initial clinical results with the AneuRx device. J Vasc Surg 2001; **33**: 927–934.

5 Greenberg RK, O'Neill S, Walker E, Haddad F, Lyden SP, Svensson LG *et al*. Endovascular repair of thoracic aortic lesions with the Zenith TX1 and TX2 thoracic grafts: Intermediate-term results. J Vasc Surg 2005; **41**: 589–596.

6 Ellozy SH, Carroccio A, Minor M, Jacobs T, Chae K, Cha A *et al*. Challenges of endovascular tube graft repair of thoracic aortic aneurysm: Midterm follow-up and lessons learned. [see comment]. J Vasc Surg 2003; **38**: 676–683.

7 Cho JS, Dillavou ED, Rhee RY, Makaroun MS. Late abdominal aortic aneurysm enlargement after endovascular repair with the Excluder device. J Vasc Surg 2004; **39**: 1236–1241.

8 Criado FJ, Clark NS, Barnatan MF. Stent graft repair in the aortic arch and descending thoracic aorta: A 4-year experience. J Vasc Surg 2002; **36**: 1121–1128.

9 Greenberg RK, Resch T, Nyman U, Lindh M, Brunkwall J, Brunkwall P *et al*. Endovascular repair of descending thoracic aortic aneurysms: An early experience with intermediate-tem follow-up. J Vasc Surg 2000; **31**: 147–156.

10 Gravereaux EC, Faries PL, Burks JA, Latessa V, Spielvogel D, Hollier LH *et al*. Risk of spinal cord ischemia after endograft repair of thoracic aortic aneurysms. J Vasc Surg 2001; **34**: 997–1003.

11 Moon MR, Mitchell RS, Dake MD, Zarins CK, Fann JI, Miller DC. Simultaneous abdominal aortic replacement and thoracic stent-graft placement for multilevel aortic disease. J Vasc Surg 1997; **25**: 332–340.

12 Gorich J, Asquan Y, Seifarth H, Kramer S, Kapfer X, Orend KH *et al*. Initial experience with intentional stent-graft coverage of the subclavian artery during endovascular thoracic aortic repairs. J Endovasc Ther 2002; **9**: 39–43.

CHAPTER 11

Medtronic *TALENT* and *VALIANT* devices: moving toward the next generation of thoracic aortic stent grafts

Ron Fairman

With the recent completion of enrollment in the three arms of The *Valor Trial* (Evaluation of the Medtronic Vascular Talent Thoracic Stent-Graft System for the Treatment of Thoracic Aortic Aneurysms), Medtronic is preparing to introduce into US clinical trials their next generation thoracic aortic endovascular stent graft, called the *Valiant* device. This technology has already been introduced in Europe through a limited market release program last spring. The *Talent* thoracic stent-graft system evaluated in *The Valor Trial* has been used extensively outside the United States for many years. In addition physicians have gained considerable experience with the *Talent* thoracic stent graft since the feasibility phase I high risk trial was performed in the United States in 1998. The evolution of the *Talent* thoracic stent graft to the *Valiant* design is a result of accumulated feedback from thousands of implants worldwide. Medtronic engineers have enhanced both the delivery system as well as the stent graft itself creating a product that promises to be vastly superior to the original *Talent* thoracic stent graft. That being said, the original *Talent* thoracic stent graft was the first endovascular device that we had available to treat thoracic aortic pathology when we began our thoracic endovascular program at the Hospital of the University of Pennsylvania in 1998. The customization features of that first generation *Talent* thoracic device presented us with our first opportunity to offer novel endovascular options to patients who were being managed

with "watchful waiting." The preliminary outcomes in our first 50 patients using that early *Talent* design were largely extraordinary. Minor changes to that original *Talent* device culminated in the *Talent* thoracic stent-graft system used in the *Valor Trial* (Fig. 11.1). The system is composed of a preloaded stent graft and the CoilTrac TDS delivery system. For the purposes of the *Valor Trial*, the delivery system was redesigned to a balloon-less system with a longer pushrod. This change was made on the basis of previous clinical trial experiences. Elimination of the integral balloon served to reduce the potential for kinking thereby reducing the deployment forces. The implanted Talent endoprosthesis is composed of a polyester graft fabric sewn to a self-expanding Nitinol wire frame. The design concept is modular and although the *Talent* stent graft has been viewed as a customized device, only catalog sizes were available in the *Valor Trial*. Proximal and distal stent-graft diameters range from 22 mm to 46 mm, and the total covered length of the device ranges from 112 mm to 116 mm. Bare Spring (proximal device diameter < 24 mm) and Freeflo (proximal device diameter ≥ 24 mm) configurations are available proximally which are indicative of terminating spring without fabric coverage. Bare Spring configurations are also available distally. Both proximal and distal Bare Spring configurations allow for crossing the great vessels of the arch as well as the celiac artery respectively. An accessory *Reliant* stent-graft balloon, packaged separately, is intended

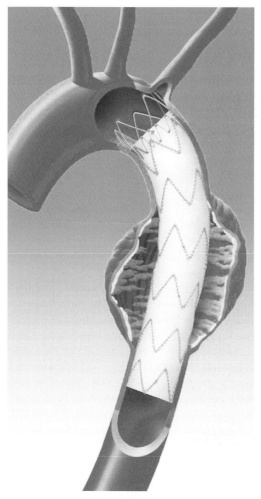

Figure 11.1 The Talent thoracic stent graft.

for use following stent-graft deployment to facilitate modeling of the covered springs and to remove fabric pleats from the graft material.

The *Valor Trial* is a prospective, multicenter, non-randomized evaluation of the safety (rate of "all cause" mortality) and efficacy (successful aneurysm treatment at 1 year) of the *Talent* thoracic stent-graft system when used in patients with thoracic aortic aneurysms (*test arm*, Fig. 11.2). The *test arm* consists of patients diagnosed with thoracic aortic aneurysms that are considered candidates for open surgical repair which is low to moderate risk based on SVS/ISCVS criteria. Additionally, two observational treatment group registries

were conducted concurrently, serving to record descriptive information that may serve as the basis for future clinical investigations. The *Registry and High Risk Arms* include patients diagnosed with dissections, traumatic injury, pseudoaneurysms, as well as aneurysms without a distinct proximal or distal aneurysm neck of >20 mm or greater in length.

Although there were 40 active sites in the *Valor Trial,* eight sites in the US trial enrolled 57% of the *test group* patients and 66% of the *high risk/registry* arm. At the time of this trial, thoracic stent grafting was performed largely in a handful of centers. Most of the pathology treated throughout all arms of the trial consisted of fusiform or saccular aneurysms; in the *high risk* arms, this pathology was present in 76% of the patients enrolled. The demographics revealed that 40% of the patients enrolled were females, a percentage not dissimilar from the phase II multicenter trial of the *Gore TAG* thoracic endoprosthesis. With a greater percentage of female patients compared to abdominal aortic aneurysmal disease, issues of iliac access assume critical importance. In the *Valor* trial, surgically placed conduits were necessary in upward of 15% of patients, demonstrating the need for delivery systems smaller than 22–24 Fr. The Bare Spring or Freeflo proximal design as well as the availability of stent-graft devices with diameters as large as 46 mm opened the door to endovascular thoracic aortic options for a broader range of patients in *Valor* than with any other industry-sponsored thoracic device trials. Due to device sizing constraints based on thoracic aortic anatomy, 35% of the patients treated with the *Talent* stent graft in the high risk arm of *Valor* could not be treated with any other industry-sponsored device. The preliminary results of the high risk arm were presented this past June at the Vascular Annual Meeting in Chicago.

The *Talent* thoracic experience has resulted in a number of consistent observations that are relevant not only to the *Talent* device, but to all endovascular therapies in the thoracic aorta. Although rigid stent grafts can function well in the abdominal aorta, flexible designs that conform to the aorta are paramount in the thoracic aorta (Fig. 11.3). Thoracic devices need to conform to the aortic arch as well as the tortuosity inherent in the atherosclerotic

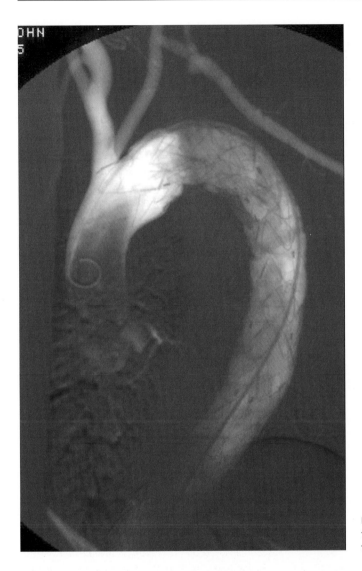

Figure 11.2 Completion angiogram following the placement of a Talent thoracic stent graft.

thoracic aorta. Although one can accurately deploy a *Talent* thoracic device in the proximal descending thoracic aorta, controlled deployment in an angulated arch or in an area of marked tortuosity is difficult. These issues are addressed with the *Xcelerant* delivery system (Fig. 11.4) which has been available to physicians in the United States for the AneuRx AAA stent graft, and has been modified for the *Valiant* device. The new thoracic version of the delivery system is smaller by 2 Fr and allows for controlled ratcheted precise deployment. Stabilization of the delivery system when deploying in the arch is

of fundamental importance in preventing embolic stroke. In order to optimize ease and accuracy of deployment as well as conformability, the long connecting bar of the *Talent* device has been removed in *Valiant*, while columnar support has been optimized through stent spacing and the exoskeleton. The removal of the connecting bar has eliminated the need to orient the device *in vivo* and results in improved flexibility. The proximal uncovered bare spring has been increased from five to eight peaks, which distributes the force of the spring over more apexes, and in addition the proximal stents have been inset into the fabric. Experience to date has shown that this change does result in more stable deployment which may prevent the rare instances of "bare spring flip" observed when deploying in an angulated arch.

Furthermore, longer stent grafts are particularly desirable when treating most pathology in the thoracic aorta. The great majority of thoracic aortic conditions require stent-graft coverage of up to 200 mm. Although shorter stent grafts are fine for treating focal disease processes such as penetrating ulcers, transections, or saccular aneurysms; in most instances we are treating fusiform longer segments of disease. Longer endografts result in less modular junctions and fewer passes of large delivery systems

through small diseased iliac arteries which can result in life-threatening iliac artery avulsions.

A consistent observation is that it is difficult to identify proximal and distal aspects of modular components once inserted. The new *Valiant* device has distinct "figure of eight" radiopaque markers proximally and "zero" markers distally which provide enhanced visibility and result in more precise overlap at modular junctions. The *Talent* and *Valiant* devices are compared side by side in Fig. 11.5. Although the preliminary outcomes of the *Valor High Risk* Arm using the *Talent* thoracic stent-graft system are encouraging and reveal high procedural success in the setting of low operative mortality, stroke incidence, and paraplegia rates,

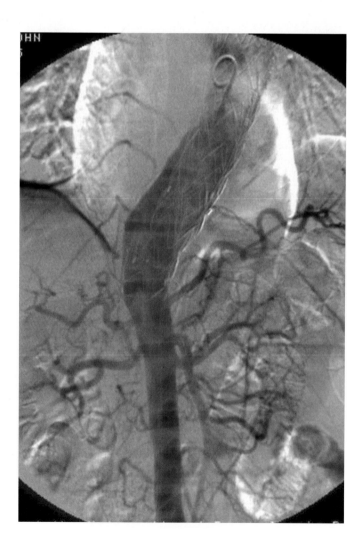

Figure 11.3 Early generation thoracic stent grafts were rigid and did not conform well to tortuous aortas; the Valiant device is more flexible.

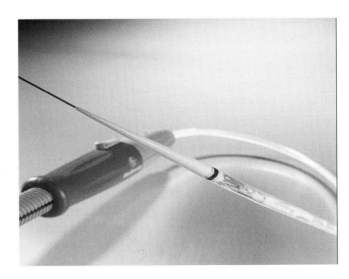

Figure 11.4 The Xcelent delivery system of the Talent thoracic stent-graft device allows stable and accurate deployment.

enhancements in stent-graft design are evolving. The delivery system and stent-graft changes culminating in the *Valiant* design will allow more precise placement of endografts and should further reduce deployment-related complications.

The *Valor Test Arm* is now in the follow-up phase and the PMA will be filed with the FDA in the early summer of 2006. Medtronic is currently finalizing their US clinical trial protocol using the *Valiant Stent-Graft System* for FDA submission.

TALENT and *VALIANT comparison*

Product features	TALENT	VALIANT
Diameters available	22-46 mm	Same
Graft material	LPS (Monofilament polyester)	Same
Suture	5-0 braided polyester	Same
Body spring	5-peak (0.020 wire)	Same
Stent material	Chemical etched nitinol	Same
Delivery system	CoilTrac TDS	Xcelerant
Maximum total length	130 mm	220 mm
Body spring attachment	Inside graft material	Outside graft material
Connecting bar	Yes	No
Proximal end configurations	Bare spring (5-peak / 0.020 wire) Open web (5-peak / 0.020 wire)	Bare spring (8-peak / 0.021 wire) Closed web (8-peak / 0.021 wire)
Distal end configurations	Closed web (5-peak / 0.020 wire) Bare spring (5-peak / 0.020 wire) Open web (5-peak / 0.020 wire)	Closed web (8-peak / 0.021 wire) Bare spring (8-peak / 0.021 wire)
Proximal radiopaque markers	2-Figure "8" Ptlr	4-Figure "8" Ptlr
Distal radiopaque markers	2-Figure "8" Ptlr	2-Circle Ptlr
Sterilization method	EtO	E-beam

Figure 11.5 Comparison of the Talent and Valiant stent grafts.

CHAPTER 12

Initial clinical experience with the Bolton Relay stent graft: a new thoracic device

Frank J. Criado

The Relay™ thoracic sten graft (Fig. 12.1) is a new endovascular device for treatment of thoracic aortic pathologies. It is composed of self-expanding nitinol stents that are sutured to a polyester graft fabric. The skeleton of the device is made up of a series of sinusoidal stents placed along the length of the graft fabric. A curved nitinol wire provides longitudinal support. This wire is attached to the graft with surgical sutures. It provides moderate column strength while, at the same time, preserving desirable flexibility and torque response. Radiopaque markers (made of platinum/iridium) have been placed in various locations to enhance fluoroscopic visualization.

The Transport™ delivery system (Fig. 12.2) is a two-stage device that consists of a series of coaxially arranged sheaths and catheters (primary introduction sheath, secondary delivery sheath, and thru lumen), handle, and apex release mechanism. The stent graft is constrained within the secondary sheath, which is further constrained within the primary sheath. The radiopaque polymeric primary (outer) sheath is introduced endovascularly via puncture of the femoral artery (or through an access conduit), tracking over a stiff guidewire. Once the system reaches the desired level within the aorta (at or just above the level of the renal arteries), the proximal handle of the delivery system is advanced to exit the secondary sheath from the primary sheath in preparation for deployment. The secondary sheath, composed of thin-wall flexible polymer, enables the thoracic endograft to be easily advanced and delivered across curved and tortuous

portions of the anatomy—such as the aortic arch. The secondary sheath, which is connected to the delivery catheter and the delivery handle, can now be retracted to deploy the constrained stent graft in a controlled fashion. The apex release mechanism constrains the Safex (uncovered) stent at the top end of the endograft. The Safex stent is released by retracting the outer control tube over the guidewire lumen. This allows for controlled apposition at the seal/fixation zone on the aortic wall.

The Relay device comes in various sizes and configurations, both tapered and nontapered. Graft lengths up to 200 mm are available, with diameters from 22 to 46 mm. The profile of the primary introducer sheath ranges from 22 to 26 F depending on graft diameter and length.

Initial clinical experience

The Phase I Feasibility study for the clinical evaluation of the Relay thoracic stent graft in the treatment of intermediate and high-risk patients with descending thoracic aortic aneurysms (TAA) and penetrating ulcers (PU) was approved (by the FDA under IDE G040175) on December 2, 2004. It was initially limited to 30 patients and 5 clinical sites. Regulatory approval to include two additional sites (for a total of seven) was granted on April 28, 2005 (G040175/S3). The first implant (in the USA) took place at Union Memorial Hospital in Baltimore on January 5, 2005 (Figs.12. 3 and 12.4). To date (August 21, 2006), 27 patients (15 males, 12 females) have been treated (implanted) during the

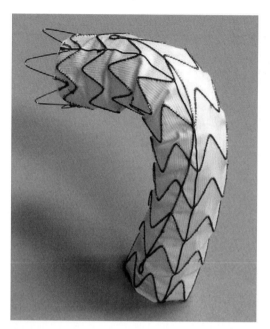

Figure 12.1 Bolton Relay thoracic stent graft.

stances except 3—all by the same physician at the same study site—where it was noted that the proximal end of the device had a tendency to "wind-sock" and migrate distally when the deployment sequence included a stop-and-go maneuver with initial expansion of the first two to three stent segments before proceeding to full uncovering and expansion along its full length. These observations were reproduced on bench testing, leading to a modification of the IFU vis-à-vis deployment technique. No further occurrences were recorded following such modifications.

Technical success rate was 96.3% in that all procedures could be completed, with delivery and deployment of the device as intended, and with complete angiographic exclusion of the target lesion with only one exception (26/27). There have been no 30-day mortalities. One endoleak (3.7%) has been uncovered on follow-up CT scans. To date, there have been no unanticipated device-related adverse events or surgical conversions. Completion of the Phase I study will be followed by the pivotal clinical trial, set to begin in late 2006 or early 2007.

Phase I study. Twenty-four (81.5%) had TAA and three had PU. Patients' demographics and comorbidities are summarized in Table 12.1. Salient procedural parameters appear in Table 12.2. Delivery and deployment of the device was judged (by the implanting investigator) to be satisfactory in all in-

In summary, the Relay thoracic stent graft emerges as a promising new endovascular device for treatment of thoracic aortic pathologies. Its performance appears satisfactory, as reflected in the early results from the Phase I clinical trial in the USA. A larger clinical experience in Europe tends to

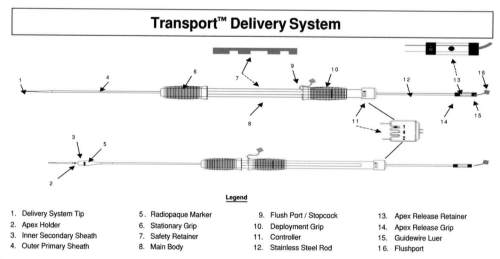

Figure 12.2 Detailed drawing of the Bolton stent-graft device.

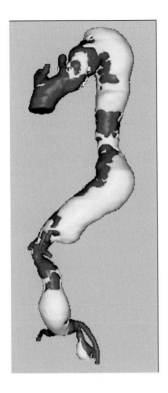

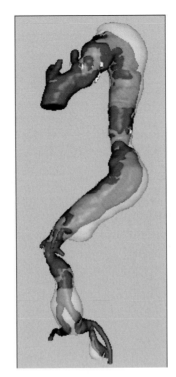

Figure 12.3 Extensive aneurysmal disease throughout aorta, with large TAA and smaller AAA.

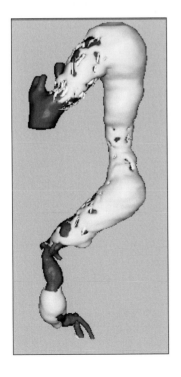

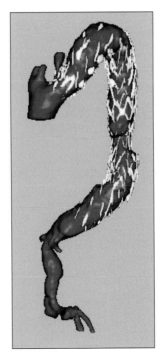

Figure 12.4 Postoperative CT images following endovascular exclusion of TAA with a 2-segment Bolton Relay stent graft.

Table 12.1 Demographic characteristics of Bolton thoracic stent-graft trial.

Demographics n = 27	
• Gender	Male 15, female 12
• Lesions	TAA 24, PU 3
• Coronary artery disease	63% (17/27)
• COPD	29.6% (8/27)
• Hypertension	88.9% (24/27)
• Prior AAA repair	35% (10/27)
• Tobacco abuse	85.2% (23/27)

Table 12.2 Procedural indicators.

• Duration	156.40 min (mean)
• EBL	344.60 ml (mean)
• Prophylactic CSF drainage	30% (8/27)
• Iliac access conduit	30% (8/27)
• Anesthesia type	Gen 70%, reg 30%

corroborate such impressions (nearly 500 implants on more than 300 patients worldwide). Its design and newly conceived delivery system make it uniquely capable of addressing difficult arch anatomies—a recognized limitation of currently available thoracic endograft devices. Results of ongoing clinical trials and a larger experience will hopefully substantiate such positive early impressions in the future.

CHAPTER 13

Clinical results of the EUROSTAR thoracic registry

Peter Harris, Lina Leurs, Randolph Statius van Eps, & Jacob Buth

Introduction

It is the perception of most vascular clinicians that the results of treatment of thoracic aortic disease by endovascular means are considerably superior to those of conventional surgery. Consequently, whereas endovascular treatment of abdominal aortic aneurysms has been subjected to randomized controlled trials, there seems to be a consensus that it would be inappropriate for similar trials to be conducted in respect of thoracic disease. This collective viewpoint is based upon an assumption that the much reduced physiological insult associated with endovascular interventions will translate into a lower risk of perioperative death and other major complications known to be associated with conventional surgical reconstruction of the thoracic aorta, including multiple organ failure and paraplegia. The burden of proof of this assumption rests with the medical community. Furthermore, it is essential to ascertain whether or not any early clinical advantage associated with the endovascular approach is at risk of being nullified subsequently by higher late complication and reintervention rates related to a comparatively limited durability of the technique.

Because most clinicians currently believe endovascular repair to be superior, i.e. they are not in equipoise regarding the results of endovascular and open repair for thoracic aortic disease, a randomized trial would not be ethical and this precept seems to have been accepted by the regulatory authorities in the USA and Europe. Therefore, reliance must be placed on lower levels of scientific evidence. The EUROSTAR Thoracic Registry is a voluntary observational study which was established in 2000. It is linked in terms of its administration and its protocol to the EUROSTAR Registry of Endovascular Repair of Abdominal Aortic Aneurysms. Data may be submitted on-line and center-specific reports together with an analysis of the whole database can similarly be retrieved on-line for the purpose of comparative audit.

In the UK the government-sponsored National Institute for Health and Clinical Excellence (NICE), while accepting that a randomized trial is not appropriate, at this stage, has recommended that all endovascular procedures undertaken for thoracic aortic disease and their outcomes should be audited by a national registry program. Accordingly, a Thoracic Registry was established within the UK Registry of Endovascular Treatment of Aortic Aneurysms (UK RETA). Compatibility between the EUROSTAR and UK RETA registries permits the data to be combined to create a relatively large population sample size from which reliable conclusions may be drawn sooner than would be possible from consideration of each dataset separately. Aggregated data from the EUROSTAR and UK Thoracic Registries were published in 2004 [1]. Data for this chapter are drawn exclusively from the EUROSTAR registry.

Sample population

To July 2005 a total of 581 patients were recruited onto the EUROSTAR Thoracic Registry by a total of 54 different European institutions (see the Appendix). The mean age of the patients was 63.4 years (range 13 to 91 years). There were 447 (77%) males and 134 (23%) females.

Seventeen per cent of the patients had an American Society of Anesthesiologists (ASA) Risk Score of 4 or 5, signifying that they were considered to be unfit for open surgical repair due to serious comorbidities. Cardiac and pulmonary diseases were the most frequent. Fifty seven per cent of the patients were current smokers and 69% were hypertensive.

Characterization of thoracic aortic disease

The patients were categorized into four groups:
1 Degenerative TAA ($N = 292$, 50%)
2 Aortic dissection ($N = 188$, 32%)
3 Traumatic rupture of the thoracic aorta ($N = 63$, 11%)
4 False anastomotic aneurysm ($N = 26$, 4%)

When aneurysm was the presenting feature 227 (60%) were found to involve the proximal third of the descending thoracic aorta, 173 (45%) the middle third of the descending aorta, and 115 (30%) the distal third. The arch was involved in 61 (16%) of patients and the ascending aorta in 3 (1%). The mean maximum diameter of the aneurysms was 62.1 mm (SD 16 mm, range 30–120 mm).

Of the patients classified under the heading "aortic dissection" 11 (6%) had type A extent, 144 (77%) had type B, and 37 (20%) had penetrating ulcers. The primary tear was within the proximal third of the descending aorta in 138 (73%), the middescending aorta in 50 (27%), the lower third of the descending aorta in 25 (13%) and in the arch in 22 (12%).

The procedures

Emergency procedures were defined arbitrarily as those that were undertaken within 7 days of first presentation. The following commercially available, Communauté Européenne (CE)-approved devices were used:
1 Talent (Medtronic/AVE) ($N = 393$)
2 Excluder (W. L. Gore & Associates) ($N = 124$)
3 Zenith (William Cook Europe) ($N = 28$)
4 Others ($N = 36$)

A single stent graft was deployed in 301 (52%) of cases, two were deployed in 167 (29%) and three or more in 110 (19%). General anesthesia was employed in 546 (94%) of the patients. The remainder

were treated under either regional or local anesthetics. Controlled hypotension was induced in 246 (42%) and cardiac cessation in 29 (5%). The left subclavian artery was overstented in 146 (25%) patients and some form of adjuvant extraanatomic bypass was undertaken in 57 (10%) of patients. "Critical" (T8-12) intercostals arteries were covered in at least 25% of patients (data reporting for this field were incomplete).

Outcome of the procedures

Complete technical success, judged from completion angiography, was achieved in 520 (90%) of patients. One hundred and ninety nine patients did not require intensive care unit postoperatively. The 382 patients that did spent a mean of 114.2 h (range 3–1800 h) in an intensive care unit. The mean duration of hospital admission was 11 days (range 0–100 days).

Arterial complications were encountered in 61 (10%) patients. These included rupture of the aorta, thrombo-emboli and ischemia related to exclusion of aortic side-branches.

Device-related complications were reported in 51 (9%) patients. The most common were failure to advance the delivery system and migration of the stent/graft. There was failure to complete the procedure on five occasions. In one case conversion to open repair was carried out and in another two the procedure was abandoned.

Endoleaks

An endoleak was noted on the completion angiogram in 54 (9%) patients. There were 40 (7%) type 1 endoleaks and 14 (2%) type 2. Another 10 were not characterized. The incidence of type 2 endoleak was much lower than that observed following endovascular repair of abdominal aortic aneurysms, but type 1 endoleaks were also less frequent.

Neurological sequelae

Neurological complications occurred in a total of 54 (9%) patients. Of these 33 were serious or permanent accounting for 6% of the whole of the treated population. Intracranial strokes occurred just as frequently as spinal cord injury with an incidence of 18 (3%) compared to 15 (2.5%). This finding highlights the risks associated with the manipulation of wires, catheters and introducer sheaths within the arch, which have potential to offset or even cancel out the benefit of a reduced risk of paraplegia in comparison to open surgery.

An analysis of the risk factors for paraplegia in 14 patients is shown in Table 13.1. The most important result from a clinical perspective is a highly significant increase in the risk of paraplegia when three or more stent grafts are used. This applied in nearly 20% of patients and presumably correlates with the length of aorta covered, i.e. the greater the length the higher the risk. Interestingly, there was no correlation between the length of the aneurysm and the risk of paraplegia and it may be speculated that the greatest risk relates to relatively healthy aorta being covered.

The risk of paraplegia associated with endovascular repair of degenerative thoracic aneurysms was

Table 13.1 Neurological complications following endovascular thoracic aortic repair.

	Paraplegia N = 14 N (%)	Other N = 495 N (%)	P-value
Degenerative aneurysm	12 (85.7)	300 (60.6)	0.057
Chronic	8 (66.7)	227 (75.7)	NS
Acute	4 (33.3)	56 (18.7)	NS
Unknown	—	17 (5.7)	NS
Dissection	2 (14.3)	195 (39.4)	0.057
Chronic	0 (0)	102 (52.2)	NS
Acute	2 (100)	93 (47.7)	NS
Localization			
A (prox)	5 (35.7)	189 (38.2)	NS
B (prox+mid)	2 (14.3)	38 (7.7)	NS
C (mid)	1 (7.1)	64 (12.9)	NS
D (dist)	1 (7.1)	46 (9.3)	NS
E (mid+dist)	2 (14.3)	27 (5.5)	NS
F (prox+mid+dist)	3 (21.4)	39 (7.9)	0.069
Length aneurysm (mean ± SD)	128.3 ± 116.7*	98.1 ± 63.5*	NS
Anesthesia			
General	14 (100)	460 (92.9)	NS
Regional	—	21 (4.2)	NS
Local	—	14 (2.8)	NS
Number of stent grafts			
≥ 3	7 (50.0)	101 (20.4)	<0.0001
Duration operation (mean ± SD)	159.1 ± 89.6	132.9 ± 86.7	NS
Replaced blood volume (mean ± SD)	362.5 ± 639.3	485.4 ± 5092.4	NS
Blocking side branches			
T9 – occlusion by device	5 (35.7)	124 (25.1)	
T10 – occlusion by device	7 (50.0)	99 (20.0)	
T11 – occlusion by device	5 (35.7)	76 (15.4)	
T12 – occlusion by device	4 (28.6)	45 (9.1)	
Conversion	1 (7.1)	10 (2.0)	NS
Early (30-day)	1 (7.1)	2 (0.4)	0.0012
Late (>30-day)	0 (0)	8 (1.6)	NS
Death	8 (57.1)	97 (19.6)	0.0006
Early (30-day)	6 (42.9)	43 (8.7)	<0.0001
Late (>30-day)	2 (14.3)	54 (10.9)	NS

Risk factors for paraplegia.
*N = 11 and 258.

12/312 (3%) while that associated with treatment of dissections was 2/97 (1%). Paraplegia was associated with a very high mortality risk 8/14 (67%). Most of these deaths occurred within 30 days of operation.

Follow-up

Currently follow-up extends to a maximum of 5 years. However data are available on just 10 out of a total of 34 patients in whom the procedure was carried out more than 5 years ago. A total of 108 patients have died, 67 within 30 days of their operation and 41 after this period. Fourteen have been converted to open repair, three have suffered late rupture of their aneurysm and eight patients have been lost to follow-up.

Life table analyses for survival, freedom from endoleak, freedom from persistent endoleak, persistent endoleak-free survival, freedom from secondary intervention, secondary intervention-free survival, and freedom from rupture are shown in Figs. 13.1–13.7.

Of the patients treated for aortic dissection complete or partial thrombosis of the false lumen was observed in 53% at 1 month after operation. For the whole population of patients the cumulative rate of survival at 5 years was 62%. The secondary intervention rate was lower than that associated with abdominal endovascular procedures at less than 20% at 5 years. The incidence of secondary intervention after the first year was very low. Almost 99% of the whole population of patients remained free from aortic rupture after 5 years.

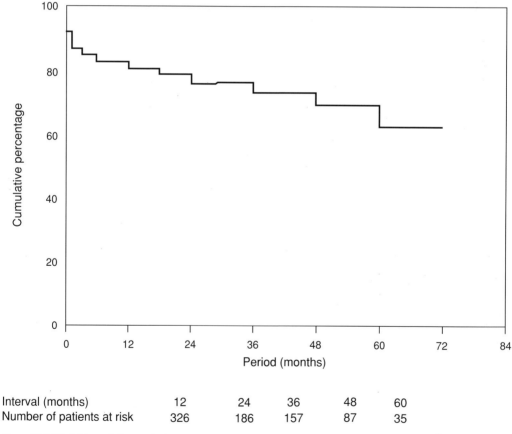

Interval (months)	12	24	36	48	60
Number of patients at risk	326	186	157	87	35

Figure 13.1 Life table analysis – survival.

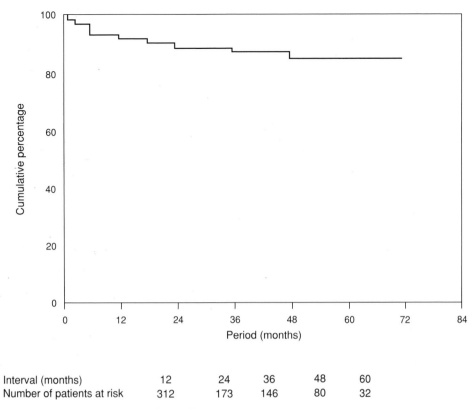

Interval (months)	12	24	36	48	60
Number of patients at risk	312	173	146	80	32

Figure 13.2 Life table analysis – freedom from endoleak.

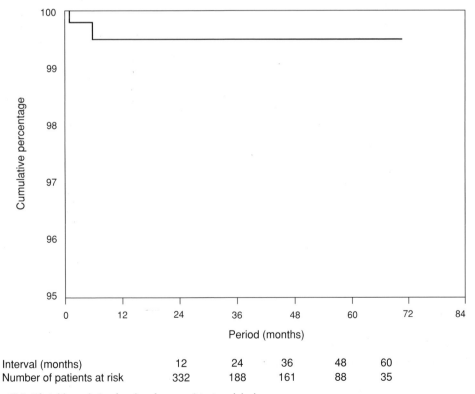

Interval (months)	12	24	36	48	60
Number of patients at risk	332	188	161	88	35

Figure 13.3 Life table analysis – freedom from persistent endoleak.

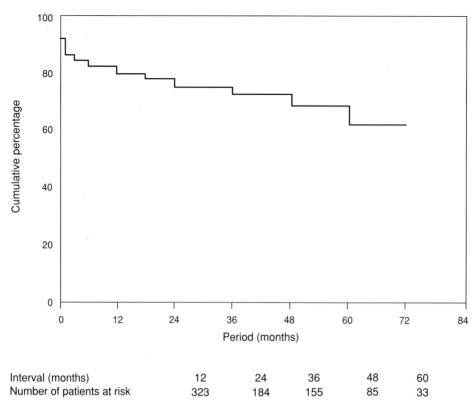

Interval (months)	12	24	36	48	60
Number of patients at risk	323	184	155	85	33

Figure 13.4 Life table analysis – freedom from death and persistent endoleak.

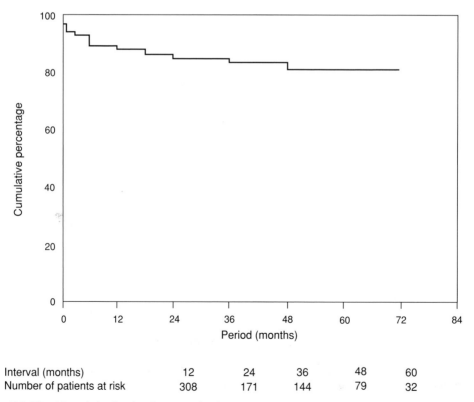

Interval (months)	12	24	36	48	60
Number of patients at risk	308	171	144	79	32

Figure 13.5 Life table analysis – freedom from secondary intervention.

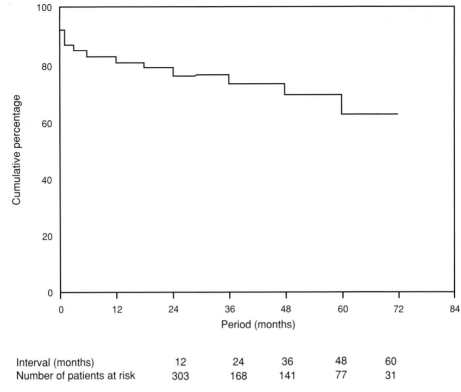

Interval (months)	12	24	36	48	60
Number of patients at risk	303	168	141	77	31

Figure 13.6 Life table analysis – freedom from death and secondary intervention.

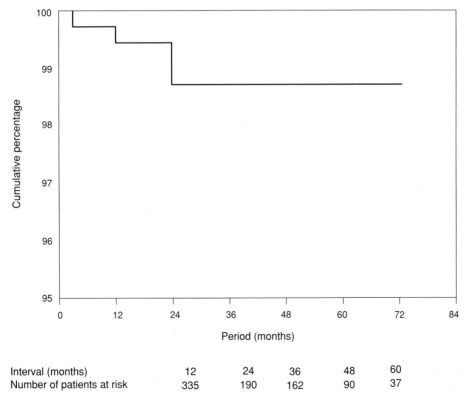

Interval (months)	12	24	36	48	60
Number of patients at risk	335	190	162	90	37

Figure 13.7 Life table analysis – freedom from rupture.

Key points

1 A variety of thoracic aortic pathologies were treated by endovascular stent/grafting.

2 Complete technical success was achieved in 90% of patients.

3 The total incidence of endoleak on completion of the procedure was 9%. Type 2 endoleak was observed in only 2% of the patients.

4 The incidence of paraplegia was low (2.5%).

5 Deployment of three or more endografts within the aorta was a highly significant risk factor for paraplegia.

6 Sixty seven per cent of patients with paraplegia died.

7 The incidence of intracranial stroke (3%) equaled that of paraplegia.

8 Partial or complete thrombosis of the false lumen occurred within 1 month in 53% of the patients treated for aortic dissection.

9 Late complications have occurred infrequently to date. Freedom from secondary intervention exceeded 80% at 5 years.

10 Durability of endovascular treatment of thoracic aortic pathologies beyond 5 years remains to be established. But, within this period late device related complications have been rare. Contrary to expectations migration of stent/grafts was reported in one patient only to date.

11 These results are consistent with the expectation of superior outcome from endovascular repair in comparison to the known results of conventional open surgery at least in the medium term.

To review updates of the EUROSTAR Thoracic and abdominal aortic aneurysm databases visit the website at:

www.eurostar-online.org

Participating institutional coordinators of the EUROSTAR Thoracic Registry

Prof A. Nevelsteen, Louvain, Belgium
Dr J. Buth, Eindhoven, The Netherlands
Prof H. Myhre, Trondheim, Norway
Dr P. Harris, Liverpool, England
Dr E. Verhoeven, Groningen, The Netherlands
Prof W. Stelter, Frankfurt, Germany
Dr M. Wyatt, Newcastle, England
Dr V. Riambau, Barcelona, Spain
Dr P. Peeters, Bonheiden, Belgium
Dr R. Balm, Amsterdam, The Netherlands
Dr R. H. Geelkerken, Enschede, The Netherlands
Dr R. Verhelst, Brussels, Belgium
Prof P. C. Maurer, Munich, Germany
Prof H. Kortmann, Hamburg, Germany
Dr A. de Smet, Rotterdam, The Netherlands
Mr S. Darke, Bournemouth, England
Dr P. Stabel, Turnhout, Belgium
Dr M. van Betsbrugge, Antwerp, Belgium
Dr H. Massin, Gilly, Belgium
Dr F. van Elst, St Truiden, Belgium
Prof. G. Shanik, Dublin, Ireland
Dr Schroë, Genk, Belgium
Dr van Sambeek, Rotterdam, The Netherlands
Dr M. Scoccianti, Rome, Italy
Dr Th. Nordh Larzon, Orebro, Sweden
Dr Sanchez-Corral, Madrid, Spain
Dr I. Degrieck, Aalst, Belgium
Dr D. de Roover, Antwerp, Belgium
Dr E. Sebrechts, Vilvoorde, Belgium
Dr H. Tubbax, Brugge, Belgium
Dr V. Pierat, Brussels, Belgium
Dr L. Verougstraete, Tongeren, Belgium
Prof M. Storck, Leipzig, Germany
Dr J. Hendriks, Edegem, Belgium
Dr J. de Letter, Brugge, Belgium
Dr J. P. Dereume, Brussels, Belgium
Dr E. Vandueren, Charleroi, Belgium
Dr M. Bosiers, Dendermonde, Belgium
Dr J. Bleyn, Deurne, Belgium
Dr F. Vermassen, Gent, Belgium
Dr J. Vandekerkhof, Hasselt, Belgium
Dr M. Buche, Mont Godine, Belgium
Dr J. Demelenne, Namur, Belgium
Dr P. Dujardin, Roeslare, Belgium
Dr P. van den Brande, Brussels, Belgium
Dr C. Choghari, Brussels, Belgium
Dr P. Dormal, Mouscron, Belgium
Dr P. van Ruyssevelt, Haint Saint Paul, Belgium
Dr A. Flamme, Gent, Belgium
Dr J. Poniewierski, La Louviere, Belgium
Dr G. Guillaume, Namur, Belgium
Dr Vahl, Amsterdam, The Netherlands
Dr Fishwick, Leicester, England
Dr Munoz, Malaga, Spain

Reference

1 Leurs LJ, Bell R, Degrieck Y, Thomas S, Hobo R, Lundboam J on behalf the EUROSTAR and UK Thoracic Endograft Registry. Endovascular treatment of thoracic aortic diseases: Combined experience from the EUROSTAR and UK Thoracic Endograft Registries. J Vasc Surg 2004; **40**(4): 670–679.

CHAPTER 14

Management of aortic aneurysms and dissections with the Zenith TX2 stent graft

W. Anthony Lee

The prevalence of thoracic aortic aneurysms is approximately 8–12 cases per 100,000. This estimate is largely based on historical data predating the endovascular era and high-speed spiral computed tomographic (CT) scans. With the more liberal use of CT scans for vascular and nonvascular diagnostic imaging, this estimate is likely to increase in the future.

TAA is a disease of the elderly with its peak incidence occurring in the eighth decade of life. There is relatively greater proportion of women presenting with TAA as compared to abdominal aortic aneurysms (AAA). Whereas in the abdominal aorta, the ratio of men to women is approximately 4:1, in the thoracic aorta it is approximately 3:2, and in some series approach 1:1.

Similar to femoral and popliteal aneurysms, the presence of a TAA is a strong marker for the presence of a concomitant AAA. Almost half of those who present with a thoracic aortic aneurysm will have or had a repair of an AAA. Conversely, those who present with an AAA have a 5% incidence of a concomitant TAA, and thus anyone being evaluated for an AAA should have a thoracic CT scan at least once during their initial workup.

The indications for treatment of TAA include symptoms of back pain, rupture, or size greater than 5.5–6.0 cm. Conventional surgical repair involves prosthetic aortic replacement under left heart bypass using variety of adjunctive measures such as distal perfusion and spinal cord drainage to minimize the risk of spinal cord ischemia. Endovascular repair involves tubular stent grafts that are delivered through the femoral or iliac arteries and deployed over uninvolved segments of the thoracic aorta proximal and distal to the aneurysm. Currently, the only FDA-approved commercially available device in the United States with this indication is the TAG thoracic endograft from W.L. Gore (Flagstaff, AZ).

In addition to thoracic aneurysm, thoracic aortic dissection is another significant disease which can affect this vasculature. Thoracic aortic dissections are primarily classified according to their chronicity and site of the primary intimal tear relative to the left subclavian artery. In the Stanford classification system, A-type refers to dissections that involve the ascending aorta, and the B-type refers to those that begin distal to the left subclavian artery with or without abdominal extension. Acute and chronic dissections are differentiated by whether onset of symptoms is older than 2 weeks. While most Stanford A dissections require urgent repair due to the risk of pericardial rupture, aortic regurgitation, and death, most Stanford B dissections are managed medically.

The clinical presentation of thoracic aortic dissections is distinctly different from atherosclerotic aneurysms. The patients are typically younger in their third and fourth decades of life and uniformly present with severe hypertension. Therefore, the mainstay of medical management is aggressive control of their blood pressure and heart rate using a combination of short acting beta-blocker and nitroprusside infusions. The physiologic aim of these two maneuvers is to reduce the *dp/dt* and prevent the risk of progression of the dissection and acute rupture.

The natural history of uncomplicated and unrepaired chronic Stanford B dissections is that of progressive aneurysmal dilation of the false lumen in up to 30–40% of cases within 5 years, most of whom will require surgical repair to prevent rupture. Currently, the only indication for endovascular or surgical intervention for acute dissections is complications refractory to medical management. These include unremitting back pain, refractory hypertension, visceral or lower extremity malperfusion, and rarely acute expansion and rupture of the false lumen.

Mortality and morbidity of surgical repair for complicated acute aortic dissections can be significant. Therefore, "minimalist" or symptom-directed approach to restore perfusion to the ischemic bed is reasonable if anatomically possible. Surgical treatments include prosthetic aortic replacement under cardiopulmonary bypass, with or without circulatory arrest, and extra-anatomic bypasses to restore lower extremity perfusion. Endovascular therapies have included percutaneous fenestrations of the dissection septum to equalize blood flow from one lumen to the other and more recently deployment of a stent graft to cover the primary tear, redirect the blood flow into the true lumen, and induce false lumen thrombosis. There are no endovascular devices currently approved in the Unted States for use in thoracic aortic dissections.

Differences between endovascular treatment of the thoracic and abdominal aorta

There are substantive differences during the execution and mechanics of endovascular treatment of the thoracic and abdominal aorta that belies the apparent similarities of the two types of devices and delivery methods. Everything in the thoracic aorta is more remote from the entry point of guidewires, catheters, and delivery systems. This means longer catheters and wires with reduced torque control and pushability. This physical distance is compounded by serial iliac, abdominal, and thoracic aortic tortuosity, most commonly present in the supradiaphragmatic segment and near the apex of the arch. (Fig. 14.1). There can also be significant motion

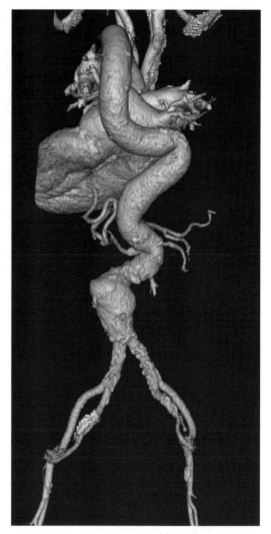

Figure 14.1 Severe abdominal and thoracic aortic tortuosity.

of the thoracic aorta that occurs during respiratory and cardiac cycles. All of these factors make precise deployment of the devices near the delimiting branch vessels (proximally: left subclavian or left common carotid arteries, distally: celiac artery) significantly more challenging than in the abdominal aorta. And lastly, thoracic devices are larger than abdominal devices and require proportionally larger access vessels. This with a relatively higher incidence of females with thoracic aortic aneurysms and their smaller iliac arteries and occlusive disease contribute to a higher incidence of local vascular

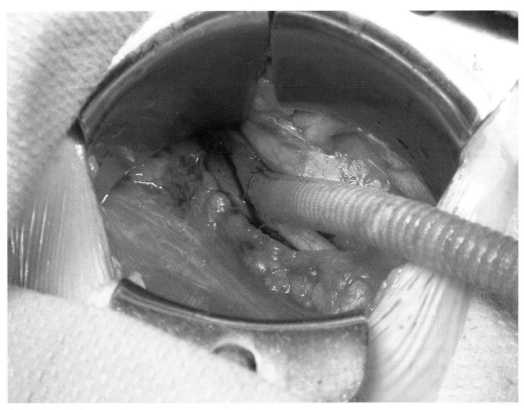

Figure 14.2 Retroperitoneal iliac conduit using a 10-mm Dacron graft anastomosed to the distal common iliac artery.

complications and need for iliac conduits for device delivery (Fig. 14.2).

Advantages of endovascular thoracic aortic repair

The advantages of endovascular thoracic aortic repair over conventional surgery parallel those of the abdominal aorta. Specifically, endovascular repair avoids the morbidity of a thoracotomy and the pleural adhesions that can occur with prior chest surgery or certain lung conditions [1–4]. The procedure typically requires only a single groin cutdown and a contralateral 5-Fr percutaneous femoral access. In the cases of small or diseased iliac arteries, a limited retroperitoneal pelvic exposure is required for an iliac conduit. Unlike open repair, endovascular repair can be performed under regional or even local anesthesia. These aspects of the procedure obviously have significant benefits in those who have compromised pulmonary function and may become ventilatory dependent with a thoracotomy and a prolonged period of general anesthesia.

Physiologically, endovascular repair offers even greater potential benefits by avoidance of cardiopulmonary bypass and need for aortic occlusion. The deleterious effects of visceral and lower extremity ischemia, reperfusion, and cytokine activation are entirely avoided. These benefits have translated into decreased early morbidity, shorter hospital length of stay, and faster recovery to baseline function.

Zenith TX2 thoracic endovascular graft

Currently, the only FDA-approved commercially available thoracic endograft in the United States is the TAG device (W.L. Gore, Flagstaff, AZ). At the time of this writing, three other devices are undergoing various stages of IDE (investigational device exemption) clinical trials including Zenith TX2 (Cook Endovascular, Bloomington, IN), Talent Thoracic

(Medtronic Vascular, Santa Rosa, CA), and the Relay Thoracic Stent Graft (Bolton Medical, Sunrise, FL). This chapter will focus on the Zenith TX2 device.

The Zenith TX2 ("TX2") is a tubular stent graft constructed of a Dacron fabric that is supported with stainless steel Z-stents [1, 2]. The device employs an active fixation mechanism with external hooks oriented in the opposite directions and designed to engage the aortic wall to decrease the risk of proximal and distal migration. The placement of the stents relative to the fabric is varied along the length of the device. At the ends of the endograft the stents are sewn inside the fabric, while in its midportion it is outside the fabric. The intent of this design was to optimize fabric apposition to the aortic lumen and fabric–fabric interstent junctions.

The TX2 system is designed as a two-piece modular system, although for focal lesions single piece repair is adequate (Fig. 14.3). The device can accommodate normal aortic outer diameters of 24 to 38 mm and requires proximal and distal landing zones with a minimum length of 30 mm. The devices are delivered through an integral introducer sheath that has an extremely lubricious outer coating that facilitates its passage through smaller and diseased access vessels. The proximal cone has a pre-shaped curve that is designed to accommodate the curvature of the aortic arch during initial positioning and deployment. The smaller half of diameters of the product matrix is housed in a 20-Fr introducer sheath and the larger half is in a 22-Fr introducer sheath.

The TX2 proximal component is a fully-covered stent graft with fixation hooks protruding outside the graft material and staggered approximately 3–5 mm from the proximal edge of the device (Fig. 14.4). The weld points of the hooks and the thickness of the Z-stent struts allow for easy visualization of the device under fluoroscopy. The device diameters range from 28 to 42 mm and lengths from 12.0 to 21.6 cm. Similar to the abdominal Zenith device, the stent graft is deployed in a staged manner for an extremely accurate and controlled deployment. After partial deployment of the device, limited longitudinal movement of the delivery catheter is allowed to fine-tune the position of the stent graft in the proximal neck with interval adjustments of the fluoroscopy gantry angle and control angiograms.

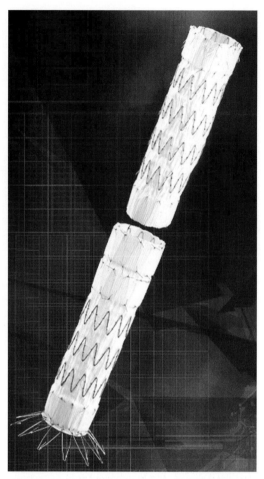

Figure 14.3 A two-piece Zenith TX2 endograft system.

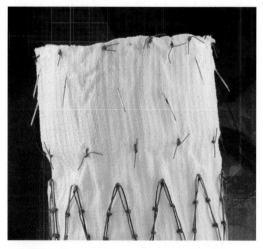

Figure 14.4 Close-up of the proximal end of the TX2 proximal component. Note the hooks protruding from the fabric.

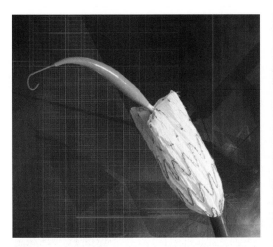

Figure 14.5 The proximal end of the proximal component is constrained in a clover-leaf pattern to allow continued aortic blood flow.

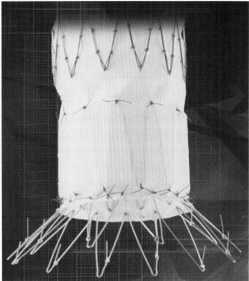

Figure 14.6 Close up of the distal end of the TX2 distal component. Note the bare stent with the retrograde-oriented hooks.

During this time, the proximal end remains partially constrained in a clover-leaf pattern to avoid a windsock effect (Fig. 14.5). Once the proximal end is positioned satisfactorily, the remainder of the device is unsheathed, and its position is secured with release of trigger wires which allows the proximal end to fully deploy and the hooks to engage the aortic wall.

The TX2 distal component has a slightly different construction from the proximal component. The distal end of the device has an uncovered bare-metal stent similar to the proximal end of the abdominal Zenith device. The hooks are on this bare stent and are oriented in a retrograde manner opposite the direction of the proximal hooks (Fig. 14.6). This bare stent configuration allows fixation of the device over the origins of the visceral vessels where it may be relatively less diseased and the covered portion to extend right to the origin of the celiac artery. Similar to the proximal component, the device diameters range from 28 to 42 mm and lengths from 12.7 to 20.7 cm. Although the minimum overlap between the proximal and distal device is two stents, there is no upper limit and nearly the entire distal component may be "tromboned" into the proximal stent. The deployment method similarly involves first unsheathing the stent graft and, after precisely positioning the distal end, releasing trigger wires to deploy the distal bare-metal stents. The product line includes 8-cm long extensions to extend proximally

or distally or bridge interstent junctions, although they are rarely necessary.

Endovascular repair of thoracic aortic aneurysms

Case planning and patient selection

Almost the entire case planning may be performed using thin-cut (≤2 mm) CT angiogram with three-dimensional multiplanar and centerline orthogonal reconstructions. Due to the intrinsic tortuosity and angulations of the thoracic aorta, anatomic sizing and length determination using plain axial imaging is nearly impossible. Conventional angiography is unnecessary in most cases as it subjects the patient to all the risks of an invasive procedure and a large contrast load.

The main determinants of anatomic eligibility are adequate proximal and distal landing zones. Proximally, the absolute limit of endograft extension is the origin of the left common carotid artery (or the innominate artery in the cases of bovine anatomy). The left subclavian artery may be covered to gain additional landing zone but preoperative evaluation of the left vertebral artery and completeness of the circle of Willis must be performed. Indications for left subclavian revascularization include left-hand dominance, a dominant left vertebral artery, and an incomplete circle of Willis. Distally, the celiac artery marks the lower limit of the landing zone. Beyond mere length of the proximal and distal necks, its quality in terms of the shape, angle, and presence of thrombus all play a role in determining the suitability for endovascular repair. For the TX2 device, the neck diameters must fall in the range of 24–38 mm in diameter and at least 30 mm in length. Secondary considerations include the size and quality of the access vessels, overall aortic tortuosity, and underlying aortic pathology.

Once the basic anatomic criteria have been met, device(s) of appropriate diameter(s) and length(s) are selected to allow coverage of the entire length of the involved thoracic aorta. The side of endograft delivery, transfemoral vs. iliac conduit, need for left subclavian coverage with or without revascularization are all determined preoperatively and are critical to the success of the procedure.

Preoperative preparation

The conduct of an endovascular thoracic aneurysm repair involves the following key points. The procedure should be performed in a sterile surgical environment with laminar airflow management. Endograft infection is a lethal complication and the meticulous sterile technique must be observed throughout the entire procedure. Any anesthetic technique can be used but because many of these patients have coexisting pulmonary insufficiency, a regional technique is favored. We have reserved general anesthetic to those patients who cannot lie flat due to back problems, are hard of hearing, or have other cognitive or medical disabilities that would impair their ability to fully cooperate by lying still and holding one's breath when asked. Use of adjunctive invasive monitoring such as Swan–Ganz catheters and transesophageal echocardiography are largely unnecessary. No attempt is made to modulate the blood pressure during endograft deployment, include adenosine-induced cardiac arrest.

Spinal drainage is not routinely performed for most cases. Consideration for prophylactic spinal drainage can be given when extensive coverage of the thoracic aorta is planned or the patient previously had an abdominal aortic replacement. However, the correlation between extent of thoracic aortic coverage and postoperative paraplegia/paraparesis has been poor. Published case reports seem to indicate that one of the most important risk factors for perioperative spinal cord ischemia is intraoperative hypotension. Therefore, maintenance of normotension or even mild hypertension with pharmacologic adjuncts is recommended. When symptoms of spinal cord ischemia are detected in the postoperative period, blood pressure is elevated and a spinal drainage catheter is expeditiously placed and left in for 48–72 h. In an overwhelming majority of cases, the paraplegia/paresis can be completely reversed if it is detected early enough. On the other hand, late onset of spinal cord ischemia up to 2 weeks postoperatively has also been reported.

Invasive arterial monitoring is typically placed in the right radial artery as coverage of the left subclavian artery may be necessary in over 20% of cases. Central venous access is unnecessary and two large bore intravenous lines are sufficient for perioperative fluid management. The prep is limited to the abdomen and thighs. The risk of emergent intraoperative conversion due to aortic rupture is less than 1% and no specific provisions are made for an emergent thoracotomy.

Excellent fluoroscopic imaging is essential to the success of the procedure. While portable C-arm fluoroscopy units may be used with relative safety, there is no substitute for a fixed unit in terms of visualization of vital structures and avoidance of overheating and system shutdown in the middle of the procedure. The procedure table should be circumferentially radiolucent to allow unimpeded imaging and EKG-leads and other radiopaque objects should be removed from the imaging field.

Technique

On the basis of preoperative studies, the side with the largest and the least diseased iliac and common femoral arteries is selected for endograft delivery. Although percutaneous access is possible using suture-mediated closure devices deployed prior to insertion of the introducer sheaths, the most common method is direct surgical exposure of the

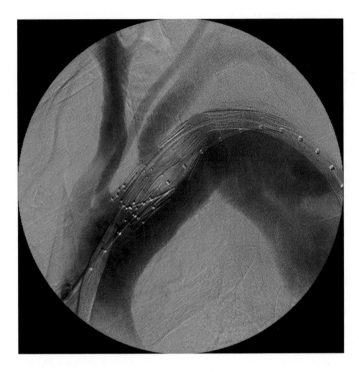

Figure 14.7 Intraoperative image of the proximal component partially deployed.

femoral arteries. In approximately 15–20% of cases, a retroperitoneal iliac conduit is required to overcome small or diseased iliac arteries. Next, the contralateral femoral artery is percutaneously accessed and a 5-Fr sheath is inserted.

Guidewire access into the ascending thoracic aorta is obtained. Occasionally in situations of severe angulation or aortic tortuosity, appropriate directional catheter support is necessary to navigate through the aorta. The initial guidewire on the side of endograft delivery is exchanged for a superstiff guidewire such as the Lunderquist Extra-Stiff (Cook Inc., Bloomington, IN), which has a preformed curve at its proximal end to conform to the curvature of the arch. A 5-Fr pigtail angiographic catheter is advanced to the proximal arch over the contralateral guidewire. The patient is systemically anticoagulated with intravenous heparin to achieve an activated clotting time of 250 s or greater.

The fluoroscope is angled approximately 30–45° in the left anterior oblique projection to "open" the aortic arch and optimally visualize the arch perpendicular to the main axis of the origins of the great vessels. An initial aortogram is performed using 15–20 ml of contrast injected at 20 ml/s to confirm preoperative CT findings. The proximal TX2 component is delivered to the proximal neck and deployed using the method described above (Fig. 14.7). While maintaining guidewire access and manual control of the femoral artery, the delivery catheter is removed and the distal component is advanced into the proximal component. The pigtail catheter is positioned in the distal thoracic aorta and the origins of the celiac and superior mesenteric arteries identified using a lateral projection. The distal end of the covered section of the distal component is positioned above the celiac artery and device is deployed as described above.

There is no obligatory ballooning required for the TX2 device. A completion aortogram is performed to confirm proper placement and exclusion of the aneurysm. Attachment site and junctional endoleaks may be treated with a compliant aortic occlusion balloon such as the Coda (Cook Inc., Bloomington, IN) to smooth any folds and ensure full expansion of the devices. All sheaths and guidewires are removed and the femoral arteriotomy is surgically repaired.

Endovascular repair of thoracic aortic dissections

Endovascular repair of Stanford B dissections is an evolving therapy whose early results hold promise for this difficult problem [1–3]. There are no devices that are currently available approved for this indication. The Zenith TX2 line of thoracic endografts has recently introduced a novel extension of the original product line to be used in conjunction with the proximal TX2 component and specially designed for the treatment of dissections. This is an investigational device and only available under an IDE in the United States.

TX2 distal bare stent component

The device is constructed of stacked Z-stents joined by polypropylene sutures (Fig. 14.8). It is introduced through a 16-Fr sheath which can be inserted through the existing TX2 proximal component sheath. A single-stent diameter accommodates aortic luminal diameters ranging from 24 to 46 mm and is available in 82-, 123-, and 164-mm lengths. Similar to the rest of the Zenith line, after unsheathing, the device is fully deployed by releasing a trigger wire. The Z-stents exert a low radial force to "gently" appose the dissection septum and reexpand the true lumen. The large open strut architecture allows maintenance of branch vessel perfusion, so that the stent can be safely deployed across the origins of intercostal, visceral, and renal arteries.

In principle, the goal of this combination construction of a covered component proximally and bare-metal component distally is to achieve true lumen reexpansion and false lumen exclusion. The size of the TX2 proximal component is based on the diameter of the most proximal uninvolved thoracic aorta, usually the segment between the left subclavian and common carotid arteries. Following deployment of this device across the primary tear, blood flow is redirected into the true lumen and the false lumen is mostly depressurized with most of the residual perfusion from distal reentry tears that are frequently present in the perivisceral aortic segment. The distal bare stent component is then used to reappose the septum against the false lumen. In the cases of persistent malperfusion due to a dissection flap into or a reentry tear near a vessel origin, the Z-stent provides structural scaffolding for placement of a bare or covered peripheral stent from the true lumen into the branch vessel bridging across the false lumen (Fig. 14.9).

Technique

The conduct of the endovascular repair of acute thoracic dissections is similar to that of thoracic aneurysms except for the following differences. The procedures are typically performed urgently or emergently due to complications from the acute dissection. Standing inventory should be available so that repair is not delayed due to lack of devices. For optimal airway control, general endotracheal anesthesia using cardiac induction techniques should be used. Wide hemodynamic fluctuations should be assiduously avoided to reduce the risk of acute extension of the dissection or even rupture of the false lumen during induction.

Right brachial arterial access is routinely obtained to maintain ready access to the true lumen for proximal thoracic angiography. The side of endograft entry is selected on the basis of preoperative CT angiography and involvement of the iliac arteries. The side that allows the best true lumen access from the femoral artery is selected. A floppy-tipped guidewire is carefully advanced into the

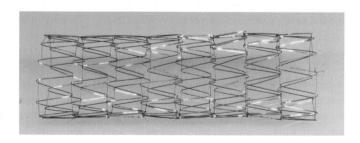

Figure 14.8 A fully-deployed TX2 distal bare stent component for treatment of aortic dissections.

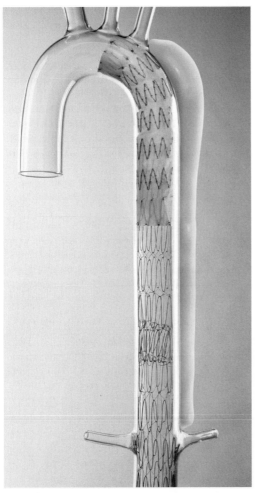

Figure 14.9 Combination repair utilizing the TX2 proximal component with the distal bare stent component. Note how the bare stent is deployed over the renal arteries in this glass model.

ascending thoracic aorta. The entire course of the guidewire is interrogated with an intravascular ultrasound (IVUS) to verify consistent true lumen passage. Occasionally, the guidewire can "weave" in and out of the dissection septum through the reentry tears. Failure to verify true lumen passage can result in mal-expansion of the stent graft with disastrous complications. Using IVUS control, the point of false lumen traversal can be visualized and the guidewire redirected into the true lumen. Ballooning is avoided unless absolutely necessary to avoid potential proximal extension of the dissection.

Following deployment of the TX2 proximal component, if the true lumen has reexpanded sufficiently and malperfusion corrected, the procedure may conclude at this point. However, if the true lumen remains collapsed distally due to persistent false lumen perfusion, the bare stent component of appropriate length is deployed. Reapposition of the septum may be sufficient to close the distal reentry tears. Additional small diameter peripheral stents may be required to tack down persistent flaps which may obstruct the branch vessels. Reversal of malperfusion is assessed angiographically and with measurements of hemodynamic gradients.

Clinical experience

The clinical experience with the Zenith TX2 stent-graft system is limited due to the current investigational nature of the device. Nearly all of the available data are from outside the United States or from individual physician-sponsored IDE single-center studies. These reports encompass a broader range of thoracic pathologies than a typical sponsored multicenter IDE clinical trial [1–6]. In a recent publication from Cleveland Clinic, Greenberg *et al.* reported the midterm results of their first 100 consecutive thoracic aortic repairs using the Zenith TX1 (1st generation) and TX2 stent-graft systems [2]. The majority of the experience comprised aneurysms (81%) and dissections. All-cause mortality in this cohort was 17% at 1 year. Spinal cord ischemia occurred in 6% and strokes in 3% of patients. Other pertinent outcomes at 1 year included 6% rate of endoleak, 15% secondary interventions, and 6% migrations. Interestingly, as previously mentioned, 55% had a prior aortic aneurysm repair and 19% required iliac conduits.

At the time of this writing, the Zenith TX2 pivotal trial has completed enrollment of the test (endovascular) arm [6]. This was a prospective, nonrandomized, multinational, IDE clinical trial involving 47 centers studying the safety and efficacy of the TX2 stent-graft system in the treatment of thoracic aortic aneurysms. Anatomic inclusion criteria included descending thoracic aortic aneurysms and penetrating ulcers with at least 3 cm of healthy, uninvolved aorta proximal, and distal to the lesion. The study design involved 135 endovascular repairs and 70 contemporary (repairs performed within 12 months of enrollment) and prospective open surgical controls. The primary safety endpoint was 30-day all-cause mortality as compared to the surgical controls and the primary efficacy endpoint was 30-day rupture-free survival. Secondary endpoints included procedural and treatment successes, adverse events, mortality, clinical utility measures, and quality of life assessment at 12 months. Detailed description and rationale of the pivotal trial can be found in the publication by Hassoun and colleagues [6].

Conclusion

Endovascular repair of thoracic aortic aneurysms and dissections may provide a less invasive alternative in the treatment of these life-threatening conditions. Although not yet FDA-approved, the Zenith TX2 thoracic endograft system holds promise as an important addition to the thoracic endovascular armamentarium. However, as in all new and emerging therapies, the long-term safety and efficacy of endovascular repair are lacking and it should be not be used with undue premature exuberance.

References

1 Appoo JJ, Moser WG, Fairman RM, Cornelius KF, Pochettino A, Woo EY, Kurichi JE, Carpenter JP, Bavaria JE. Thoracic aortic stent grafting: Improving results with newer generation investigational devices. J Thorac Cardiovasc Surg 2006; **131**: 1087–1094.

2 Greenberg RK, O'Neill S, Walker E, Haddad F, Lyden SP, Svensson LG, Lytle B, Clair DG, Ouriel K. Endovascular repair of thoracic aortic lesions with the Zenith TX1 and TX2 thoracic grafts: Intermediate-term results. J Vasc Surg 2005; **41**: 589–596.

3 Dake MD, Wang DS. Will stent-graft repair emerge as treatment of choice for acute type B dissection? Semin Vasc Surg 2006; **19**: 40–47.

4 Peterson BG, Eskandari MK, Gleason TG, Morasch MD. Utility of left subclavian artery revascularization in association with endoluminal repair of acute and chronic thoracic aortic pathology. J Vasc Surg 2006; **43**: 433–439.

5 Kasirajan K, Milner R, Chaikof EL. Late complications of thoracic endografts. J Vasc Surg 2006; **43** (Suppl) A: 94A–99A.

6 Hassoun HT, Dake MD, Svensson LG, Greenberg RK, Cambria RP, Moore RD, Matsumura JS. Multi-institutional pivotal trial of the Zenith TX2 thoracic aortic stent-graft for treatment of descending thoracic aortic aneurysms: Clinical study design. Perspect Vasc Surg Endovasc Ther 2005; **17**: 255–264.

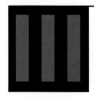

PART III

Aortic dissection and traumatic aortic injury

CHAPTER 15

Aortic dissection: evaluation and management – choosing the right intervention

David M. Williams

Contemporary treatment of aortic dissection still depends on landmark articles by DeBakey in 1955 and Wheat in 1965, which laid the groundwork for the surgical and medical treatment of acute aortic dissection observed as standard-of-care until recently [1, 2]. The approach to treatment pivoted primarily on identification of anatomical features of the dissection, namely involvement of the ascending aorta (Fig. 15.1). Identification of ascending aortic involvement depended initially on catheter-based aortography, with injection of iodinated contrast in the aortic root. The critical role of aortography was gradually replaced by computed tomography (CT) and transesophageal echocardiography (TEE).

Acute aortic dissection typically kills by tamponade or exsanguination due to false lumen rupture or by organ ischemia due to the malperfusion syndromes [1–5]. These complications comprise the targets of contemporary endovascular approaches to treating acute dissection, which include percutaneous fenestration and endograft implantation. The classical treatment algorithm asked merely: Is the ascending aorta involved? The new endovascular techniques require a more detailed anatomical description of the dissection than the classical algorithm, including on-the-spot identification of true and false lumens, location of entry and reentry tears, and sources of critical vessel perfusion. The roles and requirements of angiography, TEE, and CT have all evolved to accommodate the changing paradigms of treatment.

This presentation will discuss the pathophysiology of false lumen rupture and malperfusion, tech-

nical requirements of fenestration and endovascular treatment, and the relation of individual patient anatomy to the critical treatment decisions of open vs. endovascular treatment, endograft vs. fenestration. A detailed description of fenestration and bare stents will be presented in the second talk.

Pathoanatomy of false lumen rupture

In a model of aortic dissection with no flow and equal pressures in the true and false lumens, the true lumen immediately collapses and the false lumen immediately becomes ectatic, resulting in an overall increase in aortic cross section [6]. Consideration of the anatomy of the two lumens explains this behavior. The normal aorta expands due to blood pressure until wall tension generated by elastic recoil of the mural elastin and collagen balances blood pressure. In aortic dissection, the dissection flap typically contains the intima and 2/3 of the media, and the outer wall of the false lumen contains the remaining 1/3 of the media and the adventitia. Being thinner and less elastic than the outer wall of the undissected aorta, the outer wall of the false lumen must expand to a larger diameter in order to generate, at a given blood pressure, the same wall tension. The dissection flap, which lies between isobaric lumens, has been released from transmural pressure, and therefore undergoes radial elastic collapse. Thus, false lumen dilation and true lumen collapse are expected from purely structural considerations of the aortic wall.

Pre-fenestration and -endograft era

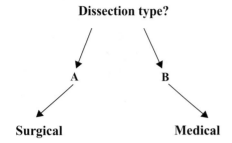

Figure 15.1 Treatment algorithm in prefenestration and preendograft era.

The availability of endografts invites us to consider the reversal of this process: What would happen if a covered endograft were deployed across the communication between the lumens, covering the tear and sequestering the false lumen? In this case, transmural pressure would be restored to the dissection flap and reduced from the outer wall of the false lumen. The dissection flap would expand, the outer wall of the false lumen would contract, and, assuming the false lumen could vent its contents, the false lumen would disappear. To what extent clinical dissections would follow this model remains to be seen. In any event, achieving this hemodynamic reversal of the dissection process requires accurate identification of the location and extent of the entry and reentry tears and judicious placement of the endograft.

Rupture of the false lumen is associated with tears in the outer wall of the false lumen. Focal partial-thickness tears in the outer wall of the false lumen are often seen in specimens resected during surgical treatment of acute type 1 or 2 dissections. These are flat, shallow, lenticulate defects in the ragged surface of the outer wall, usually without associated adventitial hemorrhage. There is no imaging correlate of these defects on CT, and so presently there is no way of studying their natural history, or of incriminating them in aortic rupture. However, because they represent areas of focal thinning, and because dehiscence of the edges of these tears suggests that local wall strain exceeds elasticity, it is reasonable to assume they are sentinel tears associated with false lumen rupture. With respect to

preventing false lumen rupture in a given patient, the inability to see these tears argues for continuing the status quo and treating all acute type 1 and 2 dissections and all acute type 3 dissections with large baseline diameters or rapid growth as high risk for rupture.

False lumen rupture at first appears to present a technical quandary. How can one seal a tear in the outer wall of the false lumen, assuming the exit tear could be identified and that the stiff delivery device could even be manipulated safely alongside it? But necropsy studies suggest that in acute dissection the location of false lumen rupture is near the entry tear of the dissection [7, 8]. Furthermore, it appears that the endograft deployed across the entry tear of an acute dissection induces localized thrombosis of the nearby false lumen [9]. Thus, there is a sound anatomical and physiological basis for treating symptomatic or leaking acute type B dissections by covering the entry tear near it, without necessarily eliminating all reentry tears throughout the aorta.

Pathoanatomy of branch artery obstruction

The Michigan classification of branch artery obstruction [10] is based on the anatomical relationship of the dissection flap to the branch artery in question (Fig. 15.2). It is an intuitively appealing classification because this anatomic distinction forms the basis of distinct treatment strategies. The causes of obstruction may be distinguished as follows:

– Static obstruction
– Dynamic obstruction
– Mixed static and dynamic
– Miscellaneous
  • Related to dissection: thrombosis, embolism
  • Unrelated to dissection: atherosclerosis, FMD

In static obstruction, the dissection flap intersects the origin of a branch and encroaches on the lumen. If the dissection enters the vessel origin but does not reenter, the true lumen of the vessel is narrowed, and a pressure gradient may be measured across the stenosis between the aorta and the arterial trunk. If the false lumen reenters through a large enough tear, then it can completely compensate for

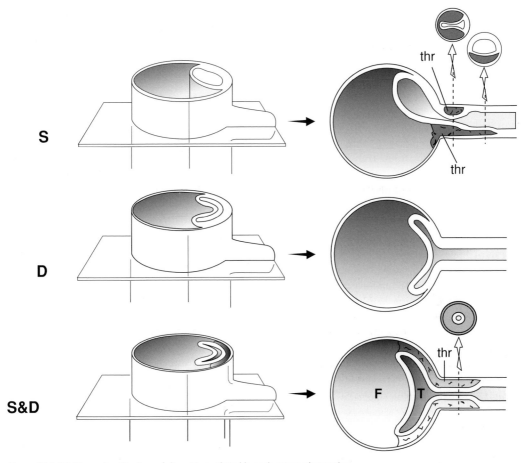

Figure 15.2 Michigan classification of dissection-related branch artery obstruction.

a narrowed true lumen, and no pressure gradient may be present. Treatment is aimed at relieving the branch artery stenosis.

In dynamic obstruction, the dissection flap spares the vessel origin, but prolapses across it like a curtain. This obstruction is dynamic in two senses. It is observed only during cross-sectional imaging with the aorta pressurized and conducting flow; it disappears when the aorta is observed at aortotomy or at necropsy. Furthermore, it may disappear during medical treatment with antihypertensives and beta-blockers, and recur when medications are discontinued. Treatment must be directed at the dissection flap in the aorta. Two approaches are feasible: covering the entry tear by means of an endograft thereby restoring true lumen flow and partially collapsing

the false lumen, and fenestrating the dissection flap thereby establishing flow across the flap into the compromised true lumen.

Identification of the true and false lumens

Identification of the true and false lumens is crucial in the endovascular treatment of aortic dissection. The true and false lumens behave differently. As noted above, the false lumen is prone to ectasia and is at risk of rupture, and the true lumen is prone to collapse and is at risk of compromise of its branch arteries. Numerous steps in the endovascular treatment of dissection require real-time knowledge of which lumen the guidewire, the diagnostic catheter, and of course treatment devices lie within. These steps include

– Deploying an endograft across the entry tear within the true lumen
– Stenting a branch artery to the aortic true lumen
– Stenting the aortic true lumen after fenestration, to reduce a prolapsing flap
– Aligning both iliac arteries with the aortic true lumen during aortoiliac stenting
– Avoid complicating future transfemoral catheter procedures, retrograde aortic perfusion, or endograft treatment because of injudicious placement of aortic or branch artery stents

In chronic dissections, the distinction between the true and false lumens is usually straightforward. For most of these patients, the interventionalist will have the benefit of a chest, abdomen, and pelvis CT. With the anatomical information garnered from the CT, and with the real-time help of intravascular ultrasound, it is easy to stay oriented with respect to true and false lumens. In acute dissections, a complete CT exam may not be available. Features identifying the false lumen include aortic cobwebs and the "beak" sign [11–13]. Aortic cobwebs are remnants of media stretching (like cobwebs) between the dissection flap and the outer wall of the false lumen. The beak sign is the acute angle (the beak) which the dissection flap meets the outer wall of the aorta. As such, it is the imaging correlate of the cleaving wedge of hematoma as it splits the medial layers to form the false lumen. These signs are highly reliable identifiers of the false lumen. Generally reliable characteristics of the true lumen are continuity with the aortic root, which remains the source of the majority of the large-diameter aortic branches, and continuity with the femoral arteries.

Once the lumens are identified, they should be traced from root to groin. A reliable anatomical rule to use while drawing a mental path within the aorta from slice to slice on a CT exam is that every time the path crosses the flap it changes the lumen. A second reliable anatomical rule is that, in acute dissections, the lumens are continuous. If two lumens are observed in the chest and two are observed in the pelvis, then two are present in the abdomen, although one of them may be difficult to identify. Sources of branch artery perfusion are identified as

exclusively true lumen, exclusively false lumen, or shared true and false lumens. Branches with shared perfusion are further characterized as with or without reentry tears.

Diagnosis of branch artery obstruction

It would be useful at this point to summarize the anatomic details required to direct endovascular treatment. These must be established by cross-sectional imaging, such as by preoperative CT or by intraoperative IVUS, and include:

Dissection type
Location of entry tear
Location of reentry tears
Identification of true and false lumens throughout the aorta
Identification of arteries at risk in malperfusion
Identification of mechanism of obstruction

Cross-sectional imaging is useful to ruling out "ischemic anatomy." If the true lumen is of reasonable caliber from entry tear to termination, and if the dissection flap spares every major branch artery, then branch artery obstruction is unlikely. However, if the flap crosses a vessel origin, or the true lumen is collapsed, then malperfusion may be present, and should be evaluated by angiography. Evaluation begins with inspection of the flap in relation to branch artery origins. This can be done most expeditiously using intravascular ultrasound. Pressure measurements are made simultaneously in the aortic root and abdominal aortic true and false lumens. If these are equal, subsequent pressurements can be made using the abdominal aortic pressure as a surrogate for root pressure. If they are unequal, then a search for a pressure drop across a coarctation-like obstruction within the aorta should be made.

Aortic pressures should be compared to arterial trunk pressures in the organ of interest clinically as well as in those branches suspected of being compromised on the basis of imaging. Equal pressures in a false lumen and a collapsed true lumen do not mean that the branch artery pressures are also equal. Pressure measurements within a branch artery should be followed by selective arteriography, to make sure that the measurement is representative of the perfusion pressure at the organ level. This precaution is necessary in instances of static obstruction, wherein the reentry tear may be several centimeters deep in the trunk; unless the measurement is distal to the reentry tear, it may underestimate the branch artery deficit in perfusion pressure.

Dynamic obstruction may be demonstrably pressure-dependent. In cases where this is suspected, especially when the clinical history suggests the patient is noncompliant with medications or clinical follow-up, a negative work-up for malperfusion is followed by reassessment after tapering down the dose of the beta-blocker. For this reason, we request patients with subacute dissection and a history suggesting sporadic episodes of malperfusion be converted to short-acting beta-blockers, antihypertensives, and sedation. Patients with acute dissection are, ordinarily, already being treated with short-acting drugs.

Management

The DeBakey and Stanford classifications provide straightforward anatomical criteria for stratifying patients into immediate surgical or medical management. Treatment of the leaking type A false lumen (impending rupture or tamponade) and florid aortic insufficiency take precedence over malperfusion, and should proceed immediately in patients with reasonable operative risk. Patients with prolonged malperfusion of gut or lower extremity may be unsuitable for immediate repair even with type A dissection, and in such cases immediate therapy is directed at restoring flow to critical vessels. The mechanism of arterial obstruction determines the appropriate treatment in a given case, and so the first principle of treatment is to define arterial anatomy and assess visceral perfusion. In particular, assuring the integrity of the superior mesenteric artery, or restoring perfusion to the compromised SMA, has the highest priority of any endovascular goal in this group of patients. Even when resection of dead bowel is necessary, preoperative endovascular restoration of SMA perfusion will give the general surgeon reliable margins between uncompromised and unsalvageable bowel.

While correcting life-threatening malperfusion is the goal of these procedures, nevertheless the endovascular physician should bear in mind that additional endovascular procedures may be necessary in the future. This is especially important when treating patients with type A dissections complicated by malperfusion, in whom aortic root reconstruction may be delayed. For example, deploying a Wallstent through a fenestration tear, from the false lumen above to the true lumen below, may effectively treat the malperfusion. However, by compressing the true lumen adjacent to the false lumen component of the Wallstent, this procedure greatly complicates future transfemoral access to the brachiocephalic vessels and precludes future cardiac bypass using retrograde transfemoral perfusion. Instead, the stent should be deployed entirely within the aortic true lumen.

In summary, four treatment algorithms or decision trees can be envisioned. The first is the conventional stratification between type A vs. type B dissections (Fig. 15.1). In the pre-endograft era, which is the current Michigan algorithm, the primary question is, "Is prolonged malperfusion suspected?" Here, patients are stratified between immediate angiography to correct malperfusion, and treatment determined by the conventional algorithm (Fig. 15.3). In the era of endografts restricted to conventional indications for surgical intervention, the first question is, "Is an endograft indicated?" followed by "Is an endograft anatomically feasible?" (Fig. 15.4). In the era of unlimited use

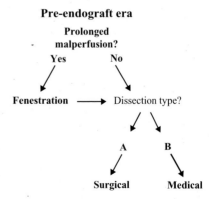

Figure 15.3 Treatment algorithm in pre-endograft era.

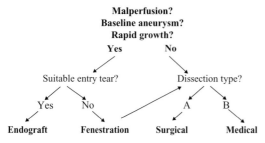

Restricted endograft era
Surgical indications for treatment

Figure 15.4 Treatment algorithm with restricted use of endografts.

of endografts, the first question is "Is an endograft anatomically feasible?" (Fig. 15.5).

Conclusion

New endovascular treatments of acute aortic dissection impose new challenges on diagnostic cross-sectional imaging to define the individual patient's vascular pathoanatomy. The integration of clinical assessment, contemporary high-resolution imaging, and new endovascular treatments suggest new

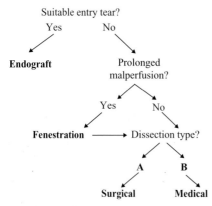

Unrestricted endograft era:
Goal of false lumen thrombosis

Figure 15.5 Treatment algorithm with unrestricted use of endografts.

algorithms or decision trees to guide treatment of dissection.

References

1 DeBakey ME, Cooley DA, Creech O. Surgical considerations of dissecting aneurysm of the aorta. Ann Surg 1955; **142**: 586–610.

2 Wheat MW, Palmer RF, Bartley TD, Seelman RC. Treatment of dissecting aneurysms of the aorta without surgery. J Thorac Cardiovasc Surg 1965; **50**: 364–373.

3 Miller DC, Mitchell RS, Oyer PE, Stinson EB, Jamieson SW, Shumway NE. Independent determinants of operative mortality for patients with aortic dissections. Circulation 1984; **70**: I153–I164.

4 Mehta RH, Suzuki T, Hagan PG *et al.* Predicting death in patients with acute type A aortic dissection. Circulation 2002; **105**: 200–206.

5 Suzuki T, Mehta RH, Ince H *et al.* Clinical profiles and outcomes of acute type B aortic dissection in the current era: Lessons from the International Registry of Aortic Dissection (IRAD). Circulation 2003; **108**(Suppl 1): II312–II317.

6 Williams DM, LePage MA, Lee DY. The dissected aorta. I. Early anatomic changes in an in vitro model. Radiology 1997; **203**: 23–31.

7 Roberts CS, Roberts WC. Aortic dissection with the entrance tear in the descending thoracic aorta. Analysis of 40 necropsy patients. Ann Surg 1991; **213**: 356–368.

8 Roberts WC. Aortic dissection: Anatomy, consequences, and causes. Am Heart J 1981; **101**: 195–214.

9 Nienaber CA, Fattori R, Lund G *et al.* Nonsurgical reconstruction of thoracic aortic dissection by stent-graft placement. N Engl J Med 1999; **340**: 1539–1545.

10 Williams DM, Lee DY, Hamilton B *et al.* The dissected aorta. III. Anatomy and radiologic diagnosis of branch-vessel compromise. Radiology 1997; **203**: 37–44.

11 Lee DY, Williams DM, Abrams GD. The dissected aorta. II. Differentiation of the true from the false lumen with intravascular US Radiol 1997; **203**: 32–36.

12 Williams DM, Joshi A, Dake MD, Deeb GM, Miller DC, Abrams GD. Aortic cobwebs: an anatomic marker identifying the false lumen in aortic dissection-imaging and pathologic correlation. Radiology 1994; **190**: 167–174.

13 LePage MA, Quint LE, Sonnad SS, Deeb GM, Williams DM. Aortic dissection: CT features that distinguish true lumen from false lumen. Am J Roentgenol 2001; **77**: 207–211.

CHAPTER 16

Aortic dissection: role of fenestration and stents in the endograft era

David M. Williams

Aortic dissections are the tornadoes of the vascular system. They are impetuous, catastrophic, and capricious. Despite their unpredictability, the complications of dissections fall into two classes: branch artery obstructions, which depend on the final anatomy of the true lumen, and aortic rupture, which depends on the final integrity of the false lumen.

Fenestration and deploying bare stents have proven to be reliable methods for treating ischemic complications of aortic dissection [1–3]. Recent articles have shown widespread acceptance of endografts for treatment of complicated as well as uncomplicated dissections [4–6]. Endografts show promise of correcting some of the ischemic complications of dissections, as well as of stabilizing the false lumen. This presentation reviews the pertinent pathoanatomy of acute and chronic dissections as related to these percutaneous treatment techniques, reviews the technical details of endografts and fenestration, and describes the complementary roles of these techniques in clinical practice.

Anatomic and hemodynamic changes in the aorta following dissection

As noted elsewhere, immediately after aortic dissection, there is variable collapse of the true lumen and growth in total aortic diameter due to the bulging false lumen [7]. The degree of true lumen collapse and false lumen expansion is related to blood pressure, circumferential extent of the dissection, and magnitude of longitudinal blood flow in the false lumen. A condition of significant longitudinal blood flow in the false lumen is the presence of sizable entry and reentry tears in the dissection flap. In such a case, false and true lumen pressures are often equal, in which case the dissection flap is in a state of elastic collapse, because there is no transmural pressure to expand it. Collapse of the true lumen is further exacerbated by the Bernoulli effect of rapid flow in the true lumen parallel to a collapsible membrane [8]. Pressures in the false and true lumens may be equal despite profound pressure deficits in branch arteries arising from the true lumen. When pressures in the lumens are unequal, false lumen pressure is usually the higher [9]. Depending on the configuration of the dissection flap, perfusion of branch arteries may be affected significantly, as discussed below.

Stability of the false lumen

The pathoanatomy of the false lumen was discussed in the previous presentation. This material will be summarized here for the sake of completeness. Autopsy data suggest that aortic ruptures associated with acute dissection occur from the false lumen near the entry tear of the dissection [10, 11]. Furthermore, preliminary observations from disparate groups of interventionalists establish that covering the entry tear of a dissection frequently induces local thrombosis in the false lumen for at least the length of the endograft.

Table 16.1 Mechanisms of branch artery obstruction.

1. Related to the dissection flap
   a. Dynamic obstruction: flap prolapses across vessel origin
   b. Static obstruction:
      i Aortic flap enters and, to a variable degree, narrows a branch artery origin
      ii Aortic occlusion due to thrombosis of large nonreentering false lumen
   c. Mixed static and dynamic
   d. Thrombosis
      i True lumen thrombosis distal to a totally obstructing flap, seen (with declining frequency) in the common iliac, renal, superior mesenteric artery, and infrarenal aortic grafts.
      ii False lumen thrombosis, seen cases of static obstruction with nonreentering false lumen.
2. Unrelated to the dissection flap
   a. Preexisting stenosis (atherosclerosis, fibromuscular dysplasia)
   b. Embolism

Table 16.2 Fenestration and stents in the era of endografts.

Indications
1. Dynamic obstruction in type A dissections with prolonged malperfusion
2. Dynamic obstruction in type A dissections persisting or developing after proximal aortic reconstruction.
3. Dynamic obstruction in type B dissections untreatable by endografts, or persisting or developing after endograft placement.
4. Arresting retrograde thrombosis in a dead-end false lumen causing aortic occlusion or spinal cord ischemia.
5. Bare stents for static obstruction
6. Covered stents for reentry tears in proximal branch arteries.
Contraindications
1. Leaking false lumen
2. Significant aortic valvular insufficiency
3. Coronary artery dissection with myocardial ischemia or heart failure

Mechanisms of branch artery obstruction

A brief review of the principal mechanisms of branch artery obstruction will be provided here for the sake of completeness, even though it is presented elsewhere and summarized below (Table 16.1). As noted earlier, branch artery obstructions are classified as dynamic or static. In dynamic obstruction, the dissection flap does not enter a vessel origin, but instead prolapses across the origin like a floating washcloth over a bathtub drain. Inspection of the aorta after aortotomy would fail to show obstruction. In static obstruction, the dissection crosses a vessel origin and directly narrows the true lumen. Whether, in a given patient, a dissection flap entering an aortic branch causes obstruction depends on the presence and size of a reentry tear within that branch. Furthermore, a dissection flap extending down the superior mesenteric artery, for example, can cause dynamic or static obstruction to jejunal or ileal branches.

Fenestration: Anatomic and hemodynamic changes

Fenestration creates a communication between the false and true lumens by tearing a hole in the dissection flap. This communication allows blood flow and pressure equilibration between the lumens. Because, at baseline, false lumen pressure either exceeds or equals true lumen pressure, fenestration does not directly reduce false lumen pressure and would, therefore, not be expected to reduce the risk of eventual aneurysmal degeneration of the false lumen. By creating a large tear in the dissection flap, fenestration may prevent adjacent false lumen thrombosis. However, it may be possible to choose the level of the fenestration at a level which allows reperfusion of compromised true lumen branches, but which can be covered by an endograft at a later time. The indications and contraindications for fenestration and stents are summarized in Table 16.2.

Endografts: Anatomic and hemodynamic changes

An endograft deployed across the entry tear of a dissection restores transmural pressure on the dissection flap, locally expands the true lumen, and locally excludes flow into the false lumen. The global effect on the true and false lumens depends on the size and number of distal reentry tears. Some retrograde flow to the false lumen may continue due to reentry tears distal in the aorta or in its branch arteries. Thus, endograft treatment can be expected to reverse dynamic obstruction in many instances, but cannot be assumed to reverse static obstruction due to dissection extending into branch arteries. Following placement of an endograft, at-risk arteries should be examined for malperfusion, such as by intravascular ultrasound and manometry.

Treating complications of aortic dissection in clinical practice

In estimating the relative role of endografts and fenestration in clinical practice of treating complicated aortic dissections, two issues are particularly important: location of the entry tear and the type of malperfusion.

The primary anatomical requirement for placing an endograft to treat aortic dissection is that the entry tear be amenable to endograft treatment. In the landmark necropsy series of aortic dissection by Hirst *et al.*, entry tears were located in the descending aorta in approximately 30% of cases [12]. Twenty years later, a notable surgical series of 125 acute and chronic type A and B dissections reported by Miller *et al.*, had virtually the same incidence of entry tears in the descending aorta [13]. It is apparent then that a significant fraction of entry tears are proximal to the descending aorta and are untreatable by current endograft technology.

Published data of the patterns of malperfusion encountered in aortic dissection are scant. In the early Michigan series reporting on 77 obstructed arteries in 24 patients, 29 vessels (38%) involved static obstruction either alone or in combination with dynamic obstruction [3]. In our subsequent (unpublished) experience with 370 obstructed arteries in 144 additional patients, nearly 50% of obstructed vessels are not expected to benefit from endografts (Table 16.3).

Table 16.3 Expectations for treating malperfusion with endografts.

Outcome (%)	RRA (N = 78)	LRA (N = 87)	SMA (N = 83)	RCIA (N = 67)	LCIA (N = 55)
Cured	45	15	48	25	9
Might benefit	14	30	17	31	29
Not helped	41	57	35	45	62

Cured = dynamic obstruction only; might benefit = some dynamic obstruction; not helped = no dynamic obstruction. N = number of obstructed vessels in 144 patient cohort.

Table 16.4 Comparison of procedures: endograft vs. fenestration and stents.

	Endograft	Fenestration and stents
Technique	Simple	Complex
Time to completion	Short (2–4 h)	Long (3–6 h)
Anatomical applicability	<40%	Nearly 100%
Fate of false lumen	Variable	Persists

As these considerations indicate, malperfusion in a significant fraction of patients cannot be corrected by endografts: either because the entry tear is currently not treatable, or because of static obstruction. Fenestration and stent placement should be considered solely a treatment of malperfusion. There is no evidence that such a treatment either exacerbates or diminishes the risk of false lumen degeneration. Endograft treatment can correct malperfusion due to dynamic obstruction, and simultaneously induce some degree of thrombosis in the false lumen, thereby diminishing the risk of late aneurysmal degeneration. A comparison of endografts and fenestration for treatment of complicated dissection is presented in Table 16.4.

Conclusion: Endografts are a promising device with wide application in treating complicated aortic dissection. In centers which have large referral practices for patients with dissection, however, fenestration and stents are complementary to endografts, and will continue to offer important options for treating malperfusion.

References

1 Chavan A, Hausmann D, Dresler C, Rosenthal H, Jaeger K, Haverich A, Borst HG, Galanski M. Intravascular ultrasound-guided percutaneous fenestration of the intimal flap in the dissected aorta. Circulation 1997; **96**: 2124–2127.

2 Slonim SM, Nyman U, Semba CP, Miller DC, Mitchell RS, Dake MD. Aortic dissection: Percutaneous management of ischemic complications with endovascular stents and balloon fenestration. J Vasc Surg 1996; **23**: 241–253.

3 Williams DM, Lee DY, Hamilton BH, Marx MV, Narasimham DL, Kazanjian SN *et al.* The dissected aorta: Percutaneous treatment of ischemic complications—Principles and results. J Vasc Interv Radiol 1997; **8**(4): 605–625.

4 Palma JH, Marcondes de Souza JA, Alves CMR, Carvalho AC, Buffolo E. Self-expandable aortic stent-grafts

for treatment of descending aortic dissections. Ann Thorac Surg 2002; **73**: 1138–1142.

5 Nienaber CA, Fattori R, Lund G, Dieckmann C, Wolf W, von Kodolitsch Y, Nicolas V, Pierangeli A. Nonsurgical reconstruction of thoracic aortic dissection by stent-graft placement. N Engl J Med 1999; **340**: 1539–1545.

6 Dake MD, Kato N, Mitchell RS, Semba CP, Razavi MK, Shimono T, Hirano T, Takeda K, Yada I, Miller DC. Endovascular stent-graft placement for the treatment of acute aortic dissection. N Engl J Med 1999; **340**: 1546–1552.

7 Williams DM, LePage MA, Lee DY. The dissected aorta. I. Early anatomic changes in an in vitro model. Radiology 1997; **203**: 23–31.

8 Chung JW, Elkins C, Sakai T, Kato N, Vestring T, Semba CP, Slonim SM, Dake MD. True-lumen collapse in aortic dissection. Part I. Evaluation of causative factors in phantoms with pulsatile flow. Radiology 2000; **214**: 87–98.

9 Williams DM, Lee DY, Hamilton B, Marx MV, Narasimham DI, Kazanjian SN, Prince MR, Cho KJ, Andrews JC, Deeb GM. The dissected aorta. III. Anatomy and radiologic diagnosis of branch-vessel compromise. Radiology 1997; **203**: 37–44.

10 Roberts WC. Aortic dissection: Anatomy, consequences, and causes. Am Heart J 1981; **101**: 195–214.

11 Roberts CS, Roberts WC. Aortic dissection with the entrance tear in abdominal aorta. Am Heart J 1991; **121**: 1834–1835.

12 Hirst AE, Johns VJ, Kime SW. Dissecting aneurysm of the aorta: A review of 505 cases. Medicine (Baltimore) 1958; **37**: 217–279.

13 Miller DC, Stinson EB, Oyer PE, Moreno-Cabral RJ, Reitz BA, Rossiter SJ, Shumway NE. Concomitant resection of ascending aortic aneurysm and replacement of the aortic valve: Operative and long-term results with "conventional" techniques in ninety patients. J Thorac Cardiovasc Surg 1980; **79**: 388–401.

17

CHAPTER 17

Blunt trauma to the thoracic aorta: current challenges

Kenneth L. Mattox, Cliff Whigham, Richard G. Fisher, &
Matthew J. Wall, Jr.

Introduction

Blunt injuries to the thoracic aorta and its branches are among the greatest challenges in surgery. Most advances in the pathophysiology, prehospital care, screening, diagnosis, and treatment of this injury have been made in the past 50 years. Nevertheless, complications and strategies of therapy continue to challenge clinicians and contribute to both debate and evolution in evaluation and therapy.

Historically, between 75% and 90% of patients with blunt thoracic injury die prior to arriving at a trauma center or being seen by a surgeon, most from exsanguination, multisystem injury, and/or airway compromise [1]. Deaths during the first 24 h, again, are secondary to multisystem injury and hemorrhage. These figures clearly demonstrate why most trauma centers will see fewer than 7–10 patients per year with an injury to the thoracic aorta [2].

While blunt injury may occur to any area of the thoracic aorta, about 80% of these injuries occur in the proximal descending thoracic aorta, probably the result of osseous pinch mechanism. Despite advances in vascular, trauma and thoracic surgery, as well as huge strides in imaging and surgical critical care, mortality rates as high as 11–40% persist [3–5]. Some selected, nonpopulation based series of treated cases report no mortality. The most dreaded complication associated with this injury, paraplegia, has been reported to occur in 13% (average) of open operated cases, although selected series report paraplegia rates ranging from 0% to over 20%. Even in the same institution, different surgeons have different approaches, techniques, preferences, and results.

Historic debates on diagnosis and treatment of thoracic aortic injury

In these complex patients with multisystem injury, it is not surprising that debates persist relating to transportation, resuscitation, timing, specific organ injury classification, and repair [6–14]. (Table 17.1)

In autopsy studies, injury location was reported at the proximal descending thoracic aorta in only 36–54%; however, in surgical cases this location is reportedly injured in 84–100% of cases. In autopsy series, 8–27% involve the ascending aorta, 8–18% involve the arch, and 11–21% involve the distal descending aorta [1, 2, 5]. In surgical series 3–10% are reported to occur in the ascending aorta, arch, or distal descending thoracic aorta. The historic autopsy and operative reported injury location distribution is important, as many radiographic and endografting series report only on injuries in the proximal descending thoracic aorta. This raises the obvious questions of selection and exclusivity of reporting.

Multisystem injury occurred in 42% of the cases presented in the classic paper by Parmley [15]. In the AAST multicenter report, 51% of patients with aortic injury had concomitant head injury, 46% had rib fractures, and 38% had lung contusions [2]. Twenty to 35% of the patients had orthopedic injury, and abdominal injury was common. Multisystem injuries sometimes make urgent aortic surgery difficult, and the use of heparin carries the potential

Table 17.1 Current debates and challenges regarding blunt injury to the thoracic aorta.

1 Patients have multisystem Injury
2 Thoracic aorta is injured at multiple locations
3 Screening strategies
4 Diagnostic strategies
5 Nonselectivity of reports in the literature
6 Delay in treatment
7 Endovascular repair
8 Complications
a Of endograft and thoracic aorta
b Of endograft portal entry site

for increased neurologic and hemorrhaging complications [16].

Although this injury is relatively uncommon, its potential lethality mandates the emergency medicine physician, general surgeon, vascular surgeon, and thoracic surgeon to have a mechanism to SCREEN for this injury, but this screen should not be so sensitive that surgery is performed on patients who have no aortic injury. Screening algorithms based on mechanism of injury, physical findings, plain chest X-ray, and various CT scanning modalities, including 3D reconstructions, have been developed [17–19]. At this time, CT and CTA scanning must be considered only a screening modality, substantiating a mediastinal hematoma, as an indirect indicator of injury to the proximal descending thoracic aorta [17]. Reports using CT as a screening modality for injury to the other areas of the thoracic aorta do not exist.

Specific diagnosis of aortic injury may be made at aortography, operation, or autopsy [17–19]. For the stable patient who has a screening test suggestive of a mediastinal hematoma or other indirect signs of aortic injury, aortogram is indicated for definitive diagnosis, to determine associated branch vessel injury, and to discern the presence of aortic arch anomalies.

Once aortic injury is diagnosed, a number of treatment options exist. For the unstable patient, immediate control of any ongoing hemorrhage requires surgical intervention. For "stable" patients or patients with multisystem injury, operative treatment may be immediate or delayed. During the operation, at least six operative strategies exist, each of which has been championed at one time or another.

During the last 10 years, the technical feasibility of catheter-based endografts has been reported.

Reports on thoracic aortic injury have been based on either autopsy series or individual hospital nonrandomized results. Population-based randomized series simply do not exist. During the past 8 years, the reports on imaging have cited imaging technical preferences and catheter-based endografts usage primarily based on nonhyper acute patients with injury to the proximal descending thoracic aorta. Even the category of "acute" repair has been extended to include patients several weeks postinjury. Expanding the "acute" injury "definition" to many days or even weeks not only eliminates many of the immediate deaths and complications, but also allows time for construction of "custom" devices. Critically ill patients who in earlier studies would have undergone operation on the night of injury or very shortly thereafter, regardless of associated injury or illness and/or the anatomic location of the aortic injury, are not included in many of the reports of thoracic endografts. This exclusivity of reporting raises questions of selection bias and whether or not the current wave of enthusiasm for CT, CTA, and even MRA imaging, as well as endografting applies to all patients with thoracic aortic injury.

In that most patients with thoracic aortic injury are seen by surgeons several hours after injury and the mean time from injury to diagnosis in major trauma centers is 8 h, such patients transferred to secondary centers are in the small group of "stable" patients from the standpoint of the aortic injury [2]. In these patients, it is no longer considered necessary to operate immediately, but rather to address the associated injuries while making specific timing plans for addressing the aortic injury. The use of afterload reduction agents to alter the dP/dT is indicated as soon as an aortic injury is suspected. Blood pressure control is aimed at keeping the systolic blood pressure lower than preinjury levels. Delay may be days, weeks, or even months in some instances. For these patients, aortic-related deaths or complications are extremely rare to nonexistent in the literature [20–25].

Since the introduction of catheter-based endograft technology in the 1990s, a small series of endografts for aortic injury have appeared in the literature, often included in a larger series of endografts used in general. Initially, such grafts were used in chronic transections, but for the last 10 years, small series reporting use in acute aortic injury have been reported [26–30]. At least 24 different custom and manufactured endografts and off-label use of components of abdominal aortic endografts have been used for thoracic aortic pathology [31]. Some radiologists and surgeons consider thoracic endografting to be as much a standard of care as open aortic reconstruction following trauma. While the average mortality for posttraumatic open thoracic aortic repair is 13% (range from 0 to 55%), and the paraplegia rates average 10% (range 0–20%), the mortality and paraplegia rate for selected blunt aortic injury treated with endografts is 3.8%, and only 1 out of 239 such cases had paraplegia (Table 17.2). Although many of the even "acute" endograft cases were treated several weeks postinjury and selectivity bias must be considered, these results mandate the risk/benefit of endografting be objectively and carefully addressed in light of current technology.

Table 17.2 Recently reported cases of injury to the proximal descending thoracic aorta treated with an endograft.

Author	Ref.	No. Cases	Deaths	Paraplegia
Amabile	[41]	9	0	0
Demers	[43]	15	1	0
Doss	[44]	16	1	0
Durham	[45]	16	1	0
Fattori	[46]	19	0	0
Kasirajan	[47]	5	1	0
Kato	[48]	6	0	0
Kuhne	[49]	5	0	0
Kwok	[50]	4	0	0
Lachat	[51]	12	1	0
Marty-Ane	[52]	9	0	0
Meites	[53]	18	0	0
Melissono	[54]	2	0	0
Neuhauser	[55]	13	0	0
Orend	[56]	11	1	0
Orford	[57]	9	1	0
Ott	[58]	6	0	0
Raupach	[59]	7	1	1
Richeux	[60]	16	0	0
Rousseau	[61]	29	0	0
Uzieblo	[62]	3	0	0
Wellons	[63]	9	1	0
Total		239	9	1

Logic for use of endovascular catheter-based therapy for thoracic aorta injury

Most of the literature relating to thoracic aortic injury and use of endografts focuses on the proximal descending thoracic aorta. For this location, there is ample potential logic to support endografts as a standard of practice. Many such patients have multiple other life-threatening injuries, particularly head, lung, abdomen, and orthopedic injury, which makes prolonged anesthesia and total body heparinization an added risk [32, 33]. Additionally, such patients often cannot tolerate one lung anesthesia. Endografting eliminates the pain from a lateral thoracotomy and the potential for recurrent laryngeal and phrenic nerve damage. The lower incidence of death and paraplegia makes further evaluation and research development essential. Especially for chronic posttraumatic thoracic aortic false aneurysms, a short endograft anchored in a relatively normal tissue has long been speculated to be the most logical indication for aortic endografting.

Concerns relating to common use of endografts in thoracic aortic injury

Thoracic aortic endografting is in its infancy, and careful, controlled, prospective and even randomized studies must be conducted. In that many trauma victims are young, long-term durability of current endografts becomes a concern. Thoracic aortic endografts have been designed for degenerative or dissecting pathology of the thoracic aorta, resulting in creation of relatively large diameter approved commercial endografts. Custom devices and off-label use of iliac artery endograft limbs or cuff extenders and abdominal aortic endografts are often not approved by IRBs and endograft manufacturers. The current CT, CTA, echocardiographic, and MRA imaging technology has resulted in use of endografts and even open surgery on aortas ultimately found to be without injury (and in most such cases, an aortogram was not obtained). The fate of endografts in the thoracic aorta has been studied only in the proximal descending thoracic aorta. During the hyperacute time period (0–3 days), the young hypotensive

Table 17.3 Gore, TAG case planning form data.

Intended aortic diameter (mm)	Recommended prosthesis diameter (mm	Prosthesis lengths (cm)
23–24	26	10
24–26	28	10, 15
26–29	31	10, 15
29–32	34	10, 15, 20
32–34	37	10, 15, 20
34–37	40	10, 15, 20

Table 17.4 Ben Taub General Hospital recent unselected cases, citing diameter of the descending thoracic aorta at the isthmus (diameters are in millimeters).

Case #	Age	Aortic diameter	Diagnosis
1	19	21.3	Lymphoma
2	32	24.6	PE
3	47	22.0	Tumor
4	34	22.7	Trauma
5	58	28.0	Tumor
6	36	25.6	Tumor
7	53	26.9	Tumor
8	56	28.7	PE
9	57	26.8	Pneumonia
10	48	22.7	Tumor
11	47	20.7	Aortic lac
12	24	21.7	Subclavian lac
13	44	20.0	Subclavian lac
14	40	24.0	Aortic lac
15	19	23.9	Aortic lac
16	23	14.9	Aortic lac

postinjury patient often has a contracted, smaller-than-normal aorta that dilates up when the patient is normovolemic.

In the young trauma patient, the average size of the thoracic aorta at the isthmus is 19.3 mm [34–37]. However, the smallest approved, commercially available thoracic endograft (in the United States) is 26 mm (Table 17.3). Physicians inserting thoracic endografts usually oversize the graft by 10–20%, although a target of 17% oversizing or less is a common practice to assure a good proximal purchase on the native uninjured aorta. With excessive oversizing, the potential for enfolding of an endograft is increased [38, 39]. For acute thoracic aortic injury treated by endografts, infolding rates up to 4% have been reported. (Formal Presentation at the Northwestern Vascular Symposium, December 2005, Dr. Brian G. Peterson). In a review of consecutive CT measurements of the aortic isthmus at the Ben Taub General Hospital, diameters of 14.9 mm to 24.0 mm in patients were found (Table 17.4). Over the past 15 years, the thoracic surgeons performing open repair have used 18 mm Dacron grafts in more than 95% of patients. Even patients ranging in age from 19 to 58 years had aortic isthmus diameters of 21.3 mm to 28.7 mm. The approved or current "under-evaluation" commercially available thoracic endografts are too large for most patients with acute thoracic aortic injury.

Angulation problems at the proximal target site add to enfolding (or windsock) deformity of the thoracic endograft, increasing the danger of endoleak and pressurization of the residual false aneurysm, resulting in expansion and possible rupture [38–40]. Any angulation of greater than 60 degrees of curvature at the aortic arch is unacceptable. Although the mean degree of curvature from the orifice of the left Subclavian artery to the descending aorta averaged 54°, the range was from −12° to 90°. To overcome the problems of angulation at the aortic arch/descending aorta interface, an endograft might need to be placed higher in the arch or lower in the descending aorta, both of which can create either occlusion of branch arteries, or have a proximal target too close to the acute aortic tear. To compensate for this angulation, cuff extenders are sometimes employed, adding complexity and cost to the procedure [31].

Even with the most detailed of current imaging, the proximal extent of an acute descending aortic tear is not always appreciated – possibly not until the aorta is opened and the tear can be directly visualized. Manufacturers currently recommend a proximal neck of 10–20 mm from the site of the subclavian artery orifice to the site of an aortic tear. In one study, only 14% of patients had a 10 mm superior neck, only 6% had a 20 mm superior neck, and 60% had a superior neck equal to or less than 5 mm [35, 41].

Aberrant anatomy reportedly occurred in 38% of patients studied [35]. At least 13 anomalies of the aorta have been reported (Table 17.5). The presence of many of these anomalies makes endografting even more challenging. Occlusion of origin of some

Table 17.5 Anomalies of the thoracic aorta.

- Common origin of innominate and left carotid arteries ("bovine arch")
- Ductus diverticulum
- Persistent left ductus arterioisus
- Aorto-pulmonary window
- Takeoff of the right subclavian artery from the descending thoracic aorta
- Dextroposition of the thoracic aorta
- Coarctation of thoracic aorta
- Origin of left vertebral artery off the aortic arch
- Pseudocoarctation of the thoracic aorta ("kinked aorta")
- Double aortic arch
- Right ductus arteriosus
- Persistent truncus arteriosus
- Cervical aortic arch (persistent complete third aortic arch)
- Absence of the internal carotid artery
- Cardio-aortic fistula

Table 17.6 Gore, TAG case planning form sheath sizes.

20 Fr (7.6 mm) for use with 26–28 size prosthesis
22 Fr (8.3 mm) for use with 31–34 size prosthesis
24 Fr (9.2 mm) for use with 37–40 size prosthesis

of these anomalies can create new problems. While such anomalies are occasionally cited in aortic trauma and endograft literature, specific cases where endografting was used in the presence of one of the major anomalies have not been reported.

Thoracic endograft and insertion site complications

Thoracic aortic endografting has not been without its complications [38–40, 42, 48–51, 54]. Issues of angulation, length of normal aorta proximal to the tear, extent of tear, coverage of the subclavian artery ostium, and other anatomic considerations are real but not insurmountable challenges from an engineering standpoint. Unless optimally addressed, they will contribute to endoleaks, enfolding of an endograft, migration, angulation, and even strut breakage. Thus, there are two different issues relating to the size of the graft and the length of the proximal purchase site. The first issue is that if the graft is too large, and/or the insertion area is too small, enfolding or parachute deformity can occur. The second issue has to do with the landing zone which is often angulated creating a proximal lip of endograft at the inner angle of the aortic arch/descending

aortic junction. The aortic arch/proximal descending thoracic aorta/left subclavian artery complex makes a secure proximal landing point for an endograft difficult. Coverage of the orifice of the left subclavian artery with consideration of carotid to subclavian bypass occurs in up to 30% of cases. At times the source of a pressurized endoleaks is from the subclavian artery.

Complications at the insertion site of a thoracic endograft have also been reported [56–60, 62]. The insertion site is either in the femoral or in the iliac artery, sometimes with a synthetic graft sutured to the iliac artery and used as a portal location. One complication relates to the size of these arteries and their ability to accommodate the introducer sheath (Table 17.6) and catheter carrying the endograft. Because of the size of the artery through which the endograft and catheter are inserted, injury to this site is not uncommon. Such injury is manifest by extravasation, false aneurysm, occlusion, stenosis, and leakage. The majority of the vascular related morbidity from thoracic endografts is from the access site.

Summary

A relatively rare, but potentially devastating injury to the thoracic aorta has been the subject of advances in prehospital treatment, screening, diagnosis, timing of intervention, and types of specific intervention. Catheter based endografting is an attractive alternative to the traditional open surgery, but concerns of enfolding, structure fracture, size disparities, coverage of the subclavian artery, and complications at the insertion sites exist. The average proximal thoracic aortic diameter of 19.3 mm in patients with aortic injury, with most open interposition grafts being 18 mm, is considerably smaller than the smallest size (26 mm) of approved commercially available thoracic endografts.

References

1 Mattox KL, Red River Anthology. J Trauma 1997; **42**: 353–368.

2 Fabian TC, Richardson JC, Croce MA *et al*. Prospective study of blunt aortic injury: Multicenter Trial of the American Association for the Surgery of Trauma. J Trauma 1997; **42**: 374–380.

3 Baguley CJ, Sibal AK, Alison PM. Repair of injuries to the thoracic aorta and great vessels: Auckland, New Zealand 1995–2004. ANZ J Surg 2005; **75**: 383–387.

4 Jamieson WR, Janusz MT, Gudas VM *et al*. Traumatic rupture of the thoracic aorta: Third decade of experience. Am J Surg 2002; **183**: 571–575.

5 Von Oppell UO, Dunne TT, De Groot MK *et al*. Traumatic aortic rupture: Twenty-year metaanalysis of mortality and risk of paraplegia. Ann Thorac Surg 1994; **58**: 585–593.

6 Finkelmeier BA, Mentzer RM, Jr., Kaiser DL *et al*. Chronic traumatic thoracic aneurysm. Influence of operative treatment on natural history: An analysis of reported cases 1950–1980. J Thorac Cardiovasc Surg 1982; **84**: 257–266

7 Javadpour H, O'Toole JJ, McEniff JN, Luke DA, Young VK. Traumatic aortic transection: Evidence for the osseous pinch mechanism. Ann Thorac Surg 2002; **73**(3): 951–953.

8 Karmy-Jones R, Hoffer E, Meissner M *et al*. Management of traumatic rupture of the thoracic aorta in pediatric patients. Ann Thorac Surg 2003; **75**: 1513–1517.

9 Mattox KL, Holzman M, Pickard LR *et al*. Clamp-repair: A safe technique for treatment of blunt injury to the descending thoracic aorta. Ann Thorac Surg 1985; **40**: 456–463.

10 Petel NH, Hahn D, Comess KA. Blunt chest trauma victims: Role of intravascular ultrasound and transesophageal echocardiography in cases of abnormal thoracic aortogram. J Trauma 2003; **55**: 330–337

11 Rogues X, Remes J, Laborde MN *et al*. Surgery of chronic traumatic aneurysm of the aortic isthmus: Benefit of direct suture. Eur J Cardiothorac Surg 2003; **23**: 46–49.

12 Santaniello JM, Miller PR, Croce MA *et al*. Blunt aortic injury with concomitant intra-abdominal solid organ injury: Treatment priorities revisited. J Trauma 2002; **53**: 442–445.

13 Sweeney MS, Young DJ, Frazier OH *et al*. Traumatic aortic transactions: Eight-year experience with the "clamp-sew" technique. Ann Thorac Surg 1997; **64**: 384–387.

14 Takach TJ, Anstadt MP, Moore HV. Pediatric aortic disruption. Tex Heart Inst J 2005; **32**: 16–20.

15 Parmley LF, Mattingly TW, Manion WC *et al*. Nonpenetrating traumatic injury of the aorta. Circulation. 1958; **17**: 1086–1101

16 Britt LD, Campbell MM. Blunt thoracic aortic injury: Old problem and new technology. J Long Term Eff Med Implants 2003; **13**: 419–427.

17 Bruckner BA, DiBardino DJ, Cumbie TC, Trinh C, Blackmon SH, Fisher RG *et al*. Critical evaluation of chest computed tomography scans for blunt descending thoracic aortic injury. Ann Thorac Surg 2006 Apr; **81**(4): 1339–1346.

18 Chen MY, Miller PR, McLaughlin CA *et al*. The trend of using computed tomography in the detection of acute thoracic aortic and branch vessel injury after blunt thoracic trauma: Single-center experience over 13 years. J Trauma 2004; **56**: 783–785.

19 Chen MY, Regan JD, D'Amore MJ *et al*. Role of angiography in the detection of aortic branch vessel injury after blunt thoracic trauma. J Trauma 2001; **51**: 1166–1171.

20 Fisher RG, Oria RA, Mattox KL *et al*. Conservative management of aortic lacerations due to blunt trauma. J Trauma 1990; **30**: 1562.

21 Galli R, Pacini D, Di Bartolomeo R *et al*. Surgical indications and timing of repair of traumatic ruptures of the thoracic aorta. Ann Thorac Surg 1998; **65**: 461–464.

22 Langanay T, Verhoye JP, Corbineau H *et al*. Surgical treatment of acute traumatic rupture of the thoracic aorta a timing reappraisal? Eur J Cardiothorac Surg 2002; **21**: 282–287.

23 Pacini D, Angeli E, Fattori R *et al*. Traumatic rupture of the thoracic aorta: Ten years of delayed management. J Thor Cardiovasc Surg 2005; **129**: 880–884.

24 Symbas PN, Sherman AJ, Silver JM *et al*. Traumatic rupture of the aorta: Immediate or delayed repair. Ann Surg 2002; **235**: 796–802.

25 Maggisano R, Nathens A, Alexandrova NA *et al*. Traumatic rupture of the thoracic aorta; should one always operate immediately? Ann Vasc Surg 1995; **9**: 44–52.

26 Kato N, Dake MD, Miller DC *et al*. Traumatic thoracic aortic aneurysm: Treatment with endovascular stent-grafts. Radiology 1997; **205**: 657–662.

27 Mitchell RS, Ishimaru S, Criado FJ *et al*. Third International Summit on Thoracic Aortic Endografting: Lessons from long-term results of thoracic stent-graft repairs. J Endovasc Ther 2005; **12**: 89–97.

28 Mitchell RS, Miller DC, Dake MD *et al*. Thoracic aortic aneurysm repair with an endovascular stent graft: The "first generation." An Thorac Surg 1999; **67**: 1971–1974.

29 Najibi S, Terramani TT, Weiss VJ *et al*. Endoluminal vs. open treatment of descending thoracic aortic aneurysms. J Vasc Surg 2002; **36**: 732–737.

30 Nishimoto M, Fukumoto H, Nishimoto Y. Surgical treatment of traumatic thoracic aorta rupture: A 7-year experience. Jpn J Thorac Cardiovasc Surg 2003; **51**: 138–143.

31 Hoffer EK, Karmy-Jones R, Bloch RD *et al*. Treatment of acute thoracic aortic injury with commercially available abdominal aortic stent grafts. J Vasc Interv Radiol 2002; **13**: 1037–1041.

32 Daenen G, Maleux G, Daenens K *et al.* Thoracic aortic endoprosthesis: The final countdown for open surgery after traumatic aortic rupture? Ann Vasc Surg 2003; **17**: 185–191.

33 Semba CP, Kato N, Kee ST *et al.* Acute rupture of the descending thoracic aorta; Repair with use of endovascular stent-grafts. J Vasc Interv Radiol 1997; **8**: 337–342.

34 Aronberg DJ, Glazer HS, Madsen K *et al.* Normal thoracic aortic diameters by computed tomography. J Comput Assist Tomogr 1984; **8**: 247–250.

35 Borsa JJ, Hoffer EK, Karmy-Jones R *et al.* Angiographic description of blunt traumatic injuries to the thoracic aorta with specific relevance to endograft repair. J Endovasc Ther 2002; **9**(Suppl 2): II84–91.

36 Hager A, Kaemmerer H, Rapp-Bernhardt U *et al.* Diameters of the thoracic aorta throughout life as measured with helical computed tomography. J Thorac Cardiovasc Surg 2002; **123**: 1060–1066.

37 Poutanen T, Tikanoja T, Sairanen H *et al.* Normal aortic dimensions and flow in 168 children and young adults. Clin Physiol Funct Imaging 2003; **23**: 224–229.

38 Grabenwoger M, Fleck T, Ehrlich M *et al.* Secondary surgical interventions after endovascular stent-grafting of the thoracic aorta. Eur J Cardiothorac Surg 2004; **26**: 608–613.

39 Idu MM, Reekers JA, Balm R *et al.* Collapse of a stent-graft following treatment of a traumatic thoracic aortic rupture. J Endovas Ther 2005; **12**: 503–507.

40 Hance KA, Hsu J, Eskew T *et al.* Secondary aortoesophageal fistula after endoluminal exclusion because of thoracic aortic transection. J Vasc Surg 2003; **37**: 886–888.

41 Amabile P, Collart F, Gariboldi V *et al.* Surgical versus endovascular treatment of traumatic thoracic aortic rupture. J Vasc Surg 2004; **40**: 873–879.

42 Bockler D, von Tengg-Kobligk H, Schumacher H *et al.* Late surgical conversion after thoracic endograft failure due to a fracture of the longitudinal support wire. J Endovasc Ther 2005; **12**: 98–102.

43 Demers P, Miller C, Scott Mitchell R *et al.* Chronic traumatic aneurysms of the descending thoracic aorta: midterm results of endovascular repair using first and second-generation stent-grafts. Eur J Cardiothorac Surg 2004; **25**: 394–400.

44 Doss M, Balzer J, Martens S *et al.* Surgical vs. endovascular treatment of acute thoracic aortic rupture: A single-center experience. Ann Thor Surg 2003; **76**: 1465–1469.

45 Dunham MB, Zygun D, Petrasek P *et al.* Endovascular stent grafts for acute blunt aortic injury. J Trauma 2004; **56**: 1173–1178.

46 Fattori R, Napoli G, Lavato, L *et al.* Indications for, timing of, and results of catheter-based treatment of traumatic injury to the aorta. AJR Am J Roentgenol 2002; **179**: 603–609.

47 Kasirajan K, Heffernana D, Langsfeld M. Acute thoracic aortic trauma: A comparison of endoluminal stent grafts with open repair and nonoperative management. Ann Vasc Surg 2003; **17**: 589–595.

48 Kato M, Yatsu S, Sato H *et al* Endovascular stent-graft treatment for blunt aortic injury. Circ J 2004; **68**: 553–557.

49 Kuhne CA, Ruchholtz S, Voggenreiter G *et al.* Traumatic aortic injuries in severely injured patients. Unfallchirurg. 2005; **108**: 279–287.

50 Kwok PC, Ho KK, Chung TK *et al.* Hong Kong Med J. 2003; **9**: 435–440.

51 Lachat M, Pfammatter T, Witzke H *et al.* Acute traumatic aortic rupture: Early stent-graft repair. Eur J Cardiothorac Surg 2002; **21**: 959–963.

52 Marty-Ane CH, Berthet JP, Branchereau P *et al.* Endovascular repair for acute traumatic rupture of the thoracic aorta. Ann Thorac Surg 2003; **75**: 1803–1807.

53 Meites G, Conil C, Rousseau H *et al.* Indication of endovascular stent grafts for traumatic rupture of the thoracic aorta. Ann Fr Anesth Reanim 2004; **23**: 700–703.

54 Melissano G, Civilini E, de Moura MR *et al.* Single center experience with a new commercially available thoracic endovascular graft. Eur J Vasc Endovasc Surg 2005; **29**: 579–585.

55 Neuhauser B, Czermak B, Jaschke W *et al.* Stent-graft repair for acute traumatic thoracic aortic rupture. Am Surg 2004; **70**: 1039–1044.

56 Orend KH, Pamler R, Kapfer X *et al.* Endovascular repair of traumatic descending aortic transection. J Endovasc Ther 2002; **9**: 573–578.

57 Orford VP, Atkinson NR, Thomson K *et al.* Blunt traumatic aortic transection: The endovascular experience. Ann Thorac Surg 2003; **75**: 106–111.

58 Ott MC, Stewart TC, Lawlor DK *et al.* Management of blunt thoracic aortic injuries: Endovascular stents vs open repair. J Trauma 2004; **56**: 565–570.

59 Raupach J, Ferko A, Lojik M *et al.* The endovascular treatment of aortic trauma. Rozhl Chir 2005; **84**: 270–276.

60 Richeux L, Dambrin C, Marcheix B *et al.* Towards a new management of acute traumatic ruptures. J Radiol 2004; **85**: 101–106.

61 Rousseau H, Dambrin C, Marcheix B *et al.* Acute traumatic aortic rupture: A comparison of surgical and stent-graft repair. J Thorac Cardiovasc Surg 2005; **129**: 1050–1055.

62 Uzieblo M, Sanchez LA, Rubin BG *et al.* Endovascular repair of traumatic descending thoracic aortic disruptions; should endovascular therapy become the gold standard? Vasc Endovascular Surg 2004; **38**: 331–337.

63 Wellons ED, Milner R, Solis M *et al.* Stent-graft repair of traumatic thoracic aortic disruptions. J Vasc Surg 2004; **40**: 1095–1100.

CHAPTER 18

Traumatic disruption of the aorta

Ross Milner, Karthik Kasirajan, & Elliot Chaikof

Introduction

Trauma is the leading cause of death in the adolescent and young adult population in the United States. A common cause of trauma is a motor vehicle collision (MVC). The severity of injuries sustained during the traumatic event dictates the extent of the morbidity and mortality for the victims involved in the MVC. A leading cause of mortality in MVC is traumatic disruption of the aorta otherwise known as blunt thoracic injury (BTI) [1]. BTI is usually associated with a spectrum of injuries that makes management of these patients very complex. The associated head, thoracic, and abdominal injuries increase the difficulty in determining appropriate timing and as well as assessing the necessity for many operative interventions.

The traditional management of BTI has been open operative repair involving a left thoracotomy and replacement of the injured portion of the aorta [2]. Some centers use adjunctive cardio-pulmonary bypass in order to decrease the risk of paraplegia [3]. The complexity of these maneuvers in the setting of a multiply-injured patient has led some to manage these patients nonoperatively [4]. The risk of this approach is potential rupture of the thoracic aorta. Antihypertensive control is the important factor in the intensive care unit care for these patients. The long-term risk is the development of a thoracic aorta pseudoaneurysm.

An evolving management paradigm is the use of endovascular techniques to treat injured patients. Aortic extension cuffs from FDA-approved abdominal aortic endografts as well as thoracic endografts have been used to treat disrupted aortas [5]. There is great promise with the minimally-invasive nature of the endovascular repair. But, as with all new management paradigms, some complications have occurred with this technique [6]. Further investigation and follow-up of the patients treated with aortic endografts will allow the true assessment of the benefit of endovascular repair in this severely injured patient population.

Background

Anatomy is the key to understanding the mechanism of injury when traumatic disruption of the aorta occurs. The underlying deceleration injury commonly occurs with ejection or crush injuries during an MVC. This leads to an aortic tear at the ligamentum arteriosum, otherwise known as the aortic isthmus. The ligamentum arteriosum is the adult structure of the embryonic connection between the pulmonary artery and the aorta, which is important in maintaining the appropriate fetal circulation. After birth and the conversion to postnatal circulation physiology, this connection fibroses and becomes the ligamentum arteriosum. This ligament is a fixation point for the thoracic aorta and causes the tear to occur at this location when the deceleration injury occurs. The tear can occur with differing complexity and can lead to complete or partial aortic disruption. A completely disrupted aorta is usually a lethal, exsanguinating event and leads to death at the scene of the trauma [7]. The survivors who make it to the hospital usually have a partial disruption of the aorta. The traditional management for these patients has been the appropriate diagnostic maneuvers to confirm the injury with urgent/emergent open repair of the aorta. As mentioned above, the traditional paradigm is being challenged with nonoperative management as well as endovascular repair.

Diagnosis and imaging

The key to appropriate diagnosis of BTI is to maintain a high level of suspicion [8]. Many of the lethal events that occur during a hospital course are from a missed diagnosis [9]. The circumstances of the traumatic event are the first clue to the possibility of a disrupted aorta. The next indicator is usually a plain chest radiograph that demonstrates a widened mediastinum. A repeat chest radiograph is likely needed as the initial trauma film is usually performed in the supine position. If the upright imaging confirms the widened mediastinum then additional imaging is required.

The additional imaging can be either a computed tomographic angiogram (CTA) of the thorax, conventional aortography, or echocardiography. A CTA is readily available and is the usual first line additional study that is obtained. The CTA can confirm the diagnosis of a disrupted aorta and identify additional injuries within the chest [10]. Three-dimensional reconstructions can be rapidly obtained and assist with the operative planning. In our experience, there is variability in which the injury to the aorta occurs in relation to the left subclavian artery. The CTA is helpful in planning the operative approach, especially from an endovascular standpoint. We usually do not perform an aortogram if the CTA confirms the diagnosis. The aortogram is reserved for the situation when the diagnosis is not clear from the CTA. This test is invasive, but does not have a high complication rate. An aortogram is always performed in the operating room during an endovascular repair.

Transesophageal echocardiography is also useful in confirming the diagnosis. It is as accurate as CTA, but availability is an issue [11]. The trained user is not always available when a patient presents with the injury. For this reason, CTA is more widely utilized.

Open operative repair

The gold standard for management of traumatic disruption of the aorta has been open repair at many centers. The open approach is performed in several different ways.

All approaches require a left thoracotomy for repair of the injured aorta. A prosthetic graft (polyester vs. PTFE) is selected for replacement of the aorta if the aorta cannot be primarily repaired. The variability in surgical management arises with the description of adjunctive maneuvers for distal aortic perfusion or repair without distal aortic perfusion.

"Clamp and sew" technique

The "clamp and sew" technique involves repair of the injured thoracic aorta without distal aortic perfusion. Exposure of the injured aorta is gained and the repair is performed as rapidly as possible. The advocates of this approach report a simplified operative management with no additional paraplegia complications or mortality [2, 12]. The detractors of this approach state that the incidence of paraplegia is higher without adjuncts for distal aortic perfusion [3].

Distal aortic perfusion

Distal aortic perfusion is an adjunct to standard thoracic aortic repair that allows perfusion while the aorta is clamped for vascular control and repair. A Gott shunt or partial left heart bypass can be used. The potential advantage is a decreased incidence of paraplegia as mentioned above [3]. The risk of repair is increased in some accounts due to the high-level of anticoagulation that is required with these adjunctive techniques. In fact, some authors have delayed operative repair in the setting of associated injuries due to the potential risk of complications [13].

Complications of open repair

The major complications of open repair are listed above in terms of mortality, paraplegia, and bleeding complications. Other reported complications include neurologic complications and intraabdominal complications including intestinal ischemia. Patients that survive the initial injury and operative repair have an excellent long-term durability of the aortic repair.

Nonoperative management

The complexity of managing the spectrum of injuries in trauma patients with BTI has prompted some authors to delay operative intervention [4].

The proponents of this philosophy believe that an operative repair that includes a left thoracotomy is too severe a physiologic stress on the multitrauma patient. The authors report improved outcomes with decreased mortality rates with nonoperative management. The gold standard of this therapy is appropriate blood pressure control. Mean arterial pressure is maintained below 70 mmHg during the acute presentation. The significant decision algorithm in this paradigm is selecting patients who are too severely injured to tolerate acute repair.

There is a spectrum of delay in this management paradigm. Nonoperative management can also be described in another way as delayed operative management [14]. These authors report the timing of repair in a selected group of patients at a mean time from injury of 8.6 months. The operative outcome was improved with decreased complication rates in the patients who were repaired in a delayed fashion as compared to early repair.

The impetus for delayed or nonoperative repair is clear. This patient population is difficult to manage due to the complexity of their spectrum of injuries and the need for a significant operation to correct the aortic injury. The advent of endovascular repair may be the solution to these issues.

Endovascular repair

The successful introduction of endovascular repair of infrarenal abdominal aortic aneurysms in 1991 by Dr Juan Parodi has led to an explosion in the field of vascular surgery. Endovascular techniques are rapidly changing the standard of care in many regions of the vascular bed. This change includes thoracic and aortic aneurysmal disease, acute and chronic aortic dissection, critical lower extremity ischemia, and carotid artery disease. The endovascular management of these disease processes has proven to be at least equivalent if not superior to several of the problems mentioned above. The limit of the success of endovascular techniques as well as the scope of its applications has not been approached as of yet. This includes the management of traumatic disruption of the aorta.

This problem is clearly complex. As written above, the optimal management of traumatic injuries of the aorta is not clearly defined. Depending on the trauma center, patients may be managed nonoperatively, operated on emergently with or without distal aortic perfusion, or repaired with an open operation in a delayed fashion. This spectrum of care allows for the possibility of innovative techniques. The advance in management of the multiply-injured trauma patient that is likely to be accepted is a less-invasive technique. This is true even in institutions where one of the management techniques listed above has been routinely utilized.

Endovascular repair of a traumatic aortic disruption is able to be performed through a small incision for femoral artery exposure and a minimal dose of systemic heparin. These two points are key advantages to the technique. Patients are able to recover in a rapid fashion with less risk of bleeding and serious wound complications. Also, there appears to be less risk of paraplegia with endovascular repair [15]. There are reports of repair of traumatic disruptions using aortic extension cuffs from FDA-approved abdominal aortic endografts [16]. In fact, it is possible to perform this repair using aortic extension cuffs without an incision [17]. In addition, thoracic endografts can be used to perform the repair. As use of thoracic endografts in the United States for traumatic injuries is considered off-label use, the experience and acceptance of this approach is more rapid in European endovascular centers of excellence [18].

Anatomic considerations

There are two key anatomic issues in the young trauma patient with a traumatic aortic disruption who is being evaluated for endovascular repair. The first is the size of the thoracic aorta. Many of these patients have a small diameter aorta that is not amenable to endovascular therapy with the current available devices. One patient referred to our institution was found on intravascular ultrasound (IVUS) to have an aortic diameter of 14 mm. Due to the concerns of significant oversizing of an endovascular device and the possibility of a poor long-term outcome, a standard operative repair was performed. The patient did well with this approach.

The second issue is the acute angulation seen in a young, healthy aortic arch. The angulation can complicate the appropriate apposition of an endograft to the aortic wall. This flared appearance of a device on imaging studies is a nidus for distal migration.

These two issues are being closely evaluated as endovascular devices are being designed to deal with traumatic aortic injuries.

Other considerations

There are several unresolved issues with the intraoperative decision-making process. One of the key issues is the coverage of the left subclavian artery. Some physicians routinely cover the left subclavian artery to treat traumatic injuries. Others intentionally attempt not to involve the artery with the endovascular repair. In our experience, the location of the injury has a 1- to 2-cm zone of variability in the location of the injury in comparison to the left subclavian artery. Therefore, we will cover the left subclavian artery when the injury approximates the artery in order to appropriately exclude the injured aorta with the endograft. The second important decision is the length of coverage of the descending thoracic aorta and the necessary seal zones for proximal and distal fixation. Once again, there is debate in this topic. Some feel that the same recommendations for treatment of thoracic aneurysmal disease apply to traumatic injuries. Others feel that the aorta is otherwise normal outside of the injured area and an endograft will have good fixation to the aorta with the use of shorter seal zones, especially when trying to avoid coverage of the left subclavian artery. The downside of this approach is the risk of migration.

The issue of migration leads to another potential problem with endovascular techniques. The follow-up of trauma patients can be a significant challenge. Although long-term complications of open repair can occur, they are small in overall number for this problem. The long-term durability of endovascular techniques is still being evaluated for traumatic injuries. Cross-sectional imaging is required to assess these patients, but they must return to clinic to be evaluated. The issue of follow-up plagues many centers that accept trauma patients from a large surrounding area. Cross-sectional imaging has already demonstrated a collapsed thoracic endograft in a patient treated for traumatic disruption [6].

Overall, the initial impression is that endovascular repair has improved the care of the multiply-injured trauma patient. The periprocedural complication rates appear to be lower and patients recover more rapidly. The long-term durability needs to be addressed.

Endovascular repair – *The Emory experience*

Over the past 2 years, we have begun to change the management paradigm of blunt thoracic aortic injury at our institution. The impression of our trauma surgeons and cardiothoracic surgeons is that there is a marked reduction in morbidity and mortality for patients treated with an endovascular approach. The experience listed here does not involve every patient who presented to our trauma center with a traumatic aortic disruption. Therefore, an accurate comparison of open versus endovascular repair can not be accomplished yet at our institution. The data given here are for the subset of patients that were referred for endovascular therapy.

We have treated 11 patients with acute injuries to the thoracic aorta over the past 2 years. Their mean age is 33 years old (range: 16–74 years old). Nine patients were male and two were female. A thoracic endograft (TAG device, W.L. Gore and Associates, Flagstaff, AZ) was used in three patients. One patient required two endografts and the other two patients only required one piece. The remaining eight patients were treated with aortic extension cuffs (see Figs. 18.1 & 18.2). Two patients had aortic cuffs from the AneuRx device (Medtronic AVE, Santa Rosa, CA) placed. The remaining six patients were treated with aortic extension cuffs from the Gore Excluder device (W.L. Gore and Associated, Flagstaff, AZ). The mean number of aortic cuffs inserted per patient was 2.9 (range: 2–5 cuffs). One patient required a laparotomy for aortic exposure in order to place aortic cuffs due to diminutive femoral and iliac vessels. One patient required a retroperitoneal incision for iliac artery exposure to place aortic cuffs due to the patient's height and the inability to reach the injured portion of the aorta from the left femoral artery. All three thoracic endografts were placed through femoral arterial access. There were no mortalities in this group.

The downside of our experience is limited follow-up. Four of the patients were treated in the last 3 months. Of the remaining seven, only five have had cross-sectional imaging performed. There are

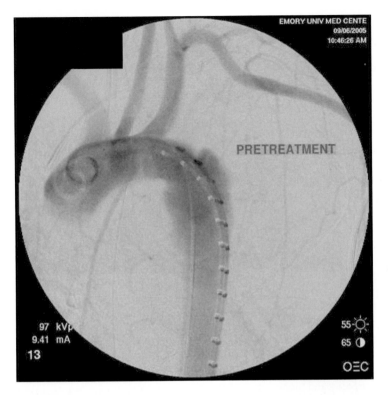

Figure 18.1 Intraoperative aortogram of a patient with a traumatic disruption of the aorta. Imaging is performed in a left anterior oblique projection with a marker pigtail catheter. The injury is approximately 1 cm from the origin of the left subclavian artery. The length of the aortic injury is approximately 4 cm.

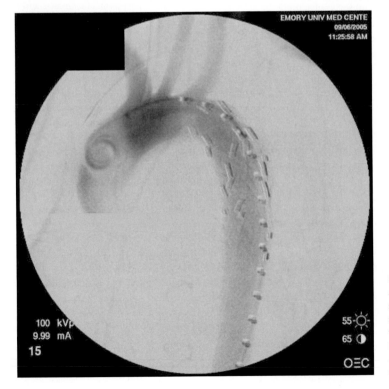

Figure 18.2 The completion arteriogram from the patient shown in Fig. 18.1. The left subclavian artery remains patent with an excellent result. The repair was performed using five aortic extension cuffs from the Gore excluder device.

no device complications noted to date in any of the patients treated. This includes device migrations or a recurrent aortic problem. The longest follow-up to date is 1 year as patients have been lost to follow-up.

Overall, we have been successful with endovascular exclusion of the acutely injured aorta in every patient treated in this manner. The recovery in this patient group has been outstanding with discharge to home or a rehabilitation facility in every patient. The downside of our experience thus far is the lack of long-term follow-up in order to ascertain the durability of this approach.

Conclusions

Traumatic disruption of the aorta is an injury with a high risk of mortality. The standard urgent surgical management has been challenged by the safety of nonoperative or delayed management in several trauma centers. The advent of endovascular therapy has questioned the need for any of these approaches with excellent initial results with endovascular devices. In addition, a decreased morbidity and mortality is seen with the endovascular approach. We have also found this to be true in our series of acutely injured patients managed with endovascular repair. The long-term durability of endovascular repair of traumatic aortic disruption needs to be fully assessed.

References

1 McGwin G, Jr., Metzger J, Moran SG, Rue LW, 3rd. Occupant- and collision-related risk factors for blunt thoracic aorta injury. J Trauma 2003 Apr; **54**(4): 655–660; discussion 660–662.

2 Razzouk AJ, Gundry SR, Wang N, del Rio MJ, Varnell D, Bailey LL. Repair of traumatic aortic rupture: A 25-year experience. Arch Surg. 2000 Aug; **135**(8): 913–918; discussion 919.

3 Hochheiser GM, Clark DE, Morton JR. Operative technique, paraplegia, and mortality after blunt traumatic aortic injury. Arch Surg 2002 Apr; **137**(4): 434–438.

4 Symbas PN, Sherman AJ, Silver JM, Symbas JD, Lackey JJ. Traumatic rupture of the aorta: Immediate or delayed repair? Ann Surg 2002 Jun; **235**(6): 796–802.

5 Nzewi O, Slight RD, Zamvar V. Management of blunt thoracic aortic injury. Eur J Vasc Endovasc Surg 2006 Jan; **31**(1): 18–27.

6 Idu MM, Reekers JA, Balm R, Ponsen KJ, de Mol BA, Legemate DA. Collapse of a stent-graft following treatment of a traumatic thoracic aortic rupture. J Endovasc Ther 2005 Aug; **12**(4): 503–507.

7 Sondenaa K, Tveit B, Kordt KF, Fossdal JE, Pedersen PH. Traumatic rupture of the thoracic aorta: A clinicopathological study. Acta Chir Scand 1990 Feb; **156**(2): 137–143.

8 O'Conor CE. Diagnosing traumatic rupture of the thoracic aorta in the emergency department. Emerg Med J 2004 Jul; **21**(4): 414–419.

9 Bajor G, Bijata W, Szczeklik M, Bohosiewicz J, Bochenek A, Daab M. Traumatic rupture of the aorta in adolescence–description of two cases. Eur J Pediatr Surg 2005 Aug; **15**(4): 287–291.

10 Alkadhi H, Wildermuth S, Desbiolles L, Schertler T, Crook D, Marincek B, Boehm T. Vascular emergencies of the thorax after blunt and iatrogenic trauma: Multi-detector row CT and three-dimensional imaging. Radiographics 2004 Sep–Oct; **24**(5): 1239–1255.

11 Cinnella G, Dambrosio M, Brienza N, Tullo L, Fiore T. Transesophageal echocardiography for diagnosis of traumatic aortic injury: An appraisal of the evidence. J Trauma 2004 Dec; **57**(6): 1246–1255.

12 Weimann S, Balogh D, Furtwangler W, Mikuz G, Flora G. Graft replacement of post-traumatic thoracic aortic aneurysm: Results without bypass or shunting. Eur J Vasc Surg 1992 Jul; **6**(4): 381–385.

13 Klena JW, Shweiki E, Woods EL, Indeck M. Purposeful delay in the repair of a traumatic rupture of the aorta with coexistent liver injury. Ann Thorac Surg 1998 Sep; **66**(3): 950–952.

14 Pierangeli A, Turinetto B, Galli R, Caldarera L, Fattori R, Gavelli G. Delayed treatment of isthmic aortic rupture. Cardiovasc Surg 2000 Jun; **8**(4): 280–283.

15 Kasirajan K, Heffernan D, Langsfeld M. Acute thoracic aortic trauma: A comparison of endoluminal stent grafts with open repair and nonoperative management. Ann Vasc Surg 2003 Nov; **17**(6): 589–595.

16 Wellons ED, Milner R, Solis M, Levitt A, Rosenthal D. Stent-graft repair of traumatic thoracic aortic disruptions. J Vasc Surg 2004 Dec; **40**(6): 1095–1100.

17 Peterson BG, Matsumura JS, Morasch MD, West MA, Eskandari MK. Percutaneous endovascular repair of blunt thoracic aortic transection. J Trauma 2005 Nov; **59**(5): 1062–1065.

18 Balm R, Hoornweg LL. Traumatic aortic ruptures. J Cardiovasc Surg (Torino) 2005 Apr; **46**(2): 101–105.

CHAPTER 19

Should endovascular repair be considered the standard treatment in traumatic thoracic aortic injury?

Peter H. Lin, Tam T. Huynh, & Eric K. Peden

Introduction

Traumatic blunt injury to the thoracic aorta is a devastating condition which can lead to immediate death at the time of injury in the majority of cases, due in part to either aortic transection or acute rupture [1]. Although blunt aortic injury accounts for less than 1% of all adult level I trauma center admissions, this condition represents the second most common cause of death due to blunt injury, second only to head trauma [2]. With an incidence of 7500 to 8000 cases of blunt aortic trauma occurring annually in North America, it is estimated that only 25% of patients who sustained aortic injuries due to blunt thoracic trauma remain alive upon arrival to the hospital [3]. Among these patients who survive the initial injury, their prognosis remains poor. Nearly 30% of them will die within the first 6 h, and 50% of these patients will not live beyond the first 24 h following the injury [4]. This high mortality rate has previously prompted traditional management of blunt aortic injury to establish early diagnosis and rapid surgical intervention in order to prevent a catastrophic rupture. This belief has been modified to allow delay of the operative intervention in order to first manage other serious concomitant injuries and lessen the high surgical mortality rate associated with emergent aortic repair [5]. Despite advances in modern trauma care, emergent operative intervention for blunt aortic injury is associated with significant cardiac, pulmonary, neurologic, and hemodynamic complications [5, 6].

The classic injury mechanism of blunt thoracic aorta is related to the combination of sudden deceleration and traction at the relatively immobile aortic isthmus, which represents the junction between the relatively mobile aortic arch and the fixed descending aorta (Fig. 19.1). The isthmus is the most common location for rupture (50–70%) followed by the ascending aorta or aortic arch (18%) and the distal thoracic aorta (14%) [4]. The objectives of this chapter are to (1) examine the role of endovascular repair of traumatic blunt aortic injury, (2) review current literatures of endovascular aortic repair of blunt injury, and (3) analyze the potential challenges of this treatment modality in blunt aortic injury.

Endovascular repair of traumatic aortic injury

Endovascular treatment of blunt thoracic aortic disruptions offers many practical benefits and technical advantages compared to conventional open repair in patients with thoracic aortic injuries. Deployment of a stent graft in the descending aorta with a focal traumatic lesion, particularly in patients with adequate proximal and distal aortic neck, can be performed in a straightforward manner. In patients with adequate femoral artery access, this procedure can even be performed under local anesthesia without incurring significant cardiopulmonary stress. Commonly encountered physiologic insults associated with an open repair, such as thoracotomy,

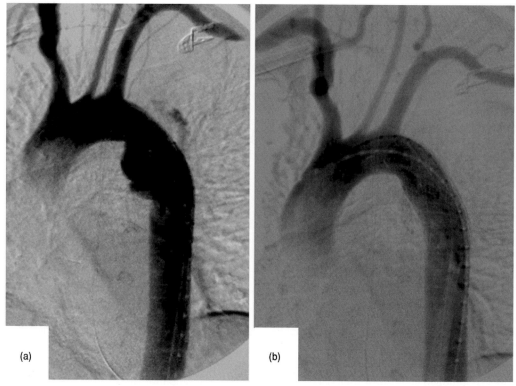

Figure 19.1 (a) Blunt aortic injury typically occurs in the proximal segment of the descending thoracic aorta, due in part to the sudden disruption of the aortic isthmus. (b) Successful repair of a blunt aortic injury can be accomplished using endoluminal treatment approach.

aortic crossclamping, extracorporeal bypass, and single lung ventilation can all be avoided in a setting of endovascular thoracic aortic endografting procedure. Exclusion of a descending aortic disruption with an endograft does not necessitate crossclamping the thoracic aorta. As a result, the avoidance of aortic crossclamping minimizes significant blood pressure shifts and coagulopathy. This also reduces operative blood loss as well as ischemic events involving the spinal cord, viscera, and kidneys. Moreover, avoidance of a thoracotomy has obvious convalescent advantages in patients who might be disabled from other multiple organ injuries.

Since the traumatic force responsible for blunt aortic disruptions frequently results in concomitant injuries involving other bodily organs, prompt endovascular exclusion of a traumatic aortic pseudoaneurysm or aortic transection can be performed without undue delay in surgical interventions of other concomitant injuries. This advantage is in

sharp contrast to an open aortic repair, which would require a patient to initially recover from any major operative intervention or intensive therapy of life-threatening complication of blunt trauma. Lastly, the use of systemic anticoagulation with heparin during an endovascular aortic procedure can be reduced to a minimum, which is particularly beneficial in patients with concomitant intracranial or abdominal injuries.

While endovascular repair has many obvious advantages compared to conventional open repair, one might keep in mind potential shortcomings of this treatment strategy. The possibility of persistent endoleak following endovascular exclusion of traumatic aortic pseudoaneurysm has been reported [7–9]. There are still concerns of late complications such as endograft migration or device infection due to fistula formation [10]. Furthermore, given the limited commercially available endovascular devices, not all patients with traumatic aortic disruptions have adequate aortic morphology to undergo this repair. Lastly, critics of this treatment strategy often cite the lack of long-term durability studies to justify the use of an aortic endograft in young trauma victims who may well tolerate the physiologic stress associated with an open repair.

Anatomical consideration in endovascular repair of traumatic aortic injury

There are several fundamental differences in the anatomical morphology between patients with atherosclerotic thoracic aortic aneurysm and traumatic aortic injuries which may impact on the choice of endograft devices and deployment techniques. In patients with descending thoracic aneurysms, adequate proximal and distal aortic neck length is critical to ensure proper device fixation and aneurysm exclusion. The diameter of aortic neck is similarly important for device selection. Because the diameter of an aortic neck may be subject to continual expansion due in part to aneurysm progression, many stent-graft devices have incorporated components such as hooks and proximal bare metal to reinforce device fixation and minimize stent-graft migration. Other pertinent factors in treating patients with thoracic aortic aneurysms include proximity to celiac artery, thrombus in the aneurysm sac, length of aneurysm involving intercostal arteries, and preexisting thrombus in the aortic landing zones. These considerations may play critical roles in subsequent aneurysm remodeling following endovascular repair, which may result in aneurysm size regression and alter stent-graft fixation. Access vessels are also an important consideration. Since a majority of patients with thoracic aneurysms are elderly male populations with underlying atherosclerotic disease, the insertion of a large thoracic endovascular device using a 21-Fr introducer may require a retroperitoneal access with the creation of an iliac artery conduit.

In treating patients with traumatic aortic disruption, many of these considerations are different. Because the majority of aortic disruptions are located in the proximal descending thoracic aorta, the proximal landing zone is generally in the proximity of the left subclavian artery. The distal landing zone, on the other hand, is usually not a critical factor due to the fact that the long segment of normal descending thoracic aorta is more than sufficient to permit proper device fixation. To ensure proper proximal device fixation in traumatic aortic injury, many have raised the concern that the left subclavian artery will be intentionally covered by the endograft in a significant number of patients. Clinical experiences have shown that critical limb-threatening ischemia of the left arm rarely occur and, if necessary, can be reversed by an elective left carotid-to-subclavian artery bypass grafting procedure [11–13]. Because the endograft device is anchored in relatively normal proximal and distal aortic segment, there is very little concern regarding the possibility of subsequent aortic neck enlargement which is the case in the aneurysm population. The possibility of device migration or late endoleak in the trauma population, while possible, is less likely and worrisome as opposed to the aneurysm cohorts. Important considerations of these anatomical features when performing endovascular thoracic repair in young trauma patients are summarized in Table 19.1.

The main anatomical challenge of endovascular treatment of traumatic aortic injury is related to the relatively small aortic diameter in these young victims, as opposed to elderly patients with thoracic aortic aneurysm. Although the GORE TAG Thoracic Endoprosthesis (W.L. Gore, Flagstaff, AZ) is currently the only device that has received the Food and Drug Administration (FDA) approval for clinical application, this device is designed for patients with thoracic aortic aneurysms who typically have larger aortic diameters. In a recent study by Borsa and associates who analyzed the angiographic

Table 19.1 Anatomical consideration of blunt aortic injury in young trauma patients.

- Smaller radius of aortic curvature, in contrast to older patients with aortic aneurysm who have wider aortic curvature
- Smaller aortic diameter, in contrast to older patients with aortic aneurysm who tend to have a larger aortic diameter
- Small iliac or femoral access vessel diameter
- Aortic disruption typically located immediately distal to the left subclavian artery, in contrast to patients with thoracic aneurysm which can occur in any segment of the thoracic aorta

morphology of 50 traumatic victims with thoracic aortic disruptions, the mean aortic diameter adjacent to the aortic injury was 19.3 mm [14]. The available Gore TAG thoracic endoprosthesis has devices ranging from 26 mm to 40 mm in diameter. Since this device was not designed in the treatment of traumatic aortic injuries, placement of even the smallest available Gore TAG device in trauma patients will likely represent a significant and inappropriate device oversize, which might lead to inadequate device fixation. This scenario was highlighted by a recent case report in which a GORE TAG device was used in a 20-year old trauma victim [15]. Because of the severe device oversize, the GORE TAG device became collapsed within the aortic lumen, and this was subsequently treated by another stent-graft insertion which unfolds the collapsed endograft [15]. Appropriately sized thoracic endografts with smaller diameters must be made available in order for endovascular therapy to be a viable treatment strategy in patients with traumatic aortic injuries.

Challenges of endovascular repair of traumatic aortic injury in young patients

Potential aortic growth in young trauma victims

Endovascular treatment of traumatic aortic injuries comes with certain challenges. Traumatic aortic injuries tend to affect younger populations, in contrast to the aneurysm population. It is not uncommon that adolescent or pediatric patients may present with this injury. Because of potential vessel expansion as a result of normal aortic growth, placement of a stent graft in young patients must be viewed with extreme caution. The possibility of stent-graft migration may occur as the aorta enlarges because of expected growth in young patients. Endovascular repair in selected pediatric patients may be considered as a temporary bridge to a more definitive operative repair at a later stage. In pediatric patients with life-threatening aortic disruption who have other concomitant injuries, it may be appropriate to perform endovascular repair to exclude the aortic injury until the patients fully recover from other injuries and can undergo an elective definitive open repair with proven long-term durability.

Challenges related to femoral artery access in young trauma patients

Femoral arterial access represents a potential challenge when considering endovascular thoracic aortic repair, particularly young trauma patients. Currently available thoracic endograft devices require a minimum 20-Fr introducer sheath. Placement of such a large introducer sheath in a diseased artery or small ileofemoral vessels less than 8 mm in diameter can result in severe iatrogenic injuries, including arterial dissection and rupture [16]. If significant resistance is encountered during the insertion of an introducer sheath, one should stop the insertion process and carefully withdraw the introducer sheath. A retroperitoneal access with the creation of an iliac or aortic conduit should be considered to limit the risk of iatrogenic rupture associated with small femoral artery access. These conduits can be converted to an ileofemoral or aortofemoral bypass graft to improve the inflow of an ischemic extremity if necessary. The potential of iatrogenic femoral artery injury in endovascular thoracic repair is highlighted in a study by White and associates who noted a 27% of access complication [16]. However, as endovascular devices undergo continual refinement and miniaturization with smaller introducer sheaths, the incidence of iatrogenic access complication will likely be decreased or possibly avoided.

Limitation in utilizing aortic endograft cuffs for treatment in descending aortic injury

Another important challenge in endovascular repair of traumatic aortic injuries is the limited availability of stent-graft devices. While several authors have reported successful usage of infrarenal aortic endograft cuffs in excluding thoracic aortic injuries, this remains a less than ideal endovascular solution [8, 17]. Current FDA-approved endovascular devices for infrarenal aortic aneurysm such as AneuRx (Medtronic, Santa Rosa, CA), Zenith (Cook, Indianapolis, IN), Endologix (Irvine, CA), and Gore Excluder endograft all have aortic extension cuffs which are designed for delivery to the infrarenal aorta. The lengths of these delivery devices ranged from 55 cm to 65 cm which may not be sufficient for juxta-subclavian artery deployment, which may be a particular concern in tall patients

Table 19.2 Delivery system lengths and diameters of aortic extender cuffs currently approved for infrarenal aneurysm repair.

Device	Delivery system shaft length (cm)	Maximum stent-graft diameter (mm)	Stent-graft length (cm)
Medtronic AneuRx	55	28	3.75
GORE Excluder	61	28.5	3.3
Cook Zenith	55	32	3.6
Endologix PowerLink	63	28	5.5–7.5

(Table 19.2). Although a retroperitoneal iliac artery conduit may provide an added advantage of delivering an endograft device to a more proximal location, these cuffs are generally short in length and will likely require multiple aortic cuff placement in order to adequately exclude an aortic disruption. Without clear evidence to demonstrate the efficacy of placing multiple aortic cuffs as an effective treatment in traumatic aortic disruptions, this treatment strategy represents an off-labeled device application and should not be widely encouraged.

Procedural-related complications due to device deployment

Delivering and deploying thoracic endovascular devices may pose certain technical challenges in young trauma victims with aortic injuries. Because younger patients with relatively normal aorta frequently have a sharp aortic angulation just distal to the left subclavian artery, it may be difficult to accurately position and deploy a thoracic stent graft in a juxta-subclavian artery location, particularly if the endograft has a rigid or relatively nonflexible device shaft. In some thoracic endovascular devices, such as the Talent endografts, the proximal bare stents need to be deployed higher in the aortic arch. The stent-graft portion of the device is then slowly pulled back in the descending thoracic aorta to allow accurate deployment. Manipulation of endograft in the vicinity of the ascending aorta not only is technically difficult, but also carries higher risk of stroke complications. Numerous complications related to manipulation of bulky devices in the aortic arch have been reported, which included cardiac perforation, aortic valve injury, arch perforation, branch vessel rupture, and cerebral embolization [18–28]. Significant device refinement, such as more flexible shaft to accommodate aortic curvature, will

undoubtedly be necessary before this technology can be widely adapted in young patients with traumatic aortic injuries.

Hemodynamic and anatomical features related to aorta in young trauma patients

An important anatomical consideration in endovascular treatment of traumatic aortic injuries in young patients relates to their tapering luminal diameter of the descending thoracic aorta. Moreover, younger patients typically have higher aortic pulsatile compliance and flow velocity when compared to elderly patients, which represents a hemodynamic factor that may destabilize aortic endograft fixation [29, 30]. Implantation of currently available nontapered thoracic endografts in young trauma victims who have relatively narrow aortic lumens will likely lead to diameter mismatch as well as endograft oversize. Gross oversizing in a relatively small diameter aorta in combination with a short radius of aortic arch curvature can result in a suboptimal conformability along the inner curve of the aortic arch, which can lead to problems including device fracture, endoleak, migration, and infolding (Fig. 19.2). It is estimated that these types of device-related complications, such as stent fracture, stent-graft compression, rate of reintervention, device explanation, or endoleak, occurred in approximately 3% when used in traumatic aortic disruptions [12, 18, 21, 31–37]. Moreover, a semirigid stent graft in a tightly curved arch may tend to lift the inferior wall of the lesser curve (Fig. 19.2). Force of cardiac pulsations pushing the stent graft against the outer curvature could further tend to push the inferior wall off the inner curvature. Some stent grafts may also adopt a fishmouth configuration with the superior–inferior diameter of the proximal graft shortening

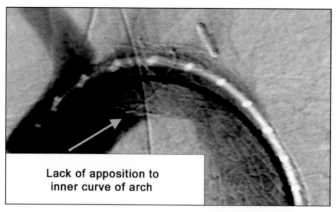

Lack of apposition to
inner curve of arch

Figure 19.2 In the clinical situation of an oversized endograft placed in a small aorta with a tight aortic curvature, the device fails to appose the inner curvature. Infolding of the lower lip of the graft can occur with catastrophic consequences. This has not occurred when the device is sized according to the directions for use.

and the lateral diameter widening, thus decreasing graft-wall apposition superiorly and inferiorly.

Endograft collapse due to significant endograft oversize in young trauma patients

Since the GORE TAG device remains the only FDA-approved thoracic endograft at the present time, available literatures demonstrated that approximately 9% of its reported applications occur in trauma patients [12, 18, 21, 31–37]. This is the scenario when significant device oversize is most likely to occur due in part to the lack of small diametered endografts to be placed in young trauma patients with relatively narrow thoracic aortic lumen. It is noteworthy that the recommended Instruction for Use (IFU) of the GORE TAG device as approved by the FDA indicates that this device should be oversized in the range of 7% to 18% in reference to patient's aortic diameter. Because the smallest diameter of the GORE TAG device is 26 mm, this device should be used in treating aortic size equal or larger than 23 mm in diameter. Deployment of a 26-mm diameter GORE TAG device in patients whose aortic diameter is less than 23 mm in diameter represents a device oversize beyond the manufacturer's recommendation, which may result in to suboptimal device performance (Fig. 19.3). All adverse events reported to date with the use of GORE TAG device were largely due to device oversize beyond the recommended IFU as approved by

the FDA (Table 19.3). Idu and colleagues recently reported a case of GORE TAG device collapse 3 months following the endovascular repair [15]. In their reported case, a 26-mm diameter GORE TAG device was implanted in a young trauma patient whose aortic diameter was only 19 mm, which represented a 37% device oversize. This significant degree of device oversize resulted in the wrinkling of the proximal segment of the thoracic endograft. While the initial aortogram revealed no gross radiograph abnormality following device deployment, the wrinkling of the proximal GORE TAG device eventually lead to device collapse, due in part to the high aortic pulsatile force. This condition was ultimately remedied by the placement of another Talent thoracic endograft to expand the collapsed GORE TAG device [15].

Results from clinical series in acute traumatic aortic injuries

The available literature on endovascular treatment of traumatic aortic injuries remains relatively scarce, in contrast to the vast body of the literature on endovascular abdominal aortic aneurysm repair. Nonetheless, nearly all reported series underscored significant advantages of endovascular treatment of blunt aortic trauma which include excellent technical success and low mortality rates (Table 19.4) [7–9, 17, 21, 26, 33, 36, 38–48].

Taylor and associates were the first to report the clinical benefit of using commercially available

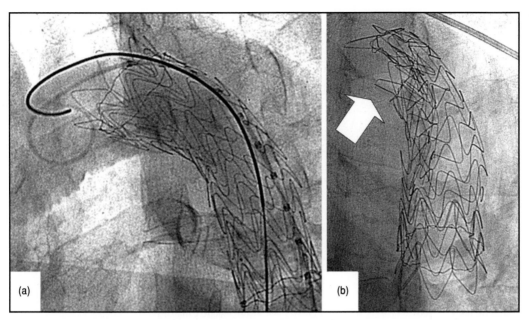

Figure 19.3 (a) Successful deployment of a GORE TAG thoracic device can be achieved when appropriate device selection was made on the basis of the recommended IFU, as evidenced by the full apposition of the stent graft in the aortic lumen. (b) When the device is inappropriately oversized relative to the aortic diameter, it can lead to device collapse in its leading segment (arrow, image courtesy of Dr Michael Dake and WL Gore Associates).

thoracic endografts in the management of blunt aortic injury in 2001 [38]. Thompson and colleagues reported on encouraging outcome following endovascular thoracic aortic repair for acute traumatic rupture in five patients. The technical success rate was 100%; no procedure-related complication or death was observed during an average

Table 19.3 Gore TAG thoracic endoprosthesis Instructions for Use (IFU) as approved by the FDA.

- Healthy neck length minimum 2 cm – may cover left subclavian artery if necessary
- The GORE TAG device has been designed to be oversized from 7–18% which has been incorporated into the sizing guide (do not oversize and follow sizing chart)
  - Measure flow lumen, do not include adventitia or calcium but include thrombus if present
  - Use case planning forms
- Neck taper must be within device sizing range – especially important around the arch transition
- Neck angles <60° recommend more than 2 cm of neck engagement

---

follow-up of 20 months [49]. Fattori and associates described 11 patients with acute and 8 with chronic thoracic traumatic injury located at the aortic isthmus treated by endovascular stent grafting [36]. All procedures resulted in successful outcome without signs of endoleaks. No death, paraplegia, or other complications were observed. The study group detected one type III endoleak during a mean follow-up period of 20 months, which showed spontaneous thrombosis within 2 months [36]. Lachat and associates reported 12 patients with acute traumatic aortic rupture treated by self-expanding stent grafts and reported a complete technical success [44]. The in-hospital mortality was 8% due to an undetected residual type I endoleak. During the mean follow-up time of 17 months, one patient experienced a perigraft leakage that was treated by an additional stent graft 12 months postoperatively [44]. Wellons and colleagues reported nine patients with traumatic aortic injuries who all underwent endovascular repair using infrarenal aortic cuff extenders [17]. There was no procedure-related mortality and technical success was achieved in all patients. Two recent studies compared the treatment outcome of

Table 19.4 Clinical series of endovascular treatment of acute traumatic aortic injuries.

Author	Year	Patient no.	Technical success (%)	Endograft type	Follow-up Paraplegia	(months)
Fujikawa [39]	2001	6	100	Home-made	None	8
Taylor [38]	2001	5	100	Gore, Talent	None	6
Bortone [50]	2002	10	100	Gore	None	14
Orend [47]	2002	11	92	Gore, Talent	None	14
Thompson [37]	2002	5	100	Gore, home-made	None	20
Fattori [36]	2002	11	100	Gore, Talent	None	20
Lachat [44]	2002	12	100	Gore, Talent	None	9
Kasirajan [42]	2003	5	100	Gore, Talent, home-made	None	10
Karmy-Jones [8]	2003	11	100	AneuRx cuff, Ancure, Talent, home-made	None	16
Iannelli [21]	2004	3	100	Gore	None	13
Wellons [17]	2004	9	100	AneuRx cuff, Excluder cuff	None	6
Kato [43]	2004	6	100	Home-made	None	6
Scheinert [48]	2004	10	100	Gore, Talent	None	17
Czermak [40]	2004	12	92	Gore, Talent	None	9
Morishita [45]	2004	7	100	Home-made	None	12
Neuhauser [46]	2004	10	100	Gore, Talent, Vanguard	None	26
Ott [7]	2004	6	100	Talent	None	16
Uzieblo [9]	2004	4	100	Talent	None	8
Bortone [33]	2004	14	100	Talent, Gore, Zenith, Endofit	None	14

traumatic thoracic aortic disruption between the conventional open repair versus endovascular therapy. Ott and colleagues reported their experience of 18 patients with blunt thoracic aortic injuries during an 11-year period [7]. The authors noted that open surgical group had a 17% early mortality rate, a paraplegic rate of 16%, and an 8.3% incidence of recurrent laryngeal nerve injury. This is in sharp contrast to the endovascular patient cohorts, who did not experience any perioperative mortality, paraplegia, or recurrent laryngeal nerve injury [7]. Similar findings regarding the benefits of endovascular treatment over open surgical repair were highlighted in another study by Kasirajan and associates [42]. These authors noted that patients who underwent endovascular repair had significantly lower perioperative mortality rates compared to those who underwent open repair. The mean procedural time and length of hospital stay were all significantly less in the endovascular group compared to the open repair cohort [42].

Paraplegia undoubtedly remains the most feared complication following repair of a traumatic aortic injury, which has a reported incidence of as high as 18% in patients following open repair for blunt aortic trauma [3]. A postulated mechanism of this complication relates to aortic crossclamp times in excess of 30 min. An overview of all available endovascular studies on traumatic aortic injuries showed that the paraplegic complication does not occur. Table 19.4 summarizes the treatment outcome of these studies. One possible explanation of this low paraplegic incidence following endovascular treatment is the avoidance of aortic crossclamping and less blood pressure variation or hemodynamic instability following endovascular repair.

Should endovascular repair be considered the new standard of treatment in traumatic aortic injury?

Because of the rarity of traumatic aortic injury, successful endovascular treatment will likely be confined to large trauma centers with a dedicated trauma team working jointly with experienced endovascular surgeons. Moreover, optimal outcome of this treatment strategy will depend on proper imaging equipment and full arrays of readily available endovascular devices. It is our belief that an emergent stent grafting is more technically demanding and conceptually challenging when compared to an elective endovascular procedure. In an elective aneurysm stent-grafting procedure, for instance, careful consideration regarding device sizing and device selection can be done in a timely fashion. In contrast, urgent endovascular repair of a traumatic aortic injury will require an experienced team of trauma surgeons, vascular surgeons, anesthesiologists, and operating room nurses ready to perform this procedure in critically injured trauma patients in an around-the-clock fashion. Physicians must rely on their expertise and skills to make critical decisions relating to device selection or arterial access both promptly and accurately. While all available clinical studies on endovascular treatment of traumatic aortic disruptions showed promising results with excellent technical success and lower mortality rates compared to conventional open repair, long-term studies will undoubtedly be necessary to prove the treatment efficacy of this minimally invasive therapy. Presently, the Achilles heel of endovascular treatment of traumatic aortic disruption relates to the limited availability of thoracic endografts in all sizes (Table 19.5). Utilizing currently approved thoracic devices in young trauma victims with aortic injuries will likely result in significant device oversize and potentially lead to late device-

Table 19.5 Examples of an inappropriate device oversize when using a Gore TAG thoracic device in patients with relatively small aortic diameters.

The Gore TAG thoracic device should not be oversized more than 18% based on the aortic diameter, as indicated by the device IFU. Given the smallest Gore TAG device has a diameter of 26 mm, placement of such a device can result in varying degree of oversize in various aortic diameters. The following description summarizes varying degree of device oversize in various scenarios of aortic diameters.

- Placement of a 26-mm thoracic endograft in a 20-mm aortic diameter would result in a 30% oversize
- Placement of a 26-mm thoracic endograft in a 18-mm aortic diameter would result in a 44% oversize
- Placement of a 26-mm thoracic endograft in a 16-mm aortic diameter would result in a 63% oversize
- Placement of a 26-mm thoracic endograft in a 14-mm aortic diameter would result in a 86% oversize

related complications (Table 19.5). Until further studies that validate this treatment durability as well as the full array of appropriately sized devices becomes available, physicians must take precautions when performing endovascular repair of traumatic aortic injuries as this therapy should only be offered in appropriately selected patients.

References

1 Williams JS, Graff JA, Uku JM, Steinig JP. Aortic injury in vehicular trauma. Ann Thorac Surg 1994; **57**: 726–730.

2 Clancy TV, Gary Maxwell J, Covington DL, Brinker CC, Blackman D. A statewide analysis of level I and II trauma centers for patients with major injuries. J Trauma 2001; **51**: 346–351.

3 Fabian TC, Richardson JD, Croce MA, Smith JS, Jr., Rodman G, Jr., Kearney PA et al. Prospective study of blunt aortic injury: Multicenter Trial of the American Association for the Surgery of Trauma. J Trauma 1997; **42**: 374–380; discussion 380–383.

4 Jamieson WR, Janusz MT, Gudas VM, Burr LH, Fradet GJ, Henderson C. Traumatic rupture of the thoracic aorta: Third decade of experience. Am J Surg 2002; **183**: 571–575.

5 Kwon CC, Gill IS, Fallon WF, Yowler C, Akhrass R, Temes RT et al. Delayed operative intervention in the management of traumatic descending thoracic aortic rupture. Ann Thorac Surg 2002; **74**: S1888–S1891; discussion S1892–S1898.

6 von Oppell UO, Dunne TT, De Groot MK, Zilla P. Traumatic aortic rupture: Twenty-year metaanalysis of mortality and risk of paraplegia. Ann Thorac Surg 1994; **58**: 585–593.

7 Ott MC, Stewart TC, Lawlor DK, Gray DK, Forbes TL. Management of blunt thoracic aortic injuries: Endovascular stents versus open repair. J Trauma 2004; **56**: 565–570.

8 Karmy-Jones R, Hoffer E, Meissner MH, Nicholls S, Mattos M. Endovascular stent grafts and aortic rupture: A case series. J Trauma 2003; **55**: 805–810.

9 Uzieblo M, Sanchez LA, Rubin BG, Choi ET, Geraghty PJ, Flye MW et al. Endovascular repair of traumatic descending thoracic aortic disruptions: Should endovascular therapy become the gold standard? Vasc Endovascular Surg 2004; **38**: 331–337.

10 Saratzis A, Saratzis N, Fillipou D, Melas N, Kiskinis D. Endovascular stent-graft repair of an aortobronchial fistula: Case report and review of the literature. Eur J Vasc Endovasc Surg 2005; **30**: 223.

11 Mattison R, Hamilton IN, Jr., Ciraulo DL, Richart CM. Stent-graft repair of acute traumatic thoracic aortic

transection with intentional occlusion of the left sub-clavian artery: Case report. J Trauma 2001; **51**: 326–328.

12 Orford VP, Atkinson NR, Thomson K, Milne PY, Campbell WA, Roberts A et al. Blunt traumatic aortic transection: The endovascular experience. Ann Thorac Surg 2003; **75**: 106–111; discussion 111–112.

13 Lin PH, Bush RL, Lumsden AB. Traumatic aortic pseudoaneurysm after airbag deployment: Successful treatment with endoluminal stent-graft placement and subclavian-to-carotid transposition. J Trauma 2005; **58**: 1282–1284.

14 Borsa JJ, Hoffer EK, Karmy-Jones R, Fontaine AB, Bloch RD, Yoon JK et al. Angiographic description of blunt traumatic injuries to the thoracic aorta with specific relevance to endograft repair. J Endovasc Ther 2002; **9**(Suppl)2: II84–II91.

15 Idu MM, Reekers JA, Balm R, Ponsen KJ, de Mol BA, Legemate DA. Collapse of a stent-graft following treatment of a traumatic thoracic aortic rupture. J Endovasc Ther 2005; **12**: 503–507.

16 White RA, Donayre CE, Walot I, Lippmann M, Woody J, Lee J et al. Endovascular exclusion of descending thoracic aortic aneurysms and chronic dissections: Initial clinical results with the AneuRx device. J Vasc Surg 2001; **33**: 927–934.

17 Wellons ED, Milner R, Solis M, Levitt A, Rosenthal D. Stent-graft repair of traumatic thoracic aortic disruptions. J Vasc Surg 2004; **40**: 1095–1100.

18 Makaroun MS, Dillavou ED, Kee ST, Sicard G, Chaikof E, Bavaria J et al. Endovascular treatment of thoracic aortic aneurysms: Results of the phase II multicenter trial of the GORE TAG thoracic endoprosthesis. J Vasc Surg 2005; **41**: 1–9.

19 Greenberg R, Resch T, Nyman U, Lindh M, Brunkwall J, Brunkwall P et al. Endovascular repair of descending thoracic aortic aneurysms: An early experience with intermediate-term follow-up. J Vasc Surg 2000; **31**: 147–156.

20 Greenberg R, Harthun N. Endovascular repair of lesions of descending thoracic aorta: Aneurysms and dissections. Curr Opin Cardiol 2001; **16**: 225–230.

21 Iannelli G, Piscione F, Di Tommaso L, Monaco M, Chiariello M, Spampinato N. Thoracic aortic emergencies: Impact of endovascular surgery. Ann Thorac Surg 2004; **77**: 591–596.

22 Fattori R, Napoli G, Lovato L, Grazia C, Piva T, Rocchi G et al. Descending thoracic aortic diseases: stent-graft repair. Radiology 2003; **229**: 176–183.

23 Semba CP, Mitchell RS, Miller DC, Kato N, Kee ST, Chen JT et al. Thoracic aortic aneurysm repair with endovascular stent-grafts. Vasc Med 1997; **2**: 98–103.

24 Mitchell RS, Miller DC, Dake MD. Stent-graft repair of thoracic aortic aneurysms. Semin Vasc Surg 1997; **10**: 257–271.

25 Kato N, Dake MD, Miller DC, Semba CP, Mitchell RS, Razavi MK et al. Traumatic thoracic aortic aneurysm: Treatment with endovascular stent-grafts. Radiology 1997; **205**: 657–662.

26 Semba CP, Kato N, Kee ST, Lee GK, Mitchell RS, Miller DC et al. Acute rupture of the descending thoracic aorta: Repair with use of endovascular stent-grafts. J Vasc Interv Radiol 1997; **8**: 337–342.

27 Dake MD, Miller DC, Mitchell RS, Semba CP, Moore KA, Sakai T. The "first generation" of endovascular stent-grafts for patients with aneurysms of the descending thoracic aorta. J Thorac Cardiovasc Surg 1998; **116**: 689–703; discussion 703–704.

28 Dake MD, Miller DC, Semba CP, Mitchell RS, Walker PJ, Liddell RP. Transluminal placement of endovascular stent-grafts for the treatment of descending thoracic aortic aneurysms. N Engl J Med 1994; **331**: 1729–1734.

29 Vulliemoz S, Stergiopulos N, Meuli R. Estimation of local aortic elastic properties with MRI. Magn Reson Med 2002; **47**: 649–654.

30 Laffon E, Marthan R, Montaudon M, Latrabe V, Laurent F, Ducassou D. Feasibility of aortic pulse pressure and pressure wave velocity MRI measurement in young adults. J Magn Reson Imaging 2005; **21**: 53–58.

31 Bell RE, Taylor PR, Aukett M, Sabharwal T, Reidy JF. Midterm results for second-generation thoracic stent grafts. Br J Surg 2003; **90**: 811–817.

32 Bell RE, Taylor PR, Aukett M, Sabharwal T, Reidy JF. Results of urgent and emergency thoracic procedures treated by endoluminal repair. Eur J Vasc Endovasc Surg 2003; **25**: 527–531.

33 Bortone AS, De Cillis E, D'Agostino D, Schinosa Lde L. Stent graft treatment of thoracic aortic disease. Surg Technol Int 2004; **12**: 189–193.

34 Cambria RP, Brewster DC, Lauterbach SR, Kaufman JL, Geller S, Fan CM et al. Evolving experience with thoracic aortic stent graft repair. J Vasc Surg 2002; **35**: 1129–1136.

35 Criado FJ, Clark NS, McKendrick C, Longway J, Domer GS. Update on the Talent LPS AAA stent graft: results with "enhanced talent." Semin Vasc Surg 2003; **16**: 158–165.

36 Fattori R, Napoli G, Lovato L, Russo V, Pacini D, Pierangeli A et al. Indications for, timing of, and results of catheter-based treatment of traumatic injury to the aorta. AJR Am J Roentgenol 2002; **179**: 603–609.

37 Thompson CS, Gaxotte VD, Rodriguez JA, Ramaiah VG, Vranic M, Ravi R et al. Endoluminal stent grafting of the

thoracic aorta: Initial experience with the Gore excluder. J Vasc Surg 2002; **35**: 1163–1170.

38 Taylor PR, Gaines PA, McGuinness CL, Cleveland TJ, Beard JD, Cooper G *et al*. Thoracic aortic stent grafts – early experience from two centres using commercially available devices. Eur J Vasc Endovasc Surg 2001; **22**: 70–76.

39 Fujikawa T, Yukioka T, Ishimaru S, Kanai M, Muraoka A, Sasaki H *et al*. Endovascular stent grafting for the treatment of blunt thoracic aortic injury. J Trauma 2001; **50**: 223–229.

40 Czermak BV, Fraedrich G, Perkmann R, Mallouhi A, Steingruber IE, Waldenberger P *et al*. Endovascular repair of thoracic aortic disease: What we have learned. Curr Probl Diagn Radiol 2004; **33**: 269–282.

41 Hausegger KA, Oberwalder P, Tiesenhausen K, Tauss J, Stanger O, Schedlbauer P *et al*. Intentional left subclavian artery occlusion by thoracic aortic stent-grafts without surgical transposition. J Endovasc Ther 2001; **8**: 472–476.

42 Kasirajan K, Heffernan D, Langsfeld M. Acute thoracic aortic trauma: A comparison of endoluminal stent grafts with open repair and nonoperative management. Ann Vasc Surg 2003; **17**: 589–595.

43 Kato M, Yatsu S, Sato H, Kyo S. Endovascular stent-graft treatment for blunt aortic injury. Circ J 2004; **68**: 553–557.

44 Lachat M, Pfammatter T, Witzke H, Bernard E, Wolfensberger U, Kunzli A *et al*. Acute traumatic aortic rupture:

Early stent-graft repair. Eur J Cardiothorac Surg 2002; **21**: 959–963.

45 Morishita K, Kurimoto Y, Kawaharada N, Fukada J, Hachiro Y, Fujisawa Y *et al*. Descending thoracic aortic rupture: Role of endovascular stent-grafting. Ann Thorac Surg 2004; **78**: 1630–1634.

46 Neuhauser B, Czermak B, Jaschke W, Waldenberger P, Fraedrich G, Perkmann R. Stent-graft repair for acute traumatic thoracic aortic rupture. Am Surg 2004; **70**: 1039–1044.

47 Orend KH, Pamler R, Kapfer X, Liewald F, Gorich J, Sunder-Plassmann L. Endovascular repair of traumatic descending aortic transection. J Endovasc Ther 2002; **9**: 573–578.

48 Scheinert D, Krankenberg H, Schmidt A, Gummert JF, Nitzsche S, Scheinert S *et al*. Endoluminal stent-graft placement for acute rupture of the descending thoracic aorta. Eur Heart J 2004; **25**: 694–700.

49 Thompson CS, Rodriguez JA, Ramaiah VG, DiMugno L, Shafique S, Olsen D *et al*. Acute traumatic rupture of the thoracic aorta treated with endoluminal stent grafts. J Trauma 2002; **52**: 1173–1177.

50 Bortone AS, Schena S, D'Agostino D, Dialetto G, Paradiso V, Mannatrizio G *et al*. Immediate versus delayed endovascular treatment of post-traumatic aortic pseudoaneurysms and type B dissections: retrospective analysis and premises to the upcoming European trial. Circulation 2002; **106**: I234– I240.

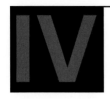

PART IV

Techniques, new devices, and surveillance

CHAPTER 20

Site-specific aortic endografting: case examples and discussion—the ascending aorta

Edward B. Diethrich

From the time of the first publication on endoluminal treatment of abdominal aortic aneurysms, investigators have made steps in applying similar technology to treat thoracic aneurysmal disease. The initial report by Dake and colleagues [1] showed encouraging results with endoluminal treatment of a typical atherosclerotic descending aortic aneurysm – both morbidity and mortality associated with the procedure were low. Later, this group described their early work with exclusion of acute dissection in the same arterial region [2]. Nevertheless, despite these and a number of other publications describing early results of endoluminal intervention in thoracic aortic pathologies [3–12], there has not been overwhelming enthusiasm or support from manufacturers. From an economic standpoint, this makes sense because abdominal aortic aneurysms are considerably more prevalent in both men and women. Additionally, corporate sponsors face an increasingly rigorous market approval process with the Food and Drug Administration (FDA). Still, the Gore thoracic aorta endoluminal graft (TAG) (W.L. Gore & Associates, Flagstaff, AZ) was approved in March 2005, and it is likely that other devices will follow it in the marketplace.

Stent-graft repair of thoracic aortic aneurysms has led to the use of grafts for the management of a wider variety of thoracic aortic pathologies, including acute and chronic dissection, intramural hematoma, penetrating ulcer, traumatic injuries, and other diseases. Relief of symptoms is frequently achieved and, when compared to the open operation in small populations or against historic controls

[13, 14], patients generally have more favorable outcomes with the endovascular procedure.

Our experience in over 300 endoluminal graft (ELG) procedures for thoracic aortic pathologies has provided us with the opportunity to extend the indications for this technology for use in more complicated aneurysmal disease. Although the entire thoracic aorta from the aortic valve to the celiac axis will undoubtedly be treated in the future with endoluminal technologies, research is presently concentrated in zones 2, 3, and 4 as illustrated in Fig. 20.1. These anatomic areas encompass all pathologies arising cephalad between the origin of the left common carotid artery and left subclavian artery to the celiac artery below the diaphragm. The majority of most thoracic aortic pathologies are encompassed within these zones, with the exception of type I and II dissections involving zones 0 and 1 in the ascending aorta and the aortic arch. It is this latter category of territory that appears to have significant potential for both endovascular and hybrid procedures. There are, however, specific challenges to ELG application in the thoracic region.

One of the unique characteristics of the thoracic aorta is its various configurations across the arch and down the descending thoracic aorta. There has been considerable experience with treatment of abdominal aortic aneurysms demonstrating a high failure rate of the endovascular procedure when there is significant angulation ($>60°$) just distal to the renal arteries (Fig. 20.2). This configuration increases the likelihood of both migration of the device and development of an endoleak. The same

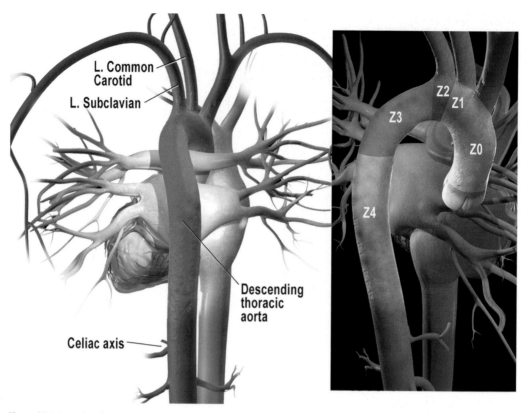

Figure 20.1 Drawing showing the zones of the thoracic aorta. Current endoluminal graft technology is concentrated on zones 2, 3, and 4. Potential exists for ELG treatment in zones 0 and 1 in the future.

right-angle configuration is frequently seen in thoracic aortic pathologies and different device designs are required to ensure proper deployment characteristics.

Another consideration unique to the thoracic aorta is fixation on a curvature in the distal aortic arch. Most abdominal aortic aneurysms have a proximal neck that is fairly straight but, as illustrated, the distal aortic arch is always on a curve that is sometimes quite steep. There is little consensus regarding an ideal fixation method in this region – barbs, hooks, and uncovered stents have all been used. One of the problems with the uncovered stent of the ELG has been erosion through the lesser curvature of the aorta proximal to the left subclavian artery (Fig. 20.3). The device in Fig. 20.3 was used to treat an acute dissection; one can legitimately question whether or not such uncovered devices should be used to treat dissections when friability of the tissue exists. Our own use of uncovered stents has not, to date, resulted in few untoward consequences and, the advantages afforded in terms of device fix-

ation, appear considerable. Even with the current limitations of equipment and the failure of industry to concentrate their efforts specifically on the thoracic area, there are ever-increasing numbers of pathologies that can be treated effectively using available endoluminal technology. The following case examples illustrate some of the advancing technologies in this exciting field of investigation.

Case examples

Case 1

Our first attempt to treat an aneurysm of the ascending thoracic aorta with an ELG was in February 2002. CW was a 48-year old male with premature atherosclerotic heart disease. He had his first quintuple CABG in 1987 at the age of 33 and then, in 1997, a redo bypass was performed to attach the gastroepiploic artery to the stub of the vein graft in the right coronary artery (RCA). Late in 2001, the patient was evaluated in Minnesota for exertional chest discomfort and dyspnea. The chest

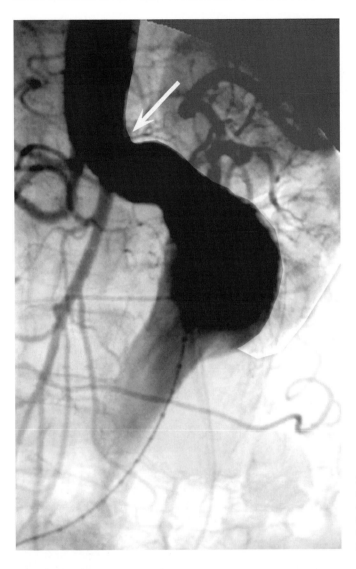

Figure 20.2 Aortogram of the abdominal aorta illustrating acute angulation at the level of the renal arteries. This anatomic/pathologic configuration often prohibits use of ELGs as a treatment modality.

X-ray demonstrated a large anterior mediastinal mass, which was confirmed by a CT scan and found to be ∼9 cm. The mass appeared full of mural thrombus, although a small area of contrast was seen coming from the ascending aorta. Left heart catheterization revealed that all vein grafts and the gastroepiploic graft were occluded, but the left internal mammary artery (LIMA) was open. The diagnosis of a large pseudoaneurysm arising from the vein graft to the RCA was made. Because the patient was considered to be at high risk for an open procedure, he was referred to the Arizona Heart Institute for further workup and treatment.

In February 2002, a repeat CT scan in Arizona demonstrated the mass to be 10 cm in diameter, with an area of contrast from the ascending aorta still visible (Fig. 20.4). The patient underwent angioplasty and stenting of a 90% lesion in the proximal circumflex artery. The following day, coil embolization of the vein graft pseudoaneurysm was performed using percutaneous techniques; however, only a single coil could be deployed in the pseudoaneurysm, and it was placed just past the anastomosis to the ascending aorta (Fig. 20.5).

Several months later in July 2002, the patient presented with persistent symptoms of chest pain, fatigue, and shortness of breath. The CT scan showed interval enlargement of the mediastinal mass to over 11 cm. The patient was taken to the operating room, where an aortogram and an intravascular

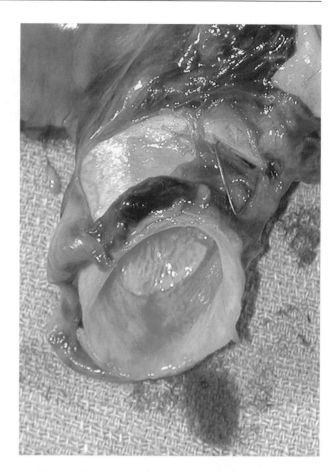

Figure 20.3 Uncovered stent erosion through the lesser curvature of the aortic arch (photo courtesy of Dr Rodney White).

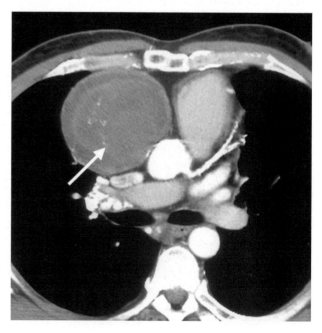

Figure 20.4 CT showing 1-cm pseudoaneurysm of the ascending aorta (arrow) secondary to a right aortocoronary vein bypass grafting procedure.

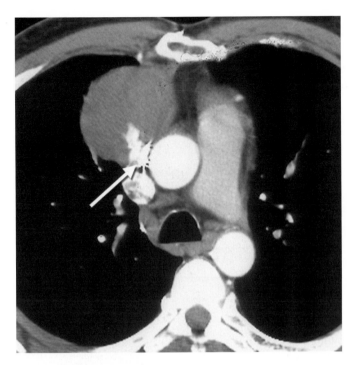

Figure 20.5 Image of single coil deployment (arrow) in an effort to close the pseudoaneurysm of the previous anastomotic site.

ultrasound were performed to determine the exact location of the pseudoaneurysm and to obtain dimensions of the ascending aorta so that a custom-made ELG could be fashioned. During this procedure, the patient experienced EKG changes and hypotension and an intraaortic balloon pump was placed. He was then taken urgently to the cardiac catheterization lab for balloon angioplasty and brachytherapy to a stenosis in the previously stented region in the circumflex artery.

During a 48-h recovery, in which the patient remained stable, a device was custom-made of PTFE and a self-expanding stainless steel stent. He was then taken back to the operating room, where the ELG was deployed in the ascending aorta (Fig. 20.6) and the vein pseudoaneurysm was excluded

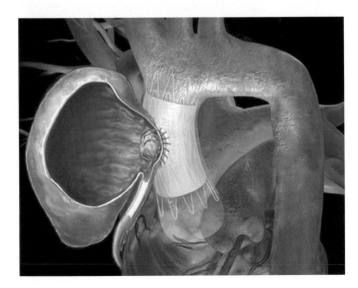

Figure 20.6 ELG deployed in the ascending aorta.

from the systemic circulation. Deployment of the 32 mm × 5 cm stent-graft was performed through a long 20-Fr sheath (Keller-Timmermans Introducer Sheath, Cook, Inc., Bloomington, IN), and was aided by pharmacologically induced hypotension and angiographic roadmapping. A temporary transvenous pacemaker and pre- and postprocedural transesophageal echocardiography (TEE) were also employed.

The postoperative CT scan showed no change in size of the pseudoaneurysm and no leaking of contrast outside the aorta. The patient was discharged in a good condition on postoperative day 3 and was essentially asymptomatic. The 1-year postoperative CT (Fig. 20.7(a)) and aortogram (Fig. 20.7(b)) showed resolution of the pseudoaneurysm complication.

Case 2

More recently, we have reported our technique for antegrade delivery of an ELG after rerouting of the aortic arch branches. Using the antegrade approach, we have extended use of this technique to treat an acute type A dissection [11].

A 50-year old white male presented to an outside facility with a painful, pulseless right lower extremity. An open thrombectomy was attempted and, when it failed to restore circulation, a computed tomography was obtained and demonstrated an aortic dissection extending from the aortic root to the aortic bifurcation and into the right common iliac artery, creating an occlusion (Fig. 20.8). The patient was transferred to the Arizona Heart Hospital for treatment of both the aortic dissection and the ischemic extremity – at the time of admission, the limb was cold and there was loss of sensation and motor function.

A femoral–femoral artery bypass and a below-the-knee, four-compartment fasciotomy were completed on the afflicted extremity. A few hours later, a median sternotomy was performed and, upon opening the pericardial sac, dark blue blood was encountered, and the dissection was verified from the ascending aorta across the aortic arch. Cardiopulmonary bypass was established after heparinization using a single, right atrial cannula and a 20-Fr femoral perfusion cannula inserted proximal to the left femoral–femoral graft. The ascending aorta was cross-clamped at the level of the brachiocephalic

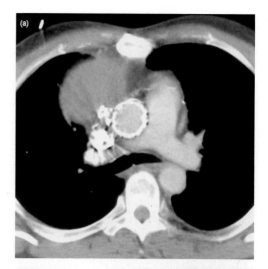

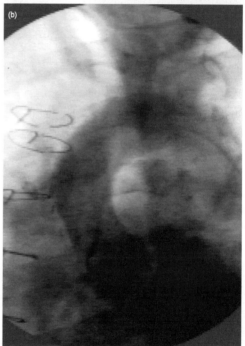

Figure 20.7 (a) CT examination at 1 year showing reduction in the aneurysm size. (b) Good angiographic confirmation of closure of the aorto-pseudoaneurysm connection.

artery, retrograde and antegrade cardiplegic solution was administered, and the patient's body temperature was lowered to 30°C. The aneurysm and dissection were opened, and the valve leaflets and coronary ostia examined. Two aortic valve

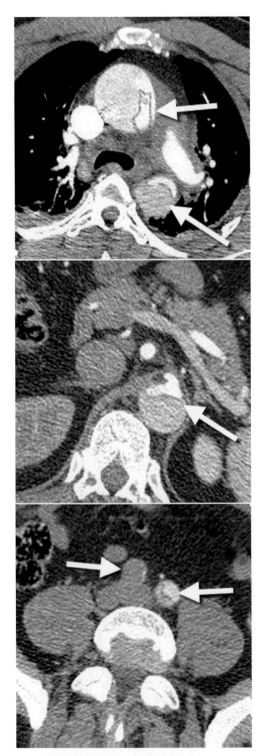

commissures were resuspended using a 2-0 Tevdek suture with pledgets. Both the proximal and distal aortic ends were reinforced with strips of felt, and the vessel layers were reunited before suturing a 30-mm Hemashield graft (Boston Scientific, Natick, MA). The suture lines were reinforced with fibrin glue. The patient was warmed, cardiopulmonary bypass was discontinued, and heparinization was partially reversed. An intraoperative transesophageal echocardiogram showed only minimal residual aortic insufficiency.

After obtaining satisfactory hemostasis, a 16 × 8 mm, branched, woven, Dacron® graft was sutured to the interposition graft over a partial occluding clamp. A third 10-mm limb was sutured to the bifurcated graft as a conduit for antegrade ELG delivery (Fig. 20.9). The left common carotid and brachiocephalic arteries were transected sequentially and then oversewn proximally, and the limbs of the bifurcated graft were attached distally (Fig. 20.10(a)). A 9-Fr sheath was attached to the conduit, and a 0.035-inch Glidewire (Medi-Tech/Boston Scientific, Watertown, MA) (Fig. 20.10(b)) was passed to the left common iliac

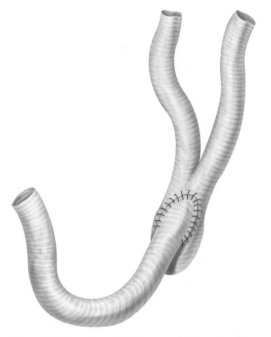

Figure 20.8 CT examination showing a type A aortic dissection from the ascending aorta to the iliac arteries with occlusion of the right common iliac artery.

Figure 20.9 Illustration of bifurcated conduit graft used for rerouting supra-aortic trunks and antegrade delivery of the ELG.

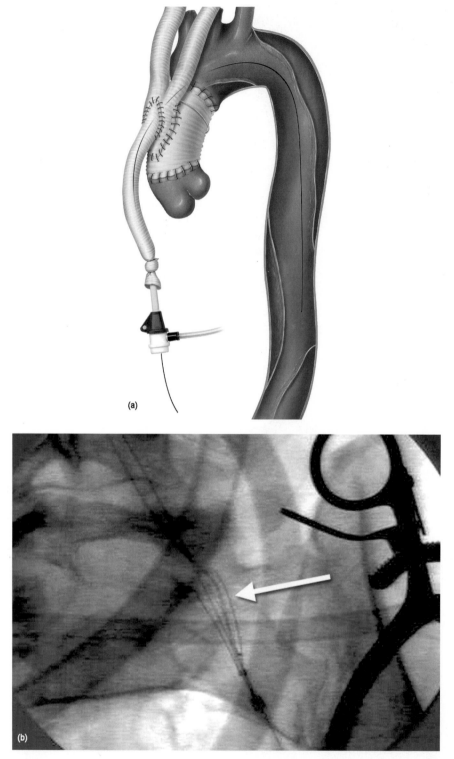

Figure 20.10 (a) A 9-Fr sheath is attached to the conduit to enable the 0.035-inch Glidewire to be passed to the left common iliac artery. (b) The guidewire was snared through a retrograde left femoral 9-Fr sheath.

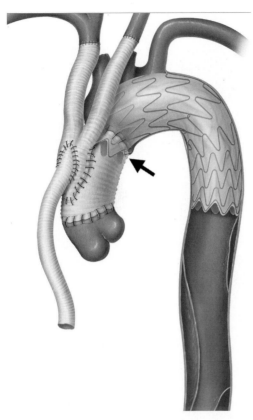

Figure 20.11 A 40 × 20 cm TAG device is deployed.

artery where, through a 9-Fr sheath, a snare was used to retrieve it.

A second wire was passed retrograde into the ascending aorta for an angiogram with roadmapping. A metal ring was placed around the conduit at its anastomosis to identify the landing zone in the ascending aorta. A 24-Fr sheath was delivered through the conduit across the aortic arch; this was made easier by pulling the left common femoral and conduit wire ends simultaneously. A 40 × 20 mm Gore thoracic aorta endoluminal graft (TAG) (W.L. Gore & Associates, Flagstaff, AZ) was deployed from the ascending aorta to the mid-descending thoracic aorta after the delivery sheath was retracted (Fig. 20.11).

An aortogram showed continued true lumen compromise distally (Fig. 20.12), and a second 40 × 20 mm TAG graft was delivered from the left common femoral approach through a 24-Fr sheath (Fig. 20.13). Aortography demonstrated complete resolution of the dissection without lumen compromise or an endoleak. The ascending conduit was clamped after sheath retrieval, transected, and then oversewn. The left common femoral artery was repaired after sheath removal.

A CT exam 1 day after the procedure showed complete resolution of the proximal arch and high descending thoracic dissection with persistent dissection into the pelvis (Fig. 20.14). The postoperative course was complicated by a left subclavian vein thrombosis secondary to catheter placement – this was treated by thrombectomy under local anesthesia. The fasciotomy sites healed without infection, and rehabilitation of neurologic complications of the ischemia to the lower extremity was begun. A 64-slice, high-resolution, contrast-enhanced CT prior to hospital discharge showed no proximal endoleak and obliteration of the false

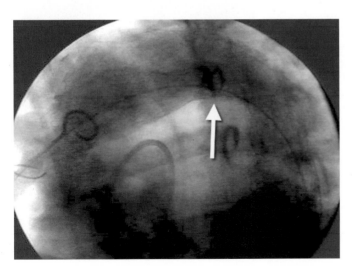

Figure 20.12 Aortogram showing continual lumen compromise distally.

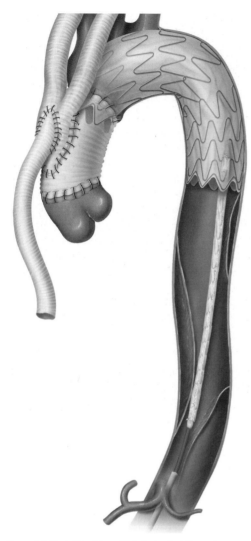

Figure 20.13 A 40 × 20 cm TAG device is delivered retrograde from the left common femoral artery.

channel (Fig. 20.15). A CT 3 months after the procedure showed patent grafts from the ascending tube grafts to the brachiocephalic and left common carotid arteries and the ELG in the descending thoracic artery (Fig. 20.16(a)). The distal abdominal aorta was also seen to have continued dissection and a patent femoral–femoral artery bypass graft (Fig. 20.16(b)).

Discussion

In general, endoluminal intervention for thoracic pathologies avoids extensive sternotomy or

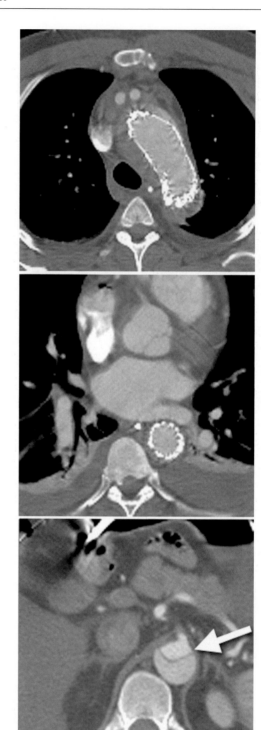

Figure 20.14 A CT examination on postoperative day 1 showing complete resolution of the dissection process down to the aortic bifurcation.

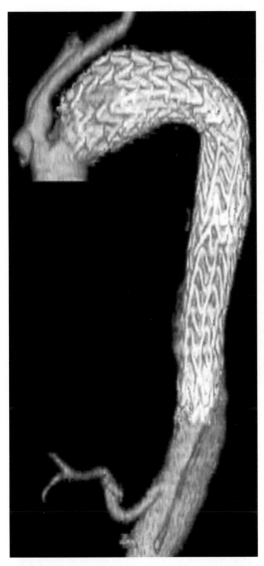

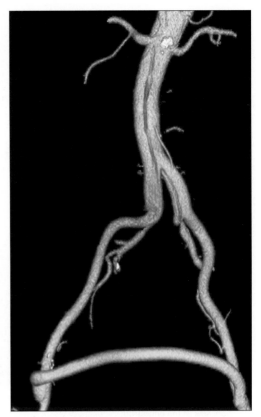

Figure 20.16 A 64-slice CT examination at 3 months showing patent grafts to the brachiocephalic and carotid arteries and satisfactory ELG position. A distal dissection of femoral–femoral bypass grafts is documented.

Figure 20.15 A 64-slice CT prior to discharge showing no proximal endoleak and obliteration of the false channel.

thoracotomy incisions, the use of chest tubes, respirators, and even general anesthesia. Blood loss is limited, ICU and hospital stays are reduced with the endoluminal procedure, and rehabilitation time is usually minimal. The rate of peripheral embolic complications, among the most dreaded problems associated with repair of thoracic pathologies, has been rare in our experience. While the rewards of endovascular intervention are apparent, the intricacy and severity of thoracic aortic pathology often requires techniques be modified to include more

than one type of approach; hybrid procedures that merge open and endovascular techniques are often obligatory in the repair of complex pathologies.

These cases illustrate extremes of thoracic aortic disease, whether caused by atherosclerosis or dissection. When treating an atherosclerotic pseudoaneurysm arising from the ascending aorta following a CABG procedure (as in case 1), the role for an ascending aortic ELG may be limited. Indeed, the saphenous vein graft from which the pseudoaneurysm arises must be already occluded, and no other vein grafts arising from the aorta can be patented because these would be covered by the graft and any perfusion would cause irreversible myocardial damage. Nevertheless, the technique described is ideal for patients without patent grafts those with conditions not associated with a previous CABG.

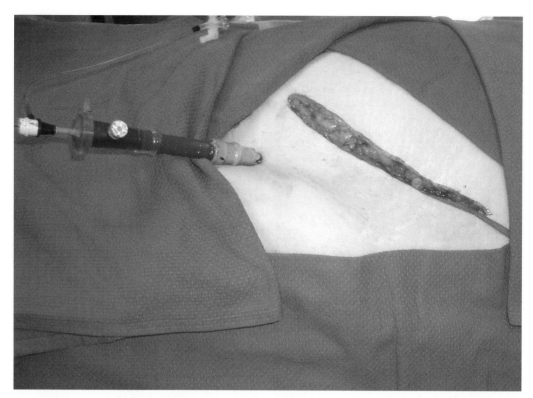

Figure 20.17 Illustration of retroperitoneal conduit used in conditions in which iliofemoral access is complicated due to large bore size of the endograft.

In terms of complexity, treatment of the ascending aorta (as described in case 2) that involves reuniting the dissected arterial wall, and interposing a graft accompanied by aortic valve suspension is the least complicated of the potential presentations. Vascular compromise with the right lower extremity viability in jeopardy shifted the usual treatment paradigm, demanding a femoral–femoral arterial bypass before the aortic procedure. At the same time, completion of the two procedures left no protection against further dissection with vascular compromise or even rupture. Appreciation of these negative consequences led to the decision for a more complete, unique, one-stage operative approach. This case also points out the fact that the delivery of the ELG across the aortic arch can be difficult due to the adverse effects of its anatomy. We have learned from our descending thoracic and abdominal aortic endografting the value of a brachial–femoral wire to assist the passage of the ELG through torturous arteries, particularly at the iliac level. The bore size

of the devices, in some cases, makes femoral access impossible. A retroperitoneal conduit attached to the common iliac artery, or even the lower abdominal aortic (particularly when accompanied by a brachial wire through the conduit as illustrated in Fig. 20.17) permits ELG delivery in most cases. In our ascending aorta and arch endografting program, we have incorporated techniques developed for some of these difficult situations and applied them with newer concepts of delivery.

Conclusions

These case examples demonstrate the potential for treatment of aneurysmal disease in the ascending aorta and arch whether caused by atherosclerosis or dissection. Thoracic pathologies are, in many cases, potentially fatal, and successful intervention is extremely important. Medical management is rarely appropriate, and conventional surgical repair is associated with a number of risks and a prolonged recuperation period; thus, interest in thoracic endoluminal grafting is significant, particularly since the approval of the TAG endograft. However, not all patients have lesions amenable to endovascular repair with an available device, and determining favorable anatomy for device placement is imperative during the screening process. Although these new techniques are advancing gradually, the potential for endovascular intervention in these regions appears quite favorable.

References

1 Dake MD, Miller DC, Semba CP, Mitchell RS, Walker PJ, Liddell RP. Transluminal placement of endovascular stent-grafts for the treatment of descending thoracic aortic aneurysms. N Engl J Med 1994; 331:1729–1734.

2 Dake MD, Kato N, Mitchell RS, Semba CP, Razavi MK, Shimono T, Hirano T, Takeda K, Yada I, Miller DC. Endovascular stent-graft placement for the treatment of acute aortic dissection. N Engl J Med 1999; 340: 1546–1552.

3 Thompson CS, Rodriguez JA, Ramaiah VG, DiMugno L, Shafique S, Olsen D, Diethrich EB. Acute traumatic rupture of the thoracic aorta treated with endoluminal stent grafts. J Trauma 2002; 52: 1173–1177.

4 Thompson CS, Gaxotte VD, Rodriguez JA, Ramaiah VG, Vranic M, Ravi R, DiMugno L, Shafique S, Olsen D, Diethrich EB. Endoluminal stent grafting of the thoracic aorta: Initial experience with the Gore Excluder. J Vasc Surg 2002; 35: 1163–1170.

5 Ramaiah V, Rodriguez-Lopez J, Diethrich EB. Endografting of the thoracic aorta. J Card Surg 2003; 18: 444–454.

6 Rodriguez JA, Olsen DM, Diethrich EB. Thoracic aortic dissections: Unpredictable lesions that may be treated using endovascular techniques. J Card Surg 2003; 18: 334–350.

7 Diethrich EB. Symposium on thoracic aortic endovascular stents: Part I. Editorial comment. J Card Surg 2003; 18: 333.

8 Diethrich EB. Endovascular thoracic aortic repairs: Greater experience brings rewards and new problems to challenge us. J Endovasc Ther 2004; 11: 168–169.

9 Diethrich EB. Endovascular surgery and pathology of the thoracic aorta. Am Heart Hosp J 2004; 2: 89–92.

10 Nathanson DR, Rodriguez-Lopez JA, Ramaiah VG, Williams J, Olsen DM, Wheatley GH, Diethrich EB. Endoluminal stent-graft stabilization for thoracic aortic dissection. J Endovasc Ther 2005; 12:354–359.

11 Diethrich EB, Ghazoul M, Wheatley GH, Alpern JB, Rodriguez-Lopez JA, Ramaiah VG. Great vessel transposition for antegrade delivery of the TAG endoprosthesis in the proximal aortic arch. J Endovasc Ther 2005; 12: 583–587.

12 Diethrich EB, Ghazoul M, Wheatley GH et al. Surgical correction of an ascending type A dissection: Simultaneous endoluminal exclusion of the arch and distal aorta. J Endovasc Ther 2005; 12: 660–666.

13 Najibi S, Terramani TT, Weiss VJ, Mac Donald MJ, Lin PH, Redd DC, Martin LG, Chaikof EL, Lumsden AB. Endoluminal versus open treatment of descending thoracic aortic aneurysms. J Vasc Surg 2002; 36: 732–737.

14 Bergeron P, De Chaumaray T, Gay J, Douillez V. Endovascular treatment of thoracic aortic aneurysms. J Cardiovasc Surg (Torino) 2003; 44: 349–361.

CHAPTER 21

Improved endograft fixation—a role for aortic endostapling?

Brian R. Hopkinson

One of the requirements of an endovascular graft is that it should stay where it has been put and it should stay sealed. The first generation of endovascular grafts such as the Vanguard produced very good initial results for seal but after 1–2 years they started migrating down the neck and developed subsequent type I endoleaks and had a high risk of rupture. Modular junctions also tended to migrate and disrupt causing a sudden increase in tension in the aneurysm with a high risk of rupture [1–4].

Devices such as the Ancure and the Zenith sought to correct the risk of migration at the aneurysm neck by incorporating spikes and hooks to hold the stent graft in place. This seemed to be quite satisfactory in practice but sometimes the hooks and spikes fractured and then migration could take place. The fact that the hooks and spikes fractured showed that there was a continuing downward force and that a stronger method of fixation was required. In Nottingham our first experience of endovascular grafting for abdominal aortic aneurysms was in 1994 using the Cook-Meadox Chuter graft. The initial results were very pleasing but after 1 year migration started to be a serious problem. We tried various ways of correcting this migration by using extension pieces but these too tended to slip as they were not fixed adequately with spikes or hooks. It was around 1995 we joined forces with Anson Medical, engineers in the UK, to devise an endovascular stapling device that would fix the graft and the extension pieces together and fix the extension piece to the wall. Previously described endostaples are one shot only [5] or require a prior to deployment drill hole [6]. Pullout tests in Sweden showed that the best fixation was for the Zenith graft at about 24 Newtons [7].

The requirements for this new staple were as follows.

1 That it should be very sharp so that it passed easily through the graft and the aortic wall without any preliminary drill holes.

2 That it should have a good pullout strength of at least 5 Newtons per staple when it was properly in place.

3 That the staple should be retractable and reloadable so that it could be refired if it did not deploy correctly in the first instance.

4 The system should be durable and biocompatible.

5 The whole system should be deployable under C-Arm X-ray intensification via a 14-Fr sheath and long enough to reach from the femoral artery up to the arch of the aorta.

Description of the device

The staple itself is made of Nitinol. It was used for its super elasticity as well as its thermal memory and biocompatibility. Its preformed shape is like a "seagull" with a loop in the wire forming its "body" and 2 "wings" with sharp points at their tips to pierce through the graft and the aortic wall as they arch outward and laterally to hold the graft circumferentially against the aortic wall. This is illustrated in Fig. 21.1. There is a thread loop passing through the body of the clip, which goes down the central delivery tube. By pulling on the thread the staple can be reloaded back into the delivery tube ready for redeployment in a different position. This redeployable function of the staple is very important

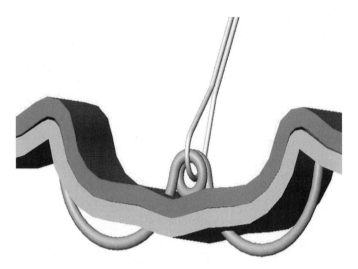

Figure 21.1 This figure shows the staple placed with the loop on the inside of the graft and two arms holding the outside of the aorta. The thread loop passing through the endostaple loop is used to retract and reload it in the delivery tube.

because it is known from vascular surgery that a needle does not always pass through a graft and the aortic wall exactly where the surgeon would wish it to. This is particularly true when dealing when calcified patches in the aorta. The idea was to mimic the action of the surgical needle with our staple. It is also important for the device to be torquable and to have controlled flection to enable the staple to be placed precisely. Radiopaque markers from within the device are used to help with orientation as the staple moves toward its target.

Testing in vivo

The first staple device was designed for open surgical stapling. Patches of polyester graft were stapled with 2–4 endoclips to the back wall of the sheep aorta and left in place for 6 months. At explantation they were studied in the pathology lab and had no biocompatibility problems.

Mechanical bench testing

Individual staples were tested in a mechanical test rig which moved the wings and the central loop up and down at least 1 mm. After 400 million cycles there were no mechanical failures of the metal. Fabric fretting tests were also done to test the effect of the Nitinol wire on fabric wear. After 400 million cycles there was very little evidence of fabric fretting.

Testing in the acute in vivo situation?

This was done in a pig laboratory using an X-ray C-Arm for imaging. AneuRx, Talent, and Aorfix stent grafts were deployed in the abdominal of the thoracic aorta of the pig. All the stent grafts had radiopaque markers sutured to them at various points so that we could test the aim and accuracy of deployment of our endostaples. The various radiopaque markers on the delivery system were easily identified and the endostaple could be seen folded up inside the delivery system. The endostaple could be easily deployed and retracted again for redeployment and with some experience it became clear when the endostaple was in the right position. The test for this was to pull gently on the delivery system while watching the C-Arm image intensifier. If the whole stent graft moved up and down while the two arms of the endostaple remained symmetrical this was found to be a good position and the loop of thread could be cut to release the endostaple. If the endostaple was not properly in position through the stent graft, it was found that the wings of the endostaple would move separately and it could easily be displaced, reloaded and redeployed in a different position. At the end of these acute experiments the aorta and stent graft with the staples inside it were explanted. The staples could be easily seen on the outside of the aorta and there was very little evidence of hematoma at the puncture site (see

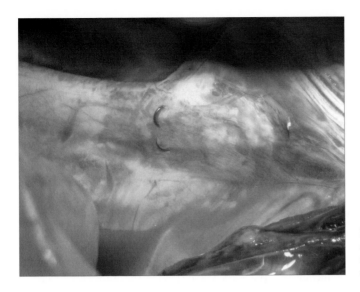

Figure 21.2 This figure shows the two arms of the endostaple on the outside of the aorta. There is very little evidence of hematoma.

Figs 21.2 & 21.3). Pullout tests found that four staples placed circumferentially required of the order of 27 Newtons. It is interesting to note that when the graft and staples had been pulled out of the aorta it was very difficult to identify the actual puncture holes that the endostaples had made and there was no evidence of any damage to structures outside the aorta.

The second stage of the in vivo acute testing was to simulate a migrating graft situation, placing two overlapping AneuRx grafts within the pig aorta. Endostaples were placed circumferentially around the top of the upper piece, fixing it to the aorta, and then four endostaples were placed through the overlapping area fixing the two grafts together. Again, it was quite easy to see that the endostaples were in the correct position when gentle traction demonstrated that both the endograft and the endostaple moved as one and the wings of the endostaple moved symmetrically. Once a satisfactory position of the staple had been achieved the retaining thread was cut and the staples released. At the end of the acute experiment the aorta, stent graft and staples were all explanted and examined. There was very

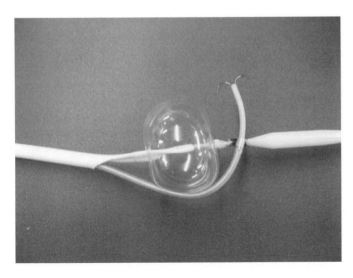

Figure 21.3 This figure shows the endovascular delivery kit with the staple in the deployed position. The curved cannula holds the staple and the hinged flexed outer cannula allows the staple to approach the target area at right angles to the stent-graft surface. The balloon helps to stabilize the whole system during deployment.

little evidence of hematoma at any of the puncture sites despite the fact that several of the staples had been deployed and redeployed several times. The pullout strength between the extension piece and the main graft with just four circumferential endostaples in place was very strong of the order of 35 Newtons.

Testing in human cadavers

This was done using fresh cadavers so that the aortic wall could be as near to the living state as possible and not influenced by embalming. We raised the aortic pressure to approximately 80 mm of mercury using a hydrostatic reservoir of warm saline so that the Nitinol could function properly at nearer to the normal 37°C. The device was easy to introduce via the femoral artery right the way up through the thoracic aorta. The markers for orientation could easily be seen. The device could be rotated appropriately and the endostaple could be identified in its loaded and deployed positions. With a little practice it was possible to deploy the staple within 2–3 mm of the declared target zone previously placed on the stent graft. AneuRx, Talent, and Aorfix commercially available stent grafts and extension pieces were placed so as to overlap within the aorta. The endostaples were used to fix the extension piece to the aorta above, then to fix the extension piece to the lower stent graft at the area of overlap. With a little practice it was possible to deploy the staples within 2–3 mm of previously identified target zones. It was quite obvious when the staple was in the correct position so that it could be released. It was also clear when the endostaple was not in a good position; it was relatively simple to withdraw it, reload it and redeploy it in a different position. At the end of the procedure we explanted the aorta, along with the stent grafts and staples and were able to observe the arms of the various staples on the outside of the aorta. The aorta and the stent graft were then divided longitudinally so that we could inspect the staple and the stent graft from the inside. The curl of the body of the staple was barely visible on the inside of the graft and was not thought likely to cause any problems by its physical size within the blood stream. There was very little evidence of damage where the staples had passed through the aorta

and been withdrawn several times. The pullout tests were done in two stages. First, we fixed the position of the extension piece and pulled on the distal stent graft to test the strength of the junction between the main stent graft and the extension piece. This proved to be quite a strong fixation with pullout forces on the order of 35 Newtons. The aorta above the extension piece was then fixed and the extension piece pulled away from it with a lower pullout strength on the order of 15–20 Newtons. The difference between the pullout strengths is thought to be due to the rather soft nature of the human aorta, which allowed the staples to pull out more easily from a single stent graft to aorta junction, as opposed to the rather stiffer stent graft to stent graft junction. Once again, inspection of the outside of the aorta at the stapling sites showed no signs of damage and it was actually very difficult to identify the actual puncture sites once the staples had been withdrawn.

Conclusion

We have produced a retractable, replaceable endostaple that can be accurately deployed and provides adequate pullout strength to attach a stent graft to the aorta.

Future progress

Although endostaples may well have a significant place in the management of migrating endovascular stent grafts in the abdominal aortic position, it is possible that endostaples could enable better fixation of patients with short and wide aortic necks. The endostaple may have an even bigger place in the management of thoracic endovascular stent grafting. The forces in the thoracic aorta that are trying to displace the primary fixation sites and the junctions of modular grafts are very much greater than the distraction forces in the abdominal aorta. Stapling together the junctions of thoracic stent grafts may well be an important application for this technology.

This preliminary work on the endostaple has shown satisfactory mechanical strength function and biocompatibility and the next step is to seek regulatory approval for appropriate clinical trials.

Acknowledgments

I would like to acknowledge the invaluable help given over the time of this project by the engineers at Lombard Medical UK (formerly Anson Medical), especially Professor Tony Anson, Dr Peter Phillips, Mr Duncan Keeble, and Mr Anthony Jones.

References

1 Marrewijk Corine J van, Leurs LJ, Vallabhanen SR *et al.* Risk adjusted outcome analysis of endovascular abdominal aortic aneurysm repair in a large population: How do stent-grafts compare? J Endovasc Ther 2005, **12**: 417–429.

2 Fransen GAJ, Desgranges P, Laheij RJF *et al.* Frequency, predictive factors and consequences of stent-graft kink following endovascular AAA repair. J Endovasc Ther 2003; **10**: 913–918.

3 Lawrence-Brown M, Semmens J, Liffman K, Sutalo I. Migration and separation of modular components in thoracic grafts: Thoughts on forces involved and prevention. J Endovasc Ther 2005; **12**: 1-1–50.

4 Beebe HG, Cronenwett JL, Katzen BT *et al.* Results of an aortic endograft trial: Impact of device failure beyond 12 months. J Vasc Surg 2001; **33**: S55–S63.

5 Bolduc LR. *United States Patent Application Publication.* Pub No: US2005/0187613 A1

6 Trout HH, Tanner HM. A new vascular endostaple: A technical description. J Vasc Surg September 2001; **34**: 3, 565–568.

7 Resch T, Malina M, Lindblad B *et al.* The impact of stent-design on proximal stent-graft fixation in the abdominal aorta: An experimental study. MD Thesis for the University of Lund 1999, ISBN 91-628-3614-5, p VI: 2–11.

CHAPTER 22

Treating smaller aneurysms: is there a rationale?

Kenneth Ouriel

Aortic aneurysms are treated to prevent rupture and rupture-associated death. Aneurysm treatment, however, cannot be accomplished without morbidity and mortality. Open surgical repair is a large operation, tolerated poorly by patients with multiple medical comorbidities. Even with endovascular treatment solutions, there exists an obligatory complication rate that occurs as a result of the procedure itself, the secondary procedures necessary to address endoleaks, migration, and other problems, as well as the rupture rate after treatment – a rate that is low but not zero. Thus, the natural history of the aneurysm must be balanced by risks of treatment and long-term treatment-associated complications.

Aneurysm diameter has been the one variable that is closely linked to the risk of rupture; the larger the aneurysm girth, the greater the risk of rupture over time. With this association in mind, there was a tendency to repair only larger aneurysms, for example 6 cm in diameter and greater, early in the evolution of the surgical procedure, when the mortality rate of the operation was high. Later on, technique improved and the mortality of the open procedure diminished to 5% or less. Without objective data, clinicians lowered the threshold for repair such that aneurysms of 5 and even 4 cm in diameter were repaired in the 1980s and 1990s.

Taken to the extreme, imagine if we had a pill that treated aneurysms, a pill that with limited side effects, would arrest the growth and therefore rupture risk of an aneurysm. Clearly, any individual with an aneurysm, regardless of how small, would be treated, analogous to the treatment of hyperlipidemia in patients with just slightly above normal lipid levels. While this example is hypothetical, it illustrates the point that the threshold diameter for which we treat an aneurysm is dependent on the risk of the intervention available.

Endovascular aneurysm repair offered a means to repair an aneurysm with the potential for markedly reduced periprocedural mortality. The European randomized trials demonstrated improved early survival in patients treated with endovascular vs. open surgical repair. Unfortunately, this mortality benefit did not hold up over longer term follow-up, likely as a result of poor device durability, a high frequency of secondary procedures, and late morbidity and mortality associated with these remedial interventions.

With more durable devices, better patient selection, and improved operator technical expertise, it is quite possible that the long-term mortality rate of patients treated with endovascular aneurysm repair will diminish. If this decrement in mortality is low enough, mortality rates after repair will compete favorably with the natural history of even smaller aneurysms. The development of improved endovascular treatment modalities will render intervention for smaller aneurysms appropriate – employing logic similar to that of the hypothetical "aneurysm pill" of the future. Until that time, we should focus on the completion of clinical trials designed to study patients with and without endovascular repair – beginning with small- to moderate-sized aneurysms of 4 to 5 cm in diameter. If we cannot demonstrate benefit in this group of patients, we should await the development of more effective treatment strategies before we lower the accepted threshold for aneurysm repair.

The data

The decision to treat an aneurysm rests on a comparison of the long-term risk of death from aneurysm rupture in patients followed medically, compared to the periprocedural risk of the repair itself and the long-term cumulative risk of death from postrepair rupture or from procedures directed at the remediation of device-associated problems (e.g. for false aneurysms after open surgery or for endoleaks after endovascular repair). Clearly, the best means to answer this question is through a large scale randomized study, allocating patients with small aneurysms to surveillance vs. early repair – with open surgical or endovascular techniques. The studies should be large enough (powered) to demonstrate a difference or the lack thereof with statistical rigor. In addition, however, the studies should be large enough to perform post-hoc subset analyses so that the general results of the overall analysis can be tailored to individual patient groups. While such post-hoc analyses lack statistical rigor, they do offer some data on which to base clinical decisions for individual patients with specific clinical presentations.

The first studies to evaluate the natural history of abdominal aortic aneurysms appeared in the early 1960s. However, due to the inability to accurately size the aneurysm with available imaging modalities at that time, the findings may not be entirely reliable. In an oft-quoted study of 24,000 patients undergoing postmortem examination at the Massachusetts General Hospital between 1952 and 1975, Darling found that approximately 25% of aneurysms between 4 and 7 cm in diameter were ruptured at the time of death [1]. This observation suggested that one-fourth of patients with aneurysms of that size would die of rupture. Of the multiple-risk factors considered, only size seemed to bear on the likelihood of aneurysm rupture. Among 52 patients followed for up to 10 years before death with known aortic aneurysms, the majority died of the ruptured aneurysms. These findings were corroborated by a study by Jensen and colleagues, published in 1989. These investigators studied 65 patients with abdominal aortic aneurysms who were not operated upon [2]. Over follow-up, 38% of patients who presented with asymptomatic aneurysms eventually died from rupture. A study by Perko and associates also evaluated patients with unrepaired aneurysms, but subdivided them into those with aneurysms less than or greater than 6 cm in diameter [3]. Patients with aneurysms greater than 6 cm in diameter had an annual rate of rupture of between 10 and 15%, while patients with smaller aneurysms had an annual risk of less than 5%.

In a study published in 1991, Guirguis and Barber examined the expansion rate of abdominal aortic aneurysms and the risk of rupture in relation to diameter [4]. This was a prospective analysis of 300 consecutive patients who presented with abdominal aortic aneurysms initially managed nonoperatively. The mean initial aneurysm diameter was 4.1 cm. Among the 208 patients who underwent more than one imaging study, the diameter of the aneurysm increased by a median of 0.3 cm per year. The 6-year cumulative incidence of rupture was only 1% in patients with aneurysms smaller than 4.0 cm in diameter. The 6-year rupture rate rose to 2% among patients with aneurysms between 4.0 and 4.9 cm in diameter, but was fully 20% among patients who presented with aneurysms greater than 5.0 cm in diameter.

Retrospective studies such as these, however, suffer from the limitations of patient selection; patients that were not offered repair may have had more medical comorbidities, advanced age, or may have been otherwise dissimilar from the larger group of patients who underwent surgical repair. A more reliable estimate of the natural history of aortic aneurysms of necessity, awaited the completion of prospective analyses. Two such studies were completed and published in 2002. Each compared early surgical repair vs. ultrasound surveillance of infrarenal abdominal aortic aneurysms.

The United Kingdom small aneurysm trial randomized 1090 patients with aortic aneurysms between 4.0 and 5.5 cm in diameter to early elective surgery (563 patients) or ultrasonographic surveillance (527 patients) [5]. The 30-day elective operative mortality rate of 5.4% was surprisingly high. After mean follow-up of 8 years, there was a trend toward a lower long-term mortality rate in the early surgery group, with a hazard ratio of 0.84 (95% confidence interval 0.70 to 1.00; $P = 0.05$, Fig. 22.1). Of note, 62% of the surveillance group underwent

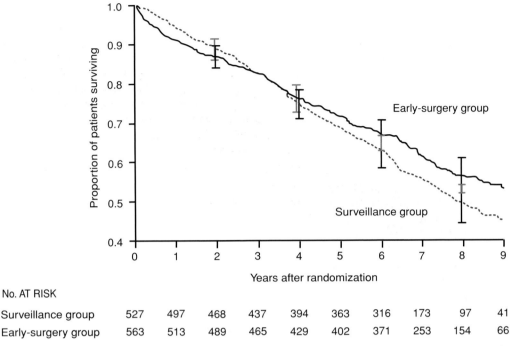

Figure 22.1 Survival after early surgery or ultrasonographic surveillance in patients with aortic aneurysms 4.0 to 5.5 cm in diameter. Reprinted with permission from the New England Journal of Medicine [5].

repair at the end of the study (mean of 8 years of follow-up). Examination of the survival curves demonstrated crossing of the curves at 3 years after randomization; in other words, the cost of the procedure was repaid after that period of time. There were more deaths from ruptured aneurysms in the surveillance group, in part accounting for the survival differences. Smoking, however, was found to be a confounding variable that may have explained the overall survival differences. While 55% of each group were current smokers at the time of randomization, over follow-up many fewer patients in the early repair group continued to smoke (28% vs. 48%, $P = 0.002$). This difference was so striking that the authors concluded that the mortality benefit of early surgery could be in part attributable to lifestyle changes adopted by the operated patients rather than repair of the aneurysm itself.

The Veteran Affairs Cooperative Study Group published the "Aneurysm Detection and Management" (ADAM) study, which randomized patients with aneurysms between 4.0 and 5.4 cm in diameter

to immediate open surgical repair (569 patients) or surveillance (567 patients). Of note, 62% of patients undergoing surveillance eventually required repair of their aneurysms; thus, the "surveillance" treatment arm might be more appropriately termed the "delayed repair" arm. The operative mortality was 2.7%, but despite this, there was no mortality benefit of early repair in this group of patients (Fig. 22.2); with a similar long-term mortality rate in the two groups, with a relative risk of 1.21 (95% confidence interval 0.95–1.54) for repair vs. surveillance. The rupture rate was 0.6% per year of follow-up for unrepaired aneurysms, a risk that was not high enough to account for any benefit in "aneurysm-related" mortality rate (contrasted to "all-cause" mortality rate) after early repair. The relative risk of aneurysm-related mortality was 1.15 (95% confidence interval 0.58–2.31) in the early repair vs. surveillance groups. These observations imply that the 2.7% "cost" of early repair is not "repaid" by the risk of rupture in a closely followed group of patients with small aneurysms.

Endovascular repair: Does it change the playing field?

We now have two well-designed, properly executed, and adequately powered prospective comparisons of early repair vs. surveillance of patients with aneurysms 4.0 to 5.5 cm in diameter. One study, the United Kingdom study, demonstrated borderline mortality benefit at 8 years in the early repair group, but this finding could be explained by smoking cessation rather than from a reduction in the risk of rupture. The other study, the Veterans Administration trial, failed to demonstrate any benefit of early repair whatsoever. Clearly, then, the risk of the repair itself was not overshadowed by the risk of rupture and aneurysm-associated death in the surveillance (or "delayed repair") group. Noting these data, should we abandon repair of small aneurysms? In the context of the low rate of rupture and the relatively substantial risk of perioperative mortality, the answer is "yes." Imagine, however, if we had a procedure with a significantly lower mortality rate. Imagine for the moment, if we had a "pill" that would prevent aneurysms from growing and rupturing – a pill without major untoward effects. Of course, we would treat every patient with the least bit of aortic ectasia with such a pill.

While we do not yet have a medication for aortic aneurysms, the decade of the 1990s introduced a minimally invasive means of treating aneurysms

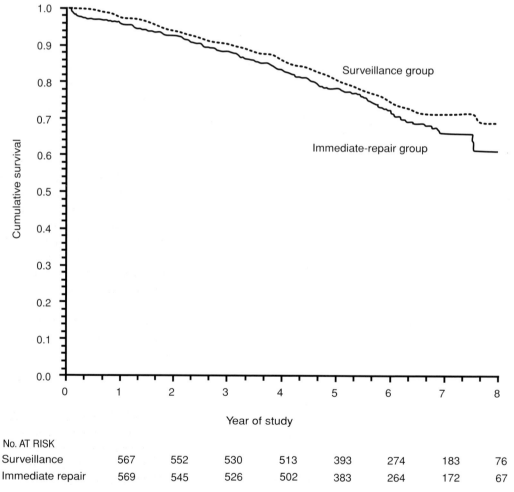

Figure 22.2 The survival rate in patients randomized to immediate surgical repair vs. surveillance of aneurysms 4.0 to 5.4 cm in diameter. Reprinted with permission from the New England Journal of Medicine [9].

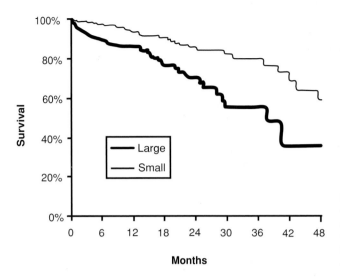

Figure 22.3 Endovascular repair of small (<5.5 cm) vs. larger abdominal aortic aneurysms. Mortality rate is significantly reduced in patients with small aneurysms. Reprinted with permission from the Journal of Vascular Surgery [7].

[6], endovascular graft repair. If endovascular repair of aortic aneurysms is associated with significantly lower periprocedural mortality than open surgical repair, and if endovascular repair protects against aneurysm-related complications over long-term follow-up, such a less invasive approach may surpass the outcome of a surveillance strategy for smaller aneurysms. In fact, there are two ongoing trials that will assess the results of endovascular repair vs. surveillance for smaller abdominal aortic aneurysms: the PIVOTAL and the CEASAR trials. These studies will not be completed, however, for several years. Until the results are available, the best we can do is compare the results of endovascular repair to open repair of small aortic aneurysms. Using principles of "transitive logic," if endovascular repair has benefits over open surgery for smaller aneurysms, and as we know, open surgical repair is associated with similar outcome to surveillance, then endovascular repair may "beat" surveillance for smaller aneurysms.

There exists a modicum of data to suggest that the endovascular repair of smaller abdominal aortic aneurysms is associated with relatively low morbidity and mortality, at least in comparison to the repair of larger aneurysms (Fig. 22.3) [7]. In a more direct analysis, Zarins and colleagues compared the outcome after (1) endovascular repair in patients treated in the AneuRx clinical trial, to (2) the surveillance group from the United Kingdom Small Aneurysm trial [8]. There was an attempt to match patients in the two groups to account for differences in baseline comorbidities. Ruptures occurred in 1.6% of endovascular patients vs. 5.1% of UK surveillance group, a difference that was not significant when adjusted for the difference in length of follow-up. Fatal aneurysm rupture rate adjusted for follow-up time, however, was four times higher in UK surveillance group (0.8/100 patient years) than in endovascular match group (0.2/100 patient years, $P < 0.001$). Aneurysm-related death rate was two times higher in UK surveillance group (1.6/100 patient years) than in the endovascular match group (0.8/100 patient years, $P = 0.03$). All-cause mortality rate was significantly higher in UK surveillance patients (8.3/100 patient years) than in endovascular group (6.4/100 patient years, $P = 0.02$). While these data do not originate from a prospective randomized analysis, they do provide some suggestion that endovascular aneurysm repair may be beneficial in patients with smaller abdominal aortic aneurysms.

Summary

In conclusion, there are no objective data on which to recommend open surgical repair of smaller abdominal aortic aneurysms. By contrast, there is some suggestion that endovascular repair may offer advantages over "watchful waiting." Resolution of this controversy, however, must await the completion of the ongoing randomized clinical trials – data that are at best several years away. Until then, practitioners must use their own clinical judgment, knowledge of the personal morbidity and mortality, and the specifics of the individual patient to arrive at rational, logical treatment strategies for patients with smaller abdominal aortic aneurysms.

References

1 Darling RC, Messina CR, Brewster DC, Ottinger LW. Autopsy study of unoperated abdominal aortic aneurysms. The case for early resection. Circulation 1977; **56** (3 Suppl): II161–II164.

2 Jensen BS, Vestersgaard-Andersen T. The natural history of abdominal aortic aneurysm. Eur J Vasc Surg 1989; **3**(2): 135–139.

3 Perko MJ, Schroeder TV, Olsen PS, Jensen LP, Lorentzen JE. Natural history of abdominal aortic aneurysm: A survey of 63 patients treated nonoperatively. Ann Vasc Surg 1993; **7**(2): 113–116.

4 Guirguis EM, Barber GG. The natural history of abdominal aortic aneurysms. Am J Surg 1991; **162**(5): 481–483.

5 The United Kingdom Small Aneurysm Trial Participants. Long-term outcomes of immediate repair compared with surveillance of small abdominal aortic aneurysms. N Engl J Med 2002; **346**(19): 1445–1452.

6 Parodi JC, Palmaz JC, Barone HD. Transfemoral intraluminal graft implantation for abdominal aortic aneurysms. Ann Vasc Surg 1991; **5**(6): 491–499.

7 Ouriel K, Srivastava SD, Sarac TP *et al.* Disparate outcome after endovascular treatment of small versus large abdominal aortic aneurysm. J Vasc Surg 2003; **37**(6): 1206–1212.

8 Zarins CK, Crabtree T, Arko FR *et al.* Endovascular repair or surveillance of patients with small AAA. Eur J Vasc Endovasc Surg 2005; **29**(5): 496–503.

9 Lederle FA, Wilson SE, Johnson GR *et al.* Immediate repair compared with surveillance of small abdominal aortic aneurysms. N Engl J Med 2002; **346**(19): 1437–1444.

CHAPTER 23

Management strategies, adjuncts, and technical tips to facilitate endovascular treatment of ruptured abdominal aortic aneurysms

Frank J. Veith, Nicholas J. Gargiulo III, & Evan C. Lipsitz

This chapter deals with the endovascular management of ruptured infrarenal abdominal aortic aneurysms (RAAAs) and ruptured aortoiliac aneurysms. By definition a RAAA is one in which the wall of the aneurysm contains a hole or a vent through which blood has leaked and is present outside the aneurysm wall. This chapter will not consider the treatment of so-called "acute aneurysms" which present with pain and even hypotension, but which show no evidence of blood outside the aneurysm wall, although some of the treatment methods presented can be used in this setting as well.

Unlike elective AAAs in which open surgery can be performed with a less than 5% operative mortality and a reasonably low morbidity, the open surgical treatment of RAAAs carries an operative mortality in the 50% range (35–70%) [1–6]. This persists despite all the technical and other adjunctive improvements that have been suggested. Moreover, the morbidity of open surgery for RAAAs remains high. Thus endovascular repair of ruptured aneurysms (EVRAR) offers considerable room for improvement.

In view of the poor results of open surgery for RAAAs, one may question why EVRAR has not been used more. One reason is that in the early days of endovascular aneurysm repair (EVAR), it took time to make the measurements required for endografting,

and it took additional time to procure the appropriate graft or grafts. The second reason is that all surgeons have traditionally advocated the need in RAAA patients to gain rapid aortic control, usually by clamp placement proximal to the aneurysm at the infrarenal or supraceliac level. This mandated emergency laparotomy.

It turns out that both these factors are not necessarily obstacles to EVAR. In 1994, we and others first began to treat RAAAs with endovascular grafts [7–9]. This was possible because the Montefiore and Nottingham groups had endografts that could be prepared rapidly and used to treat a wide variety of patients with RAAAs. It also was apparent in these early patient experiences that at least some RAAA patients remained stable or at least viable long enough for the endovascular grafting procedure to be successfully performed. EVRAR was proven feasible.

Methods

Hypotensive hemostasis

In the past, it has been noted that restricting blood transfusions and other fluid resuscitation was an effective way to control hemorrhage and improve treatment outcomes in patients who were bleeding. This was noted with patients who had upper gastrointestinal bleeding in the 1940s and subsequently those who had a variety of other conditions including vascular trauma [10–12]. In the mid-1990s, we made the observation that restricting fluid resuscitation could also be effective in the ruptured aneurysm setting, and we coined the term "hypotensive hemostasis" [13, 14]. By that we mean aggressively restricting all fluid resuscitation in RAAA patients as long as they remain conscious and able to talk and move. We accept a reduction in arterial systolic blood pressure to the 50–70 mmHg range and still minimize fluid resuscitation, as difficult as that can sometimes be. However, by doing so, bleeding will temporarily cease and time will be available to perform an endovascular graft repair (Figs. 23.1 & 23.2).

Supraceliac balloon control

Although hypotensive hemostasis can be an effective method to temporarily control bleeding in many RAAA patients, it can sometimes fail with cardiovascular collapse. Moreover, if patients are anesthetized with concomitant loss of their sympathetic nervous system compensation for a reduced blood volume, they frequently undergo cardiovascular collapse. In these circumstances emergency aortic control proximal to the rupture site becomes mandatory. As detailed in the "Current RAAA management protocol" section which follows, placement under fluoroscopic control of a guidewire via a femoral or brachial access site in the supraceliac aorta should be carried out under *local* anesthesia. This enables angiographic evaluation of the patient's arterial anatomy to determine suitability for endovascular grafting. More importantly, this guidewire can be used to enable rapid placement of a large (14–16 Fr) sheath (Cook Inc.) through which a large compliant balloon can rapidly be inserted to occlude the supraceliac aorta [13–18].

Appropriate grafts

The original endovascular grafts that were used to treat RAAAs were fabricated or assembled by surgeons so that they could be quickly inserted in the ruptured aneurysm setting [7–9, 17, 19, 20]. However, subsequently a variety of commercially-made grafts have been employed. Most of these have been of the modular bifurcated variety, although some RAAA patients have been treated with unibody

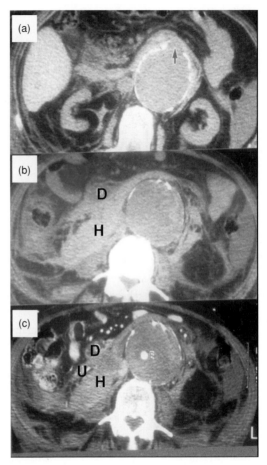

Figure 23.1 CT scan preoperatively ((a) and (b)) and 4 days after insertion of an aortounifemoral graft (MEGS) (c). Postoperatively all contrast was contained within the graft and the RAAA was excluded. Note resolution of the retroperitoneal hemorrhage (H). D is the duodenum and U is the ureter containing contrast.

devices. A key requirement is that a large inventory of devices be on hand so that anatomic variations can be properly managed and the adverse events that inevitably occur can be dealt with. Maintaining such a large inventory of devices can be expensive, particularly if modular bifurcated devices are to be used.

For that reason, there are advantages to using a unilateral aortoiliac or aortofemoral endograft in conjunction with contralateral iliac occlusion and a femorofemoral bypass, and much of the early EVRAR experience employed devices with this configuration. Such devices can be unibody or modular. They offer the additional advantage that the

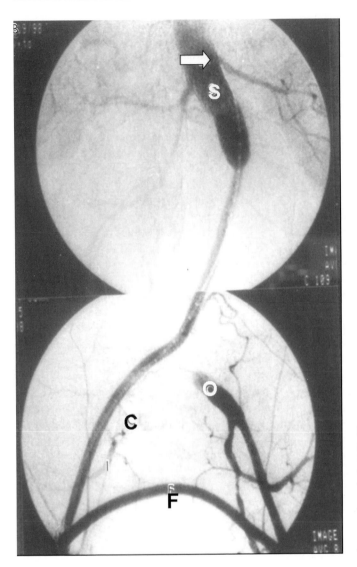

Figure 23.2 Completion arteriogram in patient shown in Fig. 23.1 after placement of an aortounifemoral endovascular graft, an occluder (O) in the left common iliac artery and coils (C) in the right hypogastric artery. A femorofemoral bypass (F) has also been performed. S is the proximal Palmaz stent. The arrow points to the top of the graft.

aneurysm will be largely depressurized once the graft is deployed.

Current RAAA management protocol

Most centers require RAAA patients to be stable enough to undergo a computerized tomographic (CT) scan to confirm the rupture and allow a decision to be made that the patient is a suitable endovascular graft candidate. We do not adhere to that requirement although more than one-half of our RAAA patients have had a CT scan performed either in our own institution or elsewhere. Our current RAAA management protocol is as follows: Once a presumed diagnosis of a RAAA is made [21], the

patient is rapidly transported to the operating room which must have full digital fluoroscopy capacity (OEC, model no. 9800), a radiolucent movable operating table and a large inventory of endovascular supplies (catheters, guidewires, sheaths, stents, and endovascular grafts). As the patient is being prepared for the procedure, fluid is restricted as outlined above. Intravenous and intraarterial lines are placed. Tubes are placed in the bladder and stomach. The patient is positioned, prepared, and draped with the right arm extended and the right antecubital fossa, lower chest, abdomen, and thighs exposed. The fluoroscope is placed on the patient's left side. Under local anesthesia, a 7-Fr sheath is placed in the femoral artery or a 5-Fr sheath is placed percutaneously in the right brachial. Through either of these sheaths a catheter and guidewire are manipulated into the supraceliac aorta. Using a pigtailed catheter in the suprarenal aorta, an abdominal aortogram is performed with posteroanterior and oblique views to define the aneurysm neck and iliac artery anatomy. A decision is made whether the patient is suitable for endovascular repair or will require an open repair. This decision is based on a number of factors including the patient's anatomy and the type of endograft available.

If an *open repair* is required, the guidewire is replaced in the supraceliac aorta. Anesthesia is induced and the open repair performed in a standard fashion. If the patient has cardiovascular collapse, a 14- or 16-Fr sheath is placed over the guidewire followed by a 33- or 40-cm compliant balloon (Meditech). Under fluoroscopic control the balloon is placed and inflated in the infrarenal neck of the aneurysm, if it is long enough. Balloon inflation is monitored fluoroscopically using dilute contrast to fill the balloon until the aorta is occluded. If the proximal neck is short, the balloon is placed and inflated in the supraceliac aorta. In this position every effort must be made to minimize balloon inflation time and to obtain infrarenal clamp control as soon as possible. Systemic heparin is administered when the aorta is occluded.

If an *endovascular repair* is to be performed, it may in some instances be carried out under local anesthesia [22]. However, we have found that RAAA patients move about on the operating table, making accurate fluoroscopic localization and graft deployment difficult. We have therefore chosen general anesthesia in most of our RAAA patients. Large sheath and balloon placement is only carried out if required by the patient's cardiovascular collapse, since these maneuvers can damage the brachial artery and the presence of the inflated balloon can complicate placement of the endograft.

Experience with EVRAR

Since 1994 we have used endovascular techniques to treat 47 patients with RAAAs. In the first 12 cases, endovascular graft repair was performed only in patients who were considered prohibitive risks for open repair because of a hostile abdomen, medical comorbidities or both. All these patients had preoperative CT scans although several were hemodynamically unstable at the time of their repair [9, 13].

In 1996 we adopted the current management protocol described above. With two exceptions when staff and facilities were unavailable, all patients with RAAAs seen by our service between 1996 and the present were managed according to this protocol. These 35 patients plus the original 12 patients constitute our total experience [13, 14]. Of these 35 patients, 8 had unsuitable anatomy for EVRAR. All eight survived their open operation. Only three required suprarenal balloon control.

The remaining 39 patients (12 plus 27) were acceptable for EVRAR and had an endograft placed. Although 25 of these patients received a Montefiore endovascular grafting system (MEGS) aortounifemoral graft (Fig. 23.2(b)) [9, 13, 14], the 14 remaining patients were treated with a commercially available graft. Of the 39 patients undergoing EVRAR, 34 survived and were discharged from the hospital with their aneurysm excluded. Only 9 of the 39 patients undergoing EVRAR required balloon control during their procedure. Three of the thirty-four survivors required evacuation of their perianeurysmal hematoma because of abdominal compartment syndrome. One surviving patient developed a late (1 year) type I endoleak that was successfully treated by placement of a second MEGS graft. There have been no other endoleaks although one patient required open conversion for endotension with an enlarging painful aneurysm.

Other experience with EVRAR

Increasing numbers of EVRARs are being performed throughout the world using a variety of grafts, mostly commercially available. We are in the process of summarizing the results of these procedures. Although there clearly is case selection in the performance of these procedures, the operative mortality of 20% is considerably below the 35–70% range reported for open RAAA repair. Clearly EVRAR avoids many of the problems which are associated with open RAAA repair and which contribute to the high mortality associated with this procedure. These problems include increased blood loss associated with release of tamponade, retroperitoneal dissection, and inadvertent venous injury; injury to other retroperitoneal structures including the duodenum and the ureters; hypothermia associated with hypotension and laparatomy and the impaired blood coagulability common in the RAAA setting.

Conclusions

1 Hypotensive hemostasis with fluid restriction is effective in many patients with a RAAA and is helpful in the management of this entity.

2 Fluoroscopically monitored proximal aortic balloon control can be obtained under local anesthesia. It is an advantageous method whether the definitive repair is performed open or with an endograft.

3 Proximal aortic control is only required in one-third of patients with a RAAA provided hypotensive hemostasis is used.

4 EVRAR is feasible.

5 Preliminary results give promise that EVRAR will lower the morbidity and mortality rates of treatment for RAAA.

6 EVRAR will likely become the gold standard for treating the majority of patients with a RAAA.

References

1 Johansen K, Kohler TR, Nicholls SC *et al*. Ruptured abdominal aortic aneurysm: The Harbor view experience. J Vasc Surg 1991; **13**: 240–247.

2 Gloviczki P, Pairolero PC, Mucha P. Ruptured abdominal aortic aneurysms: Repair should not be denied. J Vascular Surg 1992; **15**: 851–859.

3 Marty-Ane CH, Alric P, Picot MC *et al*. Ruptured abdominal aortic aneurysm: Influence of intraoperative management on surgical outcome. J Vasc Surg 1995; **22**: 780–786.

4 Darling RC, Cordero JA, Chang BB. Advances in the surgical repair of ruptured abdominal aortic aneurysms. Cardiovasc Surg 1996; **4**: 720–723.

5 Dardik A, Burleyson GP, Bowman H *et al*. Surgical repair of ruptured abdominal aortic aneurysms in the state of Maryland: Factors influencing outcome among 527 recent cases. J Vasc Surg 1998; **28**: 413–423.

6 Noel AA, Gloviczki P, Cherry KJ, Jr. *et al*. Ruptured abdominal aortic aneurysms: The excessive mortality rate of conventional repair. J Vasc Surg 2001; **34**: 41–46.

7 Marin ML, Veith FJ, Cynamon J *et al*. Initial experience with transluminally placed endovascular grafts for the treatment of complex vascular lesions. Ann Surg 1995; **222**: 1–17.

8 Yusuf SW, Whitaker SC, Chuter TA, Wenham PW, Hopkinson BR. Emergency endovascular repair of leaking aortic aneurysm. Lancet 1994; **344**: 1645.

9 Ohki T, Veith FJ, Sanchez LA *et al*. Endovascular graft repair of ruptured aorto-iliac aneurysms. J Am Coll Surg 1999; **189**: 102–123.

10 Andresen AFR. Management of gastric hemorrhage. NY State Med J 1948; **48**: 603–611.

11 Shaftan GW, Chiu CJ, Dennis C *et al*. Fundamentals of physiologic control of arterial hemorrhage. Surgery 1968; **58**: 851–856.

12 Bickell WH, Wall MJ, Jr., Pepe PE *et al*. Immediate versus delayed fluid resuscitation for hypotensive patients with penetrating torso injuries. N Engl J Med 1994; **331**: 1105–1109.

13 Veith FJ, Ohki T. Endovascular approaches to ruptured infrarenal aorto-iliac aneurysms. J Cardiovasc Surg 2002; **43**: 369–378.

14 Ohki T, Veith FJ. Endovascular grafts and other image guided catheter based adjuncts to improve the treatment of ruptured aortoiliac aneurysms. Ann Surg 2000; **232**: 466–479.

15 Hesse FG, Kletschka HD. Rupture of abdominal aortic aneurysm: Control of hemorrhage by intraluminal balloon tamponade. Ann Surg 1962; **155**: 320–322.

16 Hyde GL, Sullivan DM. Fogarty catheter tamponade of ruptured abdominal aortic aneurysms. Surg Gynecol Obstet 1982; **154**: 197–199.

17 Greenberg RK, Srivastava SD, Ouriel K *et al*. An endoluminal method of hemorrhage control and repair of ruptured abdominal aortic aneurysms. J Endovasc Ther 2000; **7**: 1–7.

18 Malina M, Veith FJ, Ivancev K, Sonesson B. Balloon occlusion of the aorta during endovascular repair of ruptured aortic aneurysm. J Endovasc Ther 2005; **12**: 556–559.

19 Yusuf SW, Whitaker SC, Chuter TAM *et al*. Early results of endovascular aortic aneurysm surgery with aortouniiliac graft, contralateral iliac occlusion, and femorofemoral bypass. J Vasc Surg 1997; **25**: 165–172.

20 Yusuf SW, Hopkinson BR. It is feasible to treat contained aortic aneurysm rupture by stent-graft combination? In: Greenhalgh RM, ed. *Indications in Vascular and Endovascular Surgery*, WB Saunders, London, 1998: 153–165.

21 Veith FJ. Emergency abdominal aortic aneurysm surgery. Compr Ther 1992; **18**: 25–29.

22 Lachat ML, Pfammatter T, Witzke HJ *et al*. Endovascular repair with bifurcated stent-grafts under local anaesthesia to improve outcome of ruptured aortoiliac aneurysms. Eur J Vasc Endovasc Surg 2002; **23**: 528–536.

CHAPTER 24

Postoperative imaging surveillance and endoleak management after endovascular repair of thoracic aortic aneurysms

S. William Stavropoulos, & Jeffrey P. Carpenter

Endovascular repair offers a subset of thoracic aortic aneurysm (TAA) patients a less invasive technique to exclude their aneurysm [1–7]. It has also altered the manner in which patients are followed after TAA repair. While minimal imaging is required after open surgical repair, patients undergoing endovascular TAA repair require life-long postoperative surveillance imaging [1–8] to detect some of the unique complications of endovascular TAA repair. These include endoleak formation, stent-graft fracture, stent-graft migration, and neck dilation [8–10]. Although the detection and management of endoleaks following endovascular abdominal aortic aneurysm repair (EVAR) has been well described, less is known about endoleaks after endovascular repair of TAAs [8–12]. This chapter discusses strategies for postoperative surveillance imaging and endoleak management in patients following endovascular repair of TAAs.

Endoleak classification

Endoleaks are defined as blood flow outside the lumen of the stent graft but within the aneurysm sac. An endoleak classification system has evolved over the last several years in which endoleaks are organized into five categories based on the source of the blood flow [13, 14].

Type 1 endoleaks have flow that originates from either the proximal or distal stent-graft attachment site. Separation between the stent graft and the native arterial wall creates a direct communication with the systemic arterial circulation. This is the most common type of endoleak seen after endovascular TAA repair. Type 2 endoleaks occur from retrograde aortic branch vessel blood flow into the aneurysm sac, when blood travels through branches from the nonstented portion of the aorta through anastomotic connections into vessels with a direct communication with the aneurysm sac. These are the most common endoleaks seen after EVAR. Type 3 endoleaks occur when there is a structural failure with the stent graft, including holes in the stent-graft fabric, stent-graft fractures, and junctional separations that can occur with modular devices. Type 4 endoleaks are identified at the time of implantation during the immediate postimplantation angiogram, when patients are fully anticoagulated. These endoleaks are caused by stent-graft porosity. They require no specific intervention except the normalization of the coagulation profile. Endotension, sometimes called a type 5 endoleak, refers to expansion of the aneurysm without the presence of an endoleak. Although the exact etiology of endotension is unknown, causes may include an undiagnosed endoleak, ultrafiltration, or thrombus providing an ineffective barrier to pressure transmission [12–14].

Imaging surveillance after endovascular TAA repair

Lifelong imaging surveillance of patients following endovascular TAA repair is critical to determine the long-term success of this procedure. Computed tomography angiography (CTA) has been the primary imaging modality for postoperative surveillance. At our institution, CTA is performed at 30 days, 6 months, and then annually for the life of the patient. Magnetic resonance angiography (MRA) may also be used for postprocedure surveillance when MR-compatible stent grafts are used for the TAA repair [15]. Ultrasound (US) is used for post-EVAR surveillance [16, 17], and can be used following endovascular TAA repair; however, US is more difficult to perform in the chest than in the abdomen due to artifact from the ribs and lungs. Transesophageal echocardiography has been used to assist in placement of thoracic aorta stent grafts and can be used to detect endoleak after the procedure [18, 19]. The technique is invasive, however, and is generally not relied upon for long-term surveillance. It is particularly useful in the case of aortic dissection. TEE is at greatest advantage in the most proximal aorta and clearly defines the true and false lumens and the separating flap with fenestration points. Guide wires can be clearly visualized on TEE images and confirmation of true lumen versus false lumen positioning of wires is helpful during these challenging cases. TEE can be used to examine the proximal attachment zone of a stent graft during the course of the procedure, and can facilitate both accurate proximal deployment and examination for adequacy of seal, using the color-Doppler capabilities of the technique. IVUS provides similar information, but can be positioned anywhere within the circulation, without the limitations of TEE, which is restricted to the more proximal aorta. IVUS is a valuable tool in the treatment of aortic dissection, and is useful in the immediate assessment of endoleak status during the initial stent grafting procedure, but it is impractical as a surveillance method owing to its invasive nature.

The primary goals of postoperative surveillance CTAs are to evaluate for aneurysm expansion or shrinkage, detect stent-graft migration or fracture, and detect endoleaks. Thin section, triple-phase CTA (images obtained before, during, and after contrast administration) is well suited for this job because it is safe, widely available, highly accurate, and fairly straightforward to interpret. The time-resolved nature of the triple-phase imaging gives important information as to when contrast enters and exits the aorta. The characteristic finding of an endoleak on CTA is a collection of contrasts outside the stent-graft lumen and inside the aneurysm sac. The delayed images often give important information, as the accumulated contrast "pools" into the endoleak while the intravascular bolus has already exited the main vessel. Because curvilinear calcifications can appear similar to contrast on some images, noncontrast CT images should be performed prior to CTA. Delayed CT images should also be performed after the CTA because some endoleaks are due to slow perigraft flow and are only seen on the delayed images [20].

MRA is another option for postoperative surveillance, particularly in patients who cannot have CTA because of decreased renal function and/or severe iodinated contrast allergy. MRA has been used to successfully detect endoleaks post-EVAR in patients with stent grafts made from materials such as Nitinol or Elgiloy, which produce little MR artifact due to their low magnetic susceptibility [21]. Because of the large MR artifacts caused by most stainless steel stent grafts, evaluation for potential endoleaks in patients with these devices is very difficult. Newer MR techniques such as blood pool imaging and time-sensitive techniques may make MRA even more sensitive than CTA for endoleak detection and classification in the future [15].

Endoleak management

Series involving stent-graft repair of TAAs have shown that endoleaks occur anywhere from 5% to 20% of patients, which is similar to endoleak incidence following endovascular repair of AAAs [1–10]. Once an endoleak has been confirmed with angiography, management has generally consisted of aggressive endovascular repair of type 1 and type 3 endoleaks, with observation of type 2 endoleaks [3–10, 22].

Type 1 endoleaks can be classified on CTA based on the location of the endoleak in contiguity with the proximal or distal attachment site, as well as early filling of the endoleak sac on the CTA. Catheter angiography is then done to confirm the diagnosis. These leaks are more prevalent in the thoracic than in the abdominal aorta, as the curved nature of the proximal attachment in the aortic arch, and the frequently short attachment zones, present a challenge to sealing. These leaks are usually observed on the initial CT scan following operative repair, but can appear later as a result of migration or failure of the metallic elements within the attachment zone. Failure of proximal or distal sealing can be expected to result in the transmission of systemic pressure to the aneurysm sac, leaving the patient unprotected from fatal rupture of the aneurysm. Therefore, it is essential that type 1 endoleaks be repaired immediately after diagnosis. These leaks can be corrected by securing the attachment sites. Initial attempts at type 1 endoleak repair are made with angioplasty balloons. These large diameter balloons are used to more fully expand the stents, encouraging them to conform to the vessel wall, producing an adequate seal. Balloon inflation in the thoracic aorta produces significant hemodynamic shifts, and careful monitoring and regulation of the blood pressure is essential during this interval. The use of a balloon which allows continual flow through the aorta by means of its trilobe design (W.L. Gore, Flagstaff, AZ) can decrease this hemodynamic effect, but does not eliminate it. If the endoleaks persist, balloon-mounted bare metal stents or stent-graft extensions can be used to secure the proximal or distal attachment sites (Fig. 24.1). Bare stents are useful when the device position is acceptable in the sealing zone, but the vessel wall contact is insufficient. Balloon expandable stents provide a greater radial force than do self-expanding stents, which are contained in the stent graft itself. If, on the other hand, the device does not fully cover the allotted seal zone, the use of a supplemental extension stent graft is preferred, to take full advantage of all available aorta in which a seal may be accomplished. Owing to the lack of available large diameter balloon expandable bare stents, the placement of stent grafts of large diameter within each other can also be performed to increasing the sealing force of a failed attachment zone. If the type 1 endoleak cannot be resolved by endovascular means, open conversion should be considered as this leak is virulent and the patient would not be expected to be protected against aneurysm rupture.

Type 2 endoleaks can be classified with CTA if the endoleak sac cannot be seen communicating with the distal or proximal attachment site or if there was delayed enhancement of the endoleak sac (Fig. 24.2). This can be a difficult diagnosis to confidently make using CTA alone, and may need to

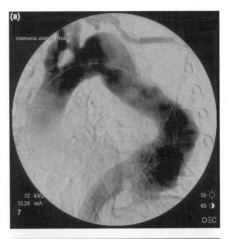

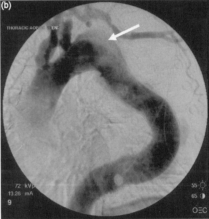

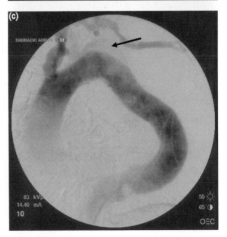

Figure 24.1 (a) DSA exam reveals TAA before stent-graft placement. (b) A stent-graft has been used to treat the TAA. There is a type 1 endoleak (white arrow) filling from the proximal attachment site. (c) A proximal stent-graft extension has been placed to treat the type 1 endoleak. DSA exam reveals a type 4 endoleak (black arrow). No endoleak was seen on 30-day CTA.

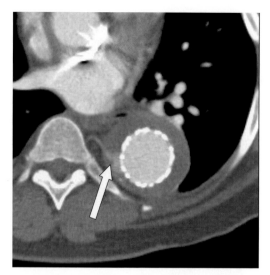

Figure 24.2 A type 2 endoleak is demonstrated on CTA with contrast filling the aneurysm sac (arrow) and in communication with an intercostals artery.

be confirmed with catheter angiography if classification is not certain. If the aneurysm is stable or shrinking in size, patients with type 2 endoleaks should be observed closely. We have not observed any late appearance of type 2 endoleaks, with all of them being appreciated on the initial CT scan following repair. Many type 2 endoleaks will spontaneously thrombose. If the aneurysm is expanding and the patient has an angiographically confirmed

type 2 endoleak, attempts can be made to embolize it. Embolization using coils and n-BCA (n-butyl cyanoacrylate) (Trufill, Cordis, Miami, FL) can be performed percutaneously through a transthoracic approach if a safe window into the aneurysm can be located. Treatment of type 2 endoleaks via transarterial or transthoracic embolization is more difficult than treatment of type 2 endoleaks following AAA repair. This is because collateral circulation in the chest involving the thoracic aorta is not as well developed as the collateral vessels of the abdomen. In addition, accessing the endoleak sac in TAA patients using a direct transthoracic puncture may involve traversing lung. This has greater risk associated with it than translumbar embolization of endoleaks in AAA patients [12, 23].

A type 3 endoleak can be diagnosed on CTA if the endoleak is associated with a junctional separation of two stent-graft sections or a hole in the stent graft diagnosed on multiplanar reformations (MPR) (Fig. 24.3). While some of these leaks are noted on the initial CT scan following repair, many appear later in time and presumably are the result of migration of components or separation of components as the result of conformational changes of the aneurysm sac after repair. Similar to type 1 endoleaks, type 3 endoleaks provide direct communication between systemic arterial blood and the aneurysm sac and are therefore fixed immediately upon diagnosis. Type 3 endoleaks can be corrected

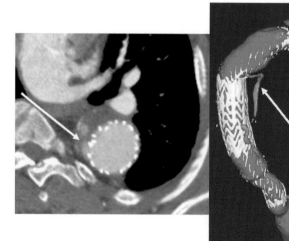

Figure 24.3 A type 3 endoleak between endograft components (arrow) is demonstrated on CTA. The aneurysm sac and contained thrombus are not included in the reconstructed image.

by covering the defect with a stent-graft extension using an endovascular approach.

Type 4 endoleaks are seen during the immediate postdeployment angiogram while a patient is fully anticoagulated with heparin. These leaks are self-limited and resolve once the patient's anticoagulation status has been corrected.

Treatment of type 5 endoleaks or endotension typically requires conversion to open aneurysm repair. Nonoperative management of endotension patients following EVAR has been described [14].

Conclusion

The occurrence of endoleaks after endovascular repair of TAAs remains one of the principal limitations of this procedure. Endoleak detection requires rigorous follow-up with high quality imaging. CTA is currently the most widely used imaging modality for endoleak detection, although MRA and TEE also have an important role, which may expand in the future. After an endoleak has been diagnosed and classified, most can be repaired using endovascular techniques.

References

1 Morishita K, Kurimoto Y, Kawaharada N *et al.* Descending thoracic aortic rupture: Role of endovascular stent-grafting. Ann Thorac Surg 2004; **78**: 1630–1634.

2 Amabile P, Collart F, Gariboldi V, Rollet G, Bartoli J, Piquet P. Surgical versus endovascular treatment of traumatic thoracic aortic rupture. J Vasc Surg 2004; **40**: 873–879.

3 Makaroun M, Dillavou E, Kee S *et al.* Endovascular treatment of thoracic aortic aneurysms: Results of the phase II multicenter trial of the GORE TAG thoracic endoprosthesis. J Vasc Surg 2005; **41**: 1–9.

4 Leurs L, Bell R, Degrieck Y, Thomas S, Hobo R, Lundbom J. Endovascular treatment of thoracic aortic diseases: Combined experience from the EUROSTAR and United Kingdom Thoracic Endograft registries. J Vasc Surg 2004; **40**: 670–680.

5 Farber M, Criado F, Hill C. Endovascular repair of non-traumatic ruptured thoracic aortic pathologies. Ann Vasc Surg 2005; **19**: 167–171.

6 Bortone A, DeCillis E, D'Agostino D, Schinosa LdLT. Endovascular treatment of thoracic aortic disease, four years of experience. Circulation. 2004; **110**(Suppl II): II-262–267.

7 Brandt M, Hussel K, Walluscheck K *et al.* Stent-graft repair versus open surgery for the descending aorta: A case-control study. J Endovasc Ther 2004; **11**(5): 535–538.

8 Hansen C, Bui H, Donayre C *et al.* Complications of endovascular repair of high-risk and emergent descending thoracic aortic aneurysms and dissections. J Vasc Surg 2004; **40**(2): 228–234.

9 Grabenwoger M, Fleck T, Ehrlich M *et al.* Secondary surgical interventions after endovascular stent-grafting of the thoracic aorta. Eur J Cardiothorac Surg 2004; **26**(3): 608–613.

10 Barkhordarian R, Kyriakides C, Mayet J, Clark M, Cheshire N. Transoesophageal echocardiogram identifying the source of endoleak after combined open/endovascular repair of a type 3 thoracoabdominal aortic aneurysm. Ann Vasc Surg 2004; **18**(2): 264–269.

11 Stavropoulos S, Baum R. Imaging modalities for the detection and management of endoleaks. Sem Vasc Surg 2004; **17**(2): 154–160.

12 Baum R, Stavropoulos S, Fairman R, Carpenter J. Endoleaks after endovascular repair of abdominal aortic aneurysms. J Vasc Interv Rad 2003; **14**: 1111–1117.

13 Veith FJ, Baum RA, Ohki T, Amor M, Adiseshiah M, Blankensteijn JD *et al.* Nature and significance of endoleaks and endotension: Summary of opinions expressed at an international conference. J Vasc Surg 2002; **35**(5): 1029–1035.

14 Mennander A, Pimenoff G, Heikkinen M, Partio T, Zeitlin R, Salenius JP. Nonoperative approach to endotension. J Vasc Surg 2005; **42**: 194–198.

15 Lookstein RA, Goldman J, Pukin L, Marin ML. Time-resolved magnetic resonance angiography as a noninvasive method to characterize endoleaks: Initial results compared with conventional angiography. J Vasc Surg 2004; **39**: 27–33.

16 McWilliams RG, Martin J, White D, Gould DA, Rowlands PC, Haycox A *et al.* Detection of endoleak with enhanced ultrasound imaging: Comparison with biphasic computed tomography. J Endovasc Ther 2002; **9**(2): 170–179.

17 Wolf YG, Johnson BL, Hill BB, Rubin GD, Fogarty TJ, Zarins CK. Duplex ultrasound scanning versus computed tomographic angiography for postoperative evaluation of endovascular abdominal aortic aneurysm repair. J Vasc Surg 2000; **32**(6): 1142–1148.

18 Swaminathan M, Lineberger CK, McCann RL, Mathew JP. The importance of intraoperative transesophageal echocardiography in endovascular repair of thoracic aortic aneurysms. Anesth Analg 2003; **97**: 1566–1572.

19 Barkhordarian R, Kyriakides C, Mayet J, Clark M, Cheshire N. Transesophageal echocardiogram identifying the source of endoleak after combined open/endovascular

repair of a type 3 thoracoabdominal aortic aneurysm. Ann Vasc Surg 2004; **18**: 246–249.

20 Rosenblitz AM, Patlas M, Rosenbaum AT *et al.* Detection of endoleaks after endovascular repair of abdominal aortic aneurysms: Value of unenhanced and delayed CT acquisitions. Radiology 2003; **227**(2): 426–433.

21 Insko EK, Kulzer LM, Fairman RM, Carpenter JP, Stavropoulos SW. MR imaging for the detection of endoleaks in recipients of abdominal aortic stent grafts with low magnetic susceptibility. Acad Radiol 2003; **10**(5): 509–513.

22 Criado FJ, Abul-Khoudoud OR, Domer GS *et al.* Endovascular repair of the thoracic aorta: Lessons learned. Ann Thorac Surg 2005; **80**: 857–863.

23 Baum R, Carpenter JP, Golden M *et al.* Treatment of type 2 endoleaks after endovascular repair of abdominal aortic aneurysms: Comparison of transarterial and translumbar techniques. J Vasc Surg 2002; **35**(2): 23–29.

CHAPTER 25

Percutaneous repair of abdominal aortic aneurysms with local anesthesia and conscious sedation

Zvonimir Krajcer, Neil E. Strickman, Ali Mortazavi, &
Kathryn Dougherty

The rapid evolution of transcatheter devices for the delivery of vascular endoprostheses has given nonsurgical interventional radiologists and cardiologists the opportunity to get involved in the vascular surgical arena. Endovascular techniques have clearly been shown to decrease operative morbidity, patient discomfort, hospital stay, intensive care unit stay, blood loss, and the time needed to return to normal activities [1].

Until recently, the major limiting factor preventing wider use of endoluminal techniques has been stiff, large-bore stent-graft systems that preclude patients with anatomical complexities. With the advent of lower profile and more flexible stent-graft systems, endovascular aneurysm repair (EVAR) can be easily performed in a greater number of patients with complex anatomy.

The standard technique of EVAR involves bilateral groin incisions to expose and repair the femoral arteries. This procedure is commonly performed with the use of general or epidural anesthesia. This increases the invasiveness of the procedure and the risks of the complications. The complications that are associated with surgical access and repair of the femoral arteries include blood loss, infection, hematoma, lypmhocele, femoral neuropathy, prolonged pain, and restricted mobility. These complications have been reported to occur in up to 17% of patients [1–5].

Percutaneous EVAR experience in the cardiac catheterization laboratory with the use of a Prostar XL^{TM} percutaneous suture device (Perclose, Inc., Menlo Park, CA) for 16 F and 22 F sheaths has previously been reported [6]. This report describes the technique and our experience with percutaneous EVAR using local anesthesia and conscious sedation in a large patient population.

EVAR stent-graft systems

Currently, there are four devices approved for endoluminal AAA repair. They include AneuRx^{TM} (Medtronic, Santa Rosa, CA), Excluder^{TM} (WL Gore & Assoc, Temple, AZ), Zenith$^{®}$ (Cook, Inc, Bloomington, IN), and Powerlink$^{®}$ (Endologix, Sunnyvale, CA). Each device is unique and offers different materials, stent designs, and delivery system diameters. They also have different modes of deployment. The Powerlink device has a unibody system, while the other three have a modular design. The modular design requires that the main body is delivered through a larger sheath, while an iliac limb endoprosthesis is delivered via a smaller sheath, using the contralateral femoral artery. The device diameters range from 18 F to 21 F for the main body, while the iliac artery limb devices range from 12 F to 18 F. Some of the delivery devices can be introduced via percutaneous femoral artery approach (AneuRx Expediant), while the others should be introduced into the femoral artery via proprietary sheaths (Zenith, Powerlink, and Excluder).

Technique of percutaneous femoral artery repair with the Prostar XL™ device

All patients receive a dose of intravenous antibiotics prior to EVAR and for 24 h after. The patients also receive aspirin 325 mg/a day and clopidogrel 75 mg/a day for 1 month following the procedure. Intraprocedural conscious sedation with midolazam (0.5–1.0 mg IV increments) and fentanyl (25–50 mcg IV increments) are administered as needed. A vascular surgeon and anesthesiologist are always on standby for EVAR procedures in the event that surgical conversion or repair is needed although neither are present thoughout the procedure.

After the patient has been prepped and draped in sterile surgical fashion, the subcutaneous groin tissue is infiltrated with 10 cc of 2% Lidocaine bilaterally. Both common femoral arteries (CFA) are then accessed percutaneously using the modified front wall puncture, with Seldinger technique and 6 F sheaths are inserted. The femoral access sites are then connected to dual 3-port manifold systems for constant arterial pressure monitoring. The manifold system also allows flushing of heparinized saline during catheter and device exchanges to minimize blood loss and controls contrast usage throughout the procedure.

Once bilateral femoral access is obtained, low dose heparinization is administered and an abdominal arteriogram is performed using calibrated pigtail catheter (1 cm radiopaque markers), nonionic contrast, and digital subtraction angiography. This allows for precise measurements with regard to the length between the lowest renal artery and the aortic bifurcation and the length between the aortic bifurcation and both internal iliac arteries. To perform total percutaneous EVAR the "preclose" sutures with a 10 F Prostar XL (Abbott Vascular Devices, Redwood City, CA) must be deployed after initial 6 F access is obtained and prior to insertion of the large bore sheaths. Each stent-graft system uses different sheaths.

The skin above the CFA access sites is widened with a scalpel to 1 cm, and the subcutaneous tissues are bluntly dissected with a hemostat. The 6 F sheath is then removed over a 0.035″ delte hydrophilic guide wire and a 10 F Prostar XL™

device is advanced into the CFA (Fig. 25.1a). When pulsatile blood flow is seen through the marker lumen, the needles are deployed and the suture is delivered through the vessel wall (Fig. 25.1b). The needles and sutures are then removed from the PVS device hub (Fig. 25.1c) and the suture is cut from needles. The sutures are secured with hemostats and laid to the side until completion of the procedure (Fig. 25.1d). The PVS device is removed from the femoral artery over a wire, and an 11 F sheath is inserted. This same procedure is performed on the contralateral CFA. Once the Prostar XL sutures have been delivered to both CFAs, additional heparin anticoagulation is given to maintain an Activated Clotting Time of 200–300 s. An exchange length super stiff Amplatz guide wire (Cook Inc., Bloomington, IN) or similar stiff wire is placed through the arterial sheath in the CFA and advanced to the descending thoracic aorta under constant fluoroscopic visualization. Either a 5 F (65 cm) multipurpose (MP) or a 4 or 5 F RDC (renal double curve) is used to facilitate guide wire exchanges (from the more flexible "J" for the stiffer guide wires used to deploy the stent-graft system). Progressive arterial dilation is then performed first on the primary (bifurcated stent-graft) femoral artery. When using the 18 F stent-graft system, a 14 F, 16 F, and 18 F dilators (Cook Inc., Bloomington, IN) are used prior to placement of the 18 F sheath. When using the larger devices a 20 F dilator may be required. The use of dilators offers gradual dilatation of the access site, therefore reducing the risk of arterial laceration. It also offers an inexpensive way to determine if the delivery device of a selected stent-graft system will accommodate the femoral and iliac arteries. The stent-graft system should only be opened after the appropriate dilator has been easily advanced through the iliac artery.

The 4 or 5 F RDC catheter is used to cannulate the lowest renal artery to ensure precise stent-graft deployment. The RDC is then pulled back down into the aorta just prior to deployment. Once the stent graft has been deployed, the attachment sites (proximal, distal bilaterally, and the gate of the contralateral limb) should be dilated with an appropriate size balloon to ensure fixation and approximation with the aortic and iliac vessel wall. An aortic occlusion balloon (20–32 mm in diameter and 2 cm in length) is inflated at low pressure (enough to

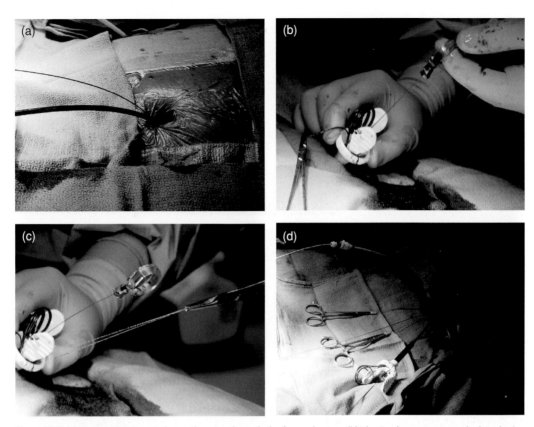

Figure 25.1 (a) Prostar XL is inserted over-the-wire through the femoral artery. (b) The Perclose sutures are deployed prior to the insertion of large bore sheaths. (c) Once the sutures have been deployed the needles are removed from the device. (d) The sutures are then placed to the side using hemostats and the Perclose device is removed over the wire.

dampen arterial pressure) at each attachment site. Note: Meticulous attention should be placed on balloon positioning keeping the edges of the balloon within the stent graft to avoid damage to the normal vessel wall. Note: Because the occlusion balloons are so large, a 70% saline: 30% contrast should be used for the inflation medium. This will allow quicker inflate and deflate times.

After the final arteriogram is performed and EVAR is complete, the subcutaneous tissue surrounding both CFA sheath entry sites is infiltrated with 10cc's of 1% lidocaine with epinephrine (1:100,000) bilaterally. The sheath is removed over the 0.035″ hydrophilic wire while guide wire position is maintained, and the Prostar XL™ sutures are tied with the sliding knot technique (Fig. 25.2(a)). A knot pusher (Perclose, Inc., Menlo Park, CA) is used to advance and secure the knots to the CFA

entry site (Fig. 25.2(b)). Once suture knots are secure, the guide wire is removed. After achieving hemostasis, the sutures are cut, and the incision edges are approximated with adhesive steri-strips (Fig. 25.3). Both CFA entry sites are cleaned and dressed with a sterile nonadhering pad and clear dressing. Five pound sandbags are placed on each entry site for 4 h following the procedure in situations of minor bleeding or hematoma. For suboptimal hemostasis an Arterial Tamper (Perclose, Inc., Menlo Park, CA, Fig. 25.4) can be inserted over the sutures and locked into position for 1–2 h or a FemoStop (RADI Medical Systems, Wilmington, MA) can be used, usually at 40 mm Hg for 2–4 h. The patient is kept at bed rest for 4–6 h with their legs straight for 4 h. After bed rest the patients can ambulate under observation. Protamine is used to reverse the effects of heparin.

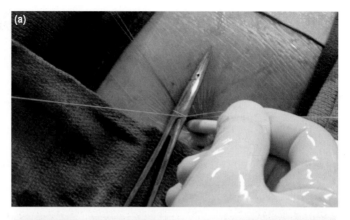

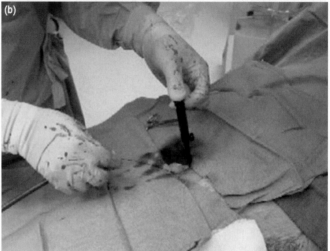

Figure 25.2 (a) Upon completion of the procedure the Perclose knots are tied using the sliding knot technique. (b) A knot pusher is used to advance and secure the sutures to the femoral artery.

Texas Heart® Institute results

A total of 913 EVAR procedures were performed in the endovascular suite of the cardiac catheterization laboratories at our institution. Percutaneous EVAR was attempted in 724 (79.2%) patients, of which local anesthesia and conscious sedation was used in 465 (64.2%). The majority (90%) of patients were male with a mean age of 72 ± 10 years. Most of the patients (98%) were Anesthesia Society

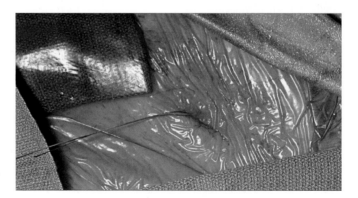

Figure 25.3 Once the knots are secure the wire is removed and the sutures are cut after hemostasis is obtained.

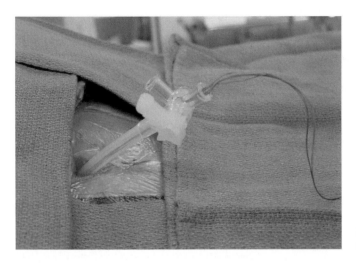

Figure 25.4 If hemostasis is inadequate then an arterial tamper can be used.

Class III and IV and suffered from multiple comorbid conditions (Table 25.1). EVAR was successful in all patients with the majority undergoing implantation of the Gore Excluder™ stent-graft system (65.1%), followed by AneuRx™ (23.2%), Zenith® (10.3%), and then Powerlink® (1.3%).

Bilateral percutaneous femoral artery closure was successful in 89.2% of the patients. There were 50 patients (10.7%) who required surgical exposure and repair of one or both femoral access sites, of which 8 (16%) suffered blood loss requiring transfusion (Table 25.2). There were three patients (0.6%) that did not tolerate local anesthesia and conscious sedation and required intubation and general anesthesia after suffering a panic attack.

All three recovered uneventfully and two were discharged from the hospital the following day.

There were four patients (0.8%) who developed psuedoaneurysms at the femoral access site, three were surgically corrected and one underwent ultrasound compression (Table 25.3). There were two patients who had worsening of their renal failure, one of whom died 4 days after the procedure the other was discharged after 3 days of fluid hydration. Another patient with known coronary artery disease and cardiomyopathy suffered a fatal arrhythmia 1 day after successful EVAR and one patient developed intestinal ischemia requiring exploratory laparotomy with bowel resection. The average length of hospital stay was 1.2 ± 2 days. On follow-up, one patient developed a groin infection that was treated with antibiotics.

Conclusion

The technique of percutaneous EVAR using local anesthesia and conscious sedation has further reduced the incidence of complications of this procedure. Further refinements, however, of percutaneous closure devices are needed. In addition, a

Table 25.1 Patient characteristics.

Prior myocardial infarction	51.1%
Congestive heart failure	22.8%
Coronary bypass / coronary angioplasty	62%
Obesity (body mass index >30)	38.6%
Hypertension	90%
Diabetes mellitus	16.2%
Chronic obstructive pulmonary disease	60.1%
Chronic renal failure	24.5%
Peripheral vascular disease	62.1%
Tobacco use	85.8%
Anesthesia society classification	
I–II	0.6%
III	29%
IV	69%

Table 25.2 Procedural complications.

Emergency intubation and general anesthesia	3 (0.6%)
Failed perclose (one or both access sites)	50 (10.7%)
Blood loss requiring transfusion	8 (1.7%)

Table 25.3 Hospital complications.

Groin infection	1 (0.2%)
Femoral psuedoaneurysm	4 (0.8%)
Worsening renal failure	2* (0.4%)
Intestinal ischemia	1 (0.2%)
Hospital mortality	2 (0.4%)
Fatal arrhythmia	1 (0.2%)
Renal failure	1* (0.2%)

further decrease in profile of the stent-graft delivery systems is also needed to simplify this procedure and offer it to a broader number of patients and to interventionalist who can perform EVAR.

References

1 Zarins C, White R, Schwarten D *et al.*, for the investigators of the Medtronic AneuRx Multicenter Clinical Trial. AneuRx stent graft versus open surgical repair of abdominal aortic aneurysms: Multicenter prospective clinical trial. J Vasc Surg 1999; **29**: 292–308.

2 May J, White G, Yu W *et al.* Concurrent comparison of endoluminal versus open repair in the treatment of abdominal aortic aneurysms: Analysis of 303 patients by life table method. J Vasc Surg 1998; **27**: 213–221.

3 Brewst D, Geller S, Kaufman J *et al.* Initial experience with endovascular aneurysm repair: Comparison of early results with outcome of conventional open repair. J Vasc Surg. 1998; **27**: 213–221.

4 Chutter TA, Wendt G, Hopkinson BR *et al.* Tranfemoral insertion of a bifurcated endovascular graft for aortic aneurysm repair: The first 22 patients. J Cardiovasc Surg 1995; **3**: 121–128.

5 Mialhe C, Amicable C, Becquemin JP. Endovascular treatment of infrarenal abdominal aortic aneurysms by the Stentor system: Preliminary results in 79 cases. J Vasc Surg 1997; **26**: 199–209.

6 Howell M, Villareal R, Krajcer Z. Percutaneous access and closure of femoral artery access sites associated with endoluminal repair of abdominal aortic aneurysms. J Endovasc Ther 2001; **8**: 68–74.

CHAPTER 26

Endoleak management in the abdominal aorta

Jennifer L. Ash, Syed M. Hussain, & Kim J. Hodgson

Introduction

Endovascular abdominal aortic aneurysm repair (EVAR) was introduced in 1990 by Parodi *et al.* [1] as a minimally invasive option for the treatment of abdominal aortic aneurysms (AAAs). Through the deployment of an indwelling interposition graft within the aneurysm sac, EVAR aims to prevent aneurysm enlargement and rupture by excluding the aneurysm from the arterial circulation. The procedure utilizes a stent-supported graft that serves as a simple blood flow conduit within the aneurysm sac while providing for attachment and seal to normal vessels proximal and distal to the aneurysm. Though simple in concept and performed with extremely high success and low complication rates, EVAR has been plagued from the outset by the need for secondary evaluations and interventions, largely to diagnose and treat endoleaks; the most common, and perhaps most debated, complication following EVAR.

The incidence of endoleak ranges from 8% to 44% in postprocedure EVAR patients [2], but since many early endoleaks resolve spontaneously, far fewer actually require invasive evaluation or retreatment. There are four primary types of endoleaks described in the literature: type I (attachment site leaks), type II (branch–vessel leaks), type III (graft integrity defects), and type IV (graft wall porosity) [3]. Regardless of the type of endoleak, all result in at least some degree of maintained aneurysm pressurization and, therefore, at least a theoretically increased risk of aneurysm rupture persists. A phenomenon called endotension, defined as an increase in the intrasac pressure after EVAR without a demonstrable endoleak, is also described in the literature. While the best management of endotension remains obscure and highly individualized, management strategies for endoleaks are more developed and depend upon the location of the leak and its type, as well as on factors such as aneurysm sac expansion. This chapter reviews current strategies available for the management of endoleaks.

Classification of endoleaks

Endoleaks after EVAR represent continued perfusion of the aneurysm sac secondary to one of a number of mechanisms that perpetuate an ongoing communication between the aneurysm sac and the systemic circulation. The previously described classification system categorizes endoleaks based on their etiology or site of origin [4, 5]. Other factors that may relate to the etiology or clinical relevance of the endoleak classify them by their time of onset, with early endoleaks occurring within the first 90 postoperative days, while late endoleaks occur after the first 90 postoperative days. Endoleaks that were first noted at the time of the initial EVAR or on the first post-EVAR CT scan are sometimes referred to as primary endoleaks, while secondary endoleaks occur after not being present at the time of the initial EVAR or initial post-EVAR imaging. The development of a secondary endoleak implies a change in the integrity of the endograft itself, or its fixation and seal to the vessel wall, and is, therefore, felt to be of greater clinical concern.

In type I endoleaks, flow into the aneurysm sac originates from around the stent-graft attachment site. Type I endoleaks are further classified as proximal (type IA), distal (type IB), or iliac occluder (type IC) in origin. Type II endoleaks occur when blood flow enters and leaves the aneurysm sac through collateral routes. Typical sources of this circuitous flow are the inferior mesenteric and lumbar arteries, as well as previously covered accessory renal arteries. Type II endoleaks may be further classified into simple "to-and-fro" (type IIA) endoleaks and complex or flow-through (type IIB) endoleaks. Type III endoleaks occur when there is a defect in the integrity of the stent graft itself. This category includes leaks from the endograft component junctions of modular endografts (type IIIA) and endograft fabric disruption (type IIIB). Type IV endoleaks occur secondary to graft wall porosity and are felt to be transient in nature, usually resolving spontaneously within the first day or so. A final condition, described as endotension, describes maintained pressurization of the aneurysm sac without the demonstrable presence of an endoleak. This puzzling condition may be related to microendoleaks from stent-graft sutures, transudation of serum through graft fabric interstices, or transmission of pressure through thrombotic seals.

Risk factors and prevention

Risk factors that have been associated with the development of type I endoleaks include short or angulated infrarenal aortic necks, a neck length less than 20 mm, and large diameter aortic necks (>28 mm) [6], reinforcing the need for careful patient selection to minimize their occurrence. Ideally, patients should have infrarenal necks longer than 15 mm and a common iliac artery diameter smaller than 18 mm over a minimum continuous length of 15 mm. Heavy or circumferential calcification and thrombus in the attachment zones are other factors that must be considered as they bear on the security of endograft fixation and achievement of a hemostatic seal. All in all, graft fixation is probably the most important factor in preventing both early and late type I endoleaks [7].

Type II endoleaks are more likely to occur and persist in the presence of a patent inferior mesenteric artery or two or more patent lumbar arteries. The IMA or large lumbar arteries can be embolized prior to EVAR to prevent type II endoleaks from occurring. However, this is rarely performed since most patients with patent branch vessels do not develop type II endoleaks and if they do their natural history is often benign. Furthermore, pre-EVAR embolization of lumbar and inferior mesenteric arteries can be quite technically challenging and the required intrasac catheter manipulation risks microembolic atheroembolization. Type III endoleaks secondary to endograft fabric defects have been primarily associated with first generation endovascular stent grafts and are not commonly seen with the endografts in current use. Type III endoleaks related to inadequate seals at modular endograft component junctions are attributed to insufficient overlap between the two components, either due to poor initial placement or due to subsequent endograft migration [8], often associated with post-EVAR aneurysm remodeling (Fig. 26.1).

Natural history of endoleaks

A number of isolated cases of patients with endoleaks who have ruptured an EVAR treated aneurysm have appeared in the literature. A EUROSTAR study published in 2000 reported an annual rupture rate of at least 1% after EVAR [9]. Proximal type I endoleaks and midgraft type II endoleaks were cited as significant risk factors for aneurysm rupture. This study reinforced several previous anecdotal case reports and clinical studies in which incomplete protection of the aneurysm sac against continued growth and rupture was observed.

In a more recent EUROSTAR study, secondary interventions (either endovascular or surgical) were required in 13% (320/2463) of endoleak patients. Ruptures of EVAR-treated aneurysms occurred in 0.52% (1/191) of the type II endoleak group, 3.37% (10/297) of the type I and III endoleak groups, and 0.25% (5/1975) of the no endoleak group at a mean postoperative follow-up of 15.7 months (range, 3–36 months). Analysis of this data demonstrated a higher incidence of conversion to open repair in the type I and III endoleak groups when compared to the other two study groups. One hundred seventy-two patients died during follow-up. Death was related to the aneurysm or to endovascular repair of the aneurysm in 7% of these patients. Causes of death in this group included rupture of the aneurysm, infected endograft, endograft thrombosis, and postoperative death following conversion

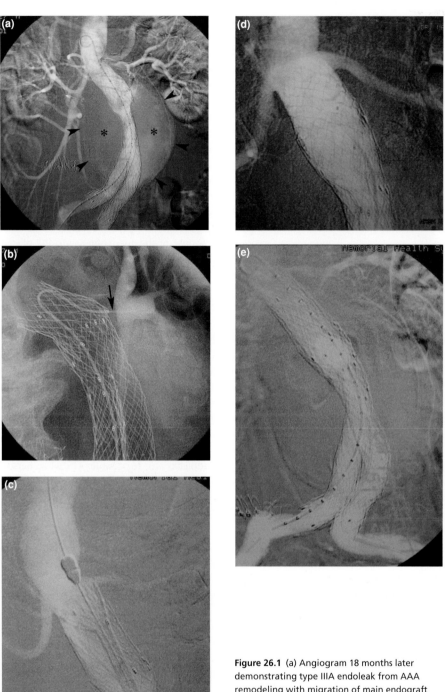

Figure 26.1 (a) Angiogram 18 months later demonstrating type IIIA endoleak from AAA remodeling with migration of main endograft component relative to aortic cuff. Black arrows define AAA wall. Asterisks define contrast within AAA sack. (b) Selective catheterization of gap between endograft components with jet of contrast marked by black arrow. (c) Deployment of an aortic cuff to bridge the endograft component gap. (d) Deployed endograft component seals the gap and leak. (e) Completion angiogram demonstrating no filling of AAA sack.

for a symptomatic, growing aneurysm. Of those patients that died of aneurysm rupture ($n = 8$), six were diagnosed with device-related (type I and III) endoleaks and two were diagnosed with no endoleaks. Secondary outcome success (defined as absence of rupture or conversion to open repair) was significantly higher in both the type II endoleak group and the no endoleak group as compared to the type I and III endoleak groups. The overall conclusion of this study was that device-related endoleaks are associated with an increased risk of aneurysmal rupture and conversion. However, the type II endoleak group, in particular, did not have an increased association with rupture or conversion [10].

Diagnosis

Endoleaks may be detected intraoperatively immediately after the stent is deployed on the intraoperative angiograms routinely performed to assess the success of the EVAR procedure. High-quality digital subtraction angiography (DSA), including high-flow power-injected runs and filming through the venous phase must be performed if endoleaks are to be reliably identified angiographically. If an endoleak is recognized, the etiology of the endoleak may remain uncertain because any type of endoleak can opacify the lumbar and inferior mesenteric arteries, either as inflow or outflow pathways. Injecting at each stent-graft attachment site may be helpful in determining the classification of the endoleak, as can multiple filming projections and high filming frame rates. A thorough review of the angiograms is then necessary to determine the direction of flow in the branch vessels. If the flow in the lumbar or inferior mesenteric arteries is antegrade, then blood is entering the aneurysm sac from another location and the patient likely has an endoleak associated with an attachment site defect. A type II endoleak is conclusively documented when inferior mesenteric and/or lumbar artery blood flow is observed to be in a retrograde direction, filling the aneurysm sac. While CT scanning can fairly reliably detect the presence of an endoleak, the exact nature of the endoleak is not always apparent. Furthermore, on occasion contrast material injected intraprocedurally may not disappear from the aneurysm sac until after the first postoperative day. Consequently, immediate postoperative CT scans can demonstrate

what appears to be an endoleak due to the residual contrast material in the aneurysm sac from the prior day's angiogram and contrast injection. Comparison with the noncontrast CT scan images will detect this condition [11].

Lifelong surveillance of EVAR patients is crucial in monitoring the long-term performance of stent-graft devices [12]. Routine postoperative spiral CT scans obtained before and after IV contrast administration are typically utilized to follow the course of EVAR patients. These studies are performed at regular intervals, customarily at 30 days, 6 months, and annually thereafter for the life of the patient. The images are primarily used to determine the response of the aneurysm sac to the placement of the stent graft. Specifically, CT scans are evaluated for aneurysm expansion or shrinkage and for the presence of endoleaks [13]. The appearance of an endoleak on CT imaging is characteristically seen as a collection of contrast outside the stent-graft lumen, but within the aortic aneurysm sac. Non-contrast images are used to differentiate between an endoleak and calcification within the aneurysm sac. Delayed CT images are also assessed because some endoleaks are caused by slow perigraft flow and are best visualized in this manner [14].

By and large, spiral CT and duplex US are the most important tools for diagnosing postoperative endoleaks [15, 16]. Duplex US, when performed in addition to spiral CT, provides useful hemodynamic information that assists in the characterization of the type of endoleak. Angiography may also be used selectively to define the source of the endoleak when it is otherwise unable to be defined or when further procedures are being considered [6].

Treatment of type I endoleaks

Type I, or attachment site endoleaks, are immediately repaired at the time of the procedure if they are recognized on completion angiography because they represent a direct communication between arterial blood under systemic pressure and the aneurysm sac and therefore, a risk for future rupture. Although spontaneous resolution of type I endoleaks has been documented, Miahle *et al.* reported 20% of type I endoleaks that spontaneously seal go on to reopen at 12 to 18 months [17]. The cause of the endoleak determines the type of intervention needed to correct the failure. If an adequate length of aortic neck has been covered but graft to aortic wall apposition is inadequate due to neck angulation, thrombus, or plaque, simple low pressure balloon angioplasty may be used to improve graft apposition at the proximal fixation site. If neck coverage has been suboptimal and there is room remaining below the renal arteries to extend the endograft cephalad with an aortic cuff, this would be the preferred initial strategy. Sometimes even with no room to extend the endograft, placement of an aortic cuff inside the aortic sealing zone of the endograft may enhance the radial expansion force and achieve a seal where one had been elusive. If a proximal type 1 endoleak persists despite all of these maneuvers, placement of a Palmaz stent across the proximal fixation zone may be effective in resolving it, and this transrenal stenting has been well tolerated (Fig. 26.2).

Other treatment options for type 1 endoleaks include coil or liquid glue embolization of the endoleak cavity and endoleak tract. Maldonado *et al.* reported success rates of 92.3% in type I endoleaks treated with n-butyl 2-cyanoacrylate embolization and of 75% in those treated with coil embolization, with or without the use of thrombin [18]. Ischemic injury to adjacent structures from nontarget embolization is a serious complication that is associated with liquid glue embolic therapy. Some authors suggest that patent outflow vessels should be coil embolized prior to the injection of liquid glue into the aneurysm sac or leak. Additionally, premature polymerization of the glue or delayed withdrawal of the catheter delivery system has resulted in gluing the catheter tip in place. While laparoscopic banding of the deficient apposition zone has been reported, most commonly, failure of the endovascular treatment options leads to conversion to traditional open repair.

Treatment of type II endoleaks

The significance, and therefore the management, of type II endoleaks (branch leaks) continues to be debated. After EVAR, many potential communications exist between aortic branch vessels and the excluded aneurysm sac. If these vessels fail to thrombose, a type II endoleak may occur. Spontaneous sealing of type II endoleaks has been reported

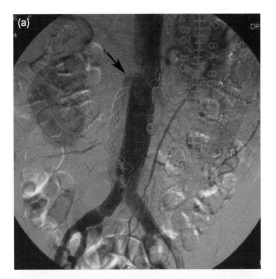

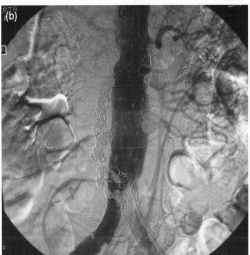

Figure 26.2 (a) Type Ia (proximal attachment zone) endoleak that has failed previous attempts at coil embolization, despite placement of coils within the endoleak cavity itself and along the track. Black arrow defines residual endoleak cavity. (b) Successful treatment by placement of a Palmaz stent across the proximal aspect of the endograft.

to occur within the first six postoperative months in as many as 53% of endoleaks [20]. Intrasac Doppler flow velocities can be used to predict spontaneous resolution of type II endoleaks. Low velocity leaks (≤80 cm/s) have been found to be more likely to seal spontaneously when compared to high velocity leaks (≥100 cm/s) [20]. Typically, high velocity endoleaks are often associated with a large number of branch vessels or with large-diameter branch vessels [19]. The formation of branch vessel endoleaks is often regarded as a dynamic process that may reflect ongoing branch vessel occlusion and recanalization.

Recent evidence, however, suggests that type II endoleaks likely have a relatively benign clinical course and may warrant no more than conservative management with close surveillance. It has been suggested that intervention for type II endoleaks is only required in the face of aneurysm enlargement. This thought process is driven by the belief that the branch vessels responsible for type II endoleaks have a high rate of spontaneous thrombosis and even if persistent, the natural history of type II endoleaks appears relatively benign. When treatment of type II endoleaks is felt to be indicated there are several treatment options, none of which are considered to be universally accepted. Treatment is generally aimed at occluding the inflow and, if possible, outflow vessels via supraselective transarterial embolization, ideally with embolization directly into the endoleak cavity itself as well. While the initial success in obliteration of type II endoleaks with this technique appeared promising, long-term follow-up revealed high rates of recanalization and/or recruitment of other collateral pathways, emphasizing the importance of intrasac endoleak cavity embolization and obliteration.

The supraselective transarterial embolization technique involves the use and manipulation of multiple coaxial catheters and guidewires, typically beginning with the placement of a 5 Fr diagnostic catheter in the origin of the arterial tree involved, the superior mesenteric (Fig. 26.3) or the hypogastric arteries. Microcatheters (3 Fr) and guidewires (0.014″) are then directed through the diagnostic catheter and manipulated through the collateral vessel branches into the terminal vessel that actually communicates with the aneurysm sac, and into the sac itself if possible. The sac and terminal vessel are then embolized, the latter near its communication with the aneurysm sac, in order that perfusion to the spine, colon, and pelvis is preserved while blood flow into and out of the sac itself is ceased. While reports of adjunctive thrombin, particulate, and cyanoacrylate injections are available in the literature, no definitively superior approach has emerged [17, 20–23].

When the pathway to the endoleak precludes successful supraselective catheterization, the endoleak can be approached directly via percutaneous translumbar puncture (Fig. 26.4), guided by the CT scan location of the endoleak relative to radiographic landmarks on the endograft and adjacent boney structures. The patient is placed in the prone position and fluoroscopy of the stent graft is performed in multiple projections for the purposes of orientation. A sheathed needle is then inserted into the aneurysm sac through the flank region at the level of the endoleak and approximately four to five fingerbreadths from the midline. The needle is advanced under fluoroscopic guidance until it passes just anterior to the vertebral body and into the aneurysm sac. Entrance of the needle into the aneurysm sac may be appreciated by tactile feedback or from fluoroscopic visualization as the needle penetrates the typically calcified and visible aortic wall. If the endoleak itself is entered, confirmation by the return of pulsatile blood may be appreciated. Entrance into the aneurysm sac may also be confirmed by opacification of the lumbar arteries or the inferior mesenteric artery on manual injection of contrast material. When the position of the catheter is confirmed under fluoroscopy, the catheter may be used to measure sac pressures. The endoleak cavity

Figure 26.3 (a) Axial CT image demonstrating type II endoleak from inferior mesenteric artery (white arrow). (b) Angiogram demonstrating filling of endoleak (black arrow) via the inferior mesenteric artery (white arrow) from a selective contrast injection into the superior mesenteric artery. (c) Supraselective catheterization of the endoleak with a 3-Fr microcatheter placed through a 5-Fr diagnostic catheter positioned in the superior mesenteric artery. (d) Completion angiogram after supra–selective coil embolization of the endoleak cavity and inferior mesenteric artery demonstrating cessation of filling of the endoleak. (e) One year after initial success at obliteration of type II endoleak, a follow-up CT scan demonstrates filling of an endoleak (black arrow) and a patent segment of inferior mesenteric artery (white arrow). The embolization coils are the bright white dots just deep to the inferior mesenteric artery. (f) Selective angiogram revealing resumed flow through the coil embolized inferior mesenteric artery (white arrow) with filling of an endoleak cavity (black arrow).

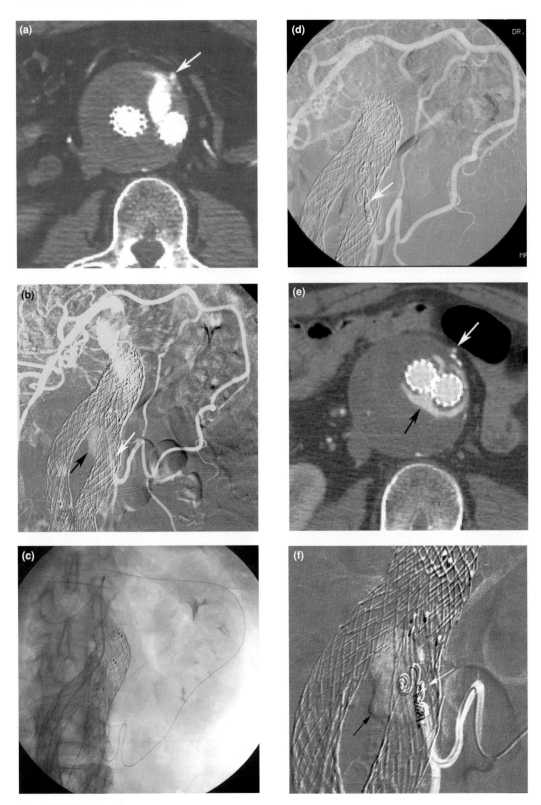

Figure 26.3 (*Continued*)

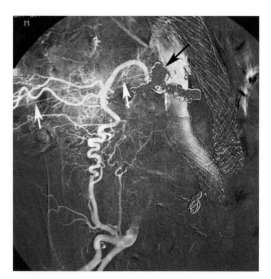

Figure 26.4 Translumbar coil embolization of a type II endoleak whose iliolumbar collateral was too tortuous to selectively catheterize for supraselective coil embolization. White arrows define translumbar needle. Black arrow defines coils placed in endoleak cavity.

may then be embolized through the catheter. Although technically challenging, the catheter may be manipulated or exchanged within the aneurysm sac for a shaped catheter in order that the inferior mesenteric and-/-or lumbar arteries may be selectively cannulated and subsequently embolized. Embolization should continue until there is no further blood return and a static column of contrast is seen on the follow-up films [24]. Commonly used embolic agents include stainless steel coils, platinum coils, thrombin, lipiodol, Gelfoam powder, and liquid embolic agents. Although n-butyl cyanoacrylate (Trufill, Cordis Neurovascular, Miami Lakes, FL) has been used with some success in the treatment of type II endoleaks, this represents an off–label use of this product, and complications with the use of this agent have been reported, typically related to the previously mentioned non–target vessel occlusions and catheter tip incorporation in the glue plug in the endoleak [25].

If all else fails, laparoscopic branch vessel clipping remains an option, but requires general anesthesia and is more invasive than the other alternative techniques and so is generally the option of last choice. The aorta and aneurysm sac are approached laparoscopically in the retroperitoneal plane. The lumbar arteries and the inferior mesenteric artery are then identified and clipped [26]. More recently, van Nes, et al, have reported a technique that combines laparoscopic clipping of the aortic branch vessels with laparoscopic fenestration of the aneurysm sac [27]. In this technique, after all of the branch vessels are clipped, the sac is fenestrated by a large incision and all of the fluid and thrombus are subsequently removed. Whenever feasible, an omental flap is then placed in the sac so that recurrent fluids can drain. Theoretically, the laparoscopic approach may also allow for the measurement of sac pressures via a laparoscopic needle.

Treatment of type III and type IV endoleaks

Type III endoleaks are associated with a high rate of aneurysm sac rupture [28] but were mostly seen with first generation endografts, being relatively uncommon with the endografts in use today. Modular limb disconnection and fabric disruption are the two primary types of type III endoleaks. Insufficient frictional force can lead to distraction at the junctional zone of the endograft, and subsequently to modular disconnection or graft separation. Migration has also been a problem commonly associated with first generation stent grafts. In addition to compromising the proximal fixation and apposition zone, distal endograft migration often causes graft distraction and can pull the limb out of its attachment zone, ultimately creating a type III endoleak. In many instances, type III endoleaks can be treated with extender cuffs to bridge the defect. Another option includes placing an entirely new endograft inside the old one, essentially relining the old endograft with a new one. If endovascular treatment of the endoleak is not an option or is unsuccessful, conversion to open repair may be the only option.

Type IV endoleaks are seen at the time of completion angiography when the patient is fully anticoagulated, and they are a consequence of either the inherent fabric porosity or suture holes created in construction of the endograft. This type of endoleak is self–limited, as it demonstrates a nearly 100-% seal rate at 1 month [29]. Therefore, no treatment or concern is warranted.

Diagnosis and treatment of endotension

Aneurysm sac enlargement despite no demonstrable endoleak implies the maintained pressurization of the aneurysm and has been termed *endotension*. Typically used thresholds are a >5 mm increase in maximal diameter or a >10% increase in volume of the post-EVAR aneurysm sac without a demonstrable endoleak. If multiple investigations fail to detect an endoleak in the face of an enlarging aneurysm, yet the proximal and distal apposition zones and all endograft component junctions are of adequate length and without significant thrombus, endotension is presumed to be present. Lumbar arteries that are patent up to the aneurysm sac wall, but that do not spill into the sac in the form of an endoleak, may still be responsible for the maintained sac pressurization and should be embolized or clipped. Lacking that or other sources to implicate, the presumption is that either "microleaks" through fabric suture holes or transudation of serum through the graft intersticies are responsible, and consideration of "relining" the endograft by placement of a new endograft inside of it may be warranted. This may require conversion from a bifurcated to an aorto-uni-iliac configuration, necessitating femoral–femoral bypass grafting and placement of an iliac artery occluder plug.

Summary

Endoleaks, and the treatment dilemmas they present, have been the major shortcoming of endovascular abdominal aortic aneurysm repair since its inception. Their evaluation and treatment are responsible for the overwhelming number of secondary interventions required after EVAR. Some of these procedures, however, would no longer be pursued as our understanding of the generally benign nature of type II endoleaks, the most common variety, becomes apparent. Furthermore, new endograft iterations may reduce the risk of type I endoleaks in future procedures, just as new fabrics and stent suturing/bonding techniques have been employed to address microleaks and endotension. As is often the case, technology is a moving target and engineering advances will likely change the incidence and treatment of endoleaks in the future.

References

1 Parodi JC, Palmaz JC, Barone HD. Transfemoral intraluminal graft implantation for abdominal aortic aneurysms. Ann Vasc Surg 1991; **5**: 491–499.

2 Choke E, Thompson M. Endoleak after endovascular aneurysm repair: Current concepts. J Cardiovasc Surg 2004; **45**: 349–366.

3 Veith FJ, Baum RA, Ohki T *et al.* Nature and significance of endoleaks and endotension: Summary of opinions expressed at an international conference. J Vasc Surg 2002; **35**: 1029–1035.

4 White GH, Yu W, May J *et al.* Endoleak as a complication of endoluminal grafting of abdominal aortic aneurysm: Classification, incidence, diagnosis, and management. J Endovasc Surg 1997; **4**: 152–168.

5 Wain RA, Marin ML, Ohki T, Sanchez LA, Lyon RT *et al.* Endoleaks after endovascular graft treatment of aortic aneurysms: Classification, risk factors, and outcomes. J Vasc Surg 27: 69–78, 1998.

6 Stanley BM, Semmens JB, Mai Q *et al.* Evaluation of patient selection guidelines for endoluminal AAA repair with the Zenith Stent-Graft: The Australasian experience. J Endovasc Ther 2001; **8**: 457–464.

7 Heikkinen MA, Arko FR, Zarins CK. What is the significance of endoleaks and endotension. Surg Clin N Am 2004; **84**: 1337–1352.

8 Hincliffe RJ, Hopkinson BR. Current concepts and controversies in endovascular repair of abdominal aortic aneurysms. J Cardiovasc Surg 2003; **44**: 481–502.

9 Harris PL, Vallabhaneni SR, Desgranges P *et al.* Incidence and risk factors of late rupture, conversion, and death after endovascular repair of infrarenal aortic aneurysms: The EUROSTAR experience. J Vas Surg 2000; **32**: 739–749.

10 Van Marrewijk C, Buth J, Haris PL *et al.* Significance of endoleaks after endovascular repair of abdominal aortic aneurysms: The EUROSTAR experience. J Vasc Surg 2002; **35**: 461–473.

11 Heikkinen MA, Arko FR, Zarins CK. What is the significance of endoleaks and endotension. Surg Clin N Am 2004; **84**: 1337–1352.

12 Thurnher S, Cejna M. Imaging of aortic stent-grafts and endoleaks. Radiol Clin North Am 2002; **40**: 799–833.

13 Stavropoulos SW, Baum RA. Imaging modalities for the detection and management of endoleaks. Semin Vasc Surg 2004; **17**: 154–160.

14 Rosenblitz AM, Patlas M, Rosenbaum AT *et al.* Detection of endoleaks after endovascular repair of abdominal aortic aneurysms: Value of unenhanced and delayed CT acquisitions. Radiology 2003; **227**: 426–433.

15 Mclafferty RB, McCrary BS, Mattos MA *et al.* The use of colour–flow duplex scan for the detection of endoleaks. J Vasc Surg 2002; **36**: 100–104.

16 Wolf YG, Johnson BL, Hill BB *et al.* Duplex ultra-sound scanning versus computed tomographic angiography for postoperative evaluation of endovascular abdominal aortic aneurysm repair. J Vasc Surg 2000; **32**: 1142–1148.

17 Miahle C, Amicabile C, Becquemin JP. Endovascular treatment of infrarenal abdominal aortic aneurysms by the Stentor system: Preliminary results of 79 cases. Stentor Retrospective Study Group. J Vasc Surg 1997; **26**: 199–209.

18 Maldonado TS, Rosen RJ, Rockman CB *et al.* Initial successful management of type I endoleak after endovascular aortic aneurysm repair with n-butyl cyanoacrylate adhesive. J Vasc Surg 2003; **38**: 664–670.

19 Arko FR, Rubin GD, Johnson BL *et al.* Type–II endoleaks following endovascular AAA repair: preoperative predictors and long-term effects. J Endovasc Ther 2003; **8**: 503–510.

20 Bush RL, Lin PH, Ronson RS *et al.* Colonic necrosis subsequent to catheter-directed thrombin embolization of the inferior mesenteric artery via the superior mesenteric artery: A complication in the management of a type II endoleak. J Vasc Surg 2001; **34**: 1119–1121.

21 Gorich J, Rilinger N, Sokiranski R *et al.* Embolization of type II endoleaks fed by the inferior mesenteric artery: Using the superior mesenteric artery approach. J Endovasc Ther 2000; **7**: 297–301.

22 Baum RA, Carpenter JP, Tuite CM *et al.* Diagnosis and treatment of inferior mesenteric arterial endoleaks after endovascular repair of abdominal aortic aneurysms. Radiology 2000; **215**: 409–413.

23 Martin ML, Dolmatch BL, Fry PD *et al.* Treatment of type II endoleaks with Onyx. J Vasc Interv Radiol 2001; **12**: 629–632.

24 Baum RA, Stavropoulos SW, Fairman RM *et al.* Endoleaks after endovascular repair of abdominal aortic aneurysms. J Vasc Interv Radiol 2003; **14**: 1111–1117.

25 Forester ND, Parry D, Kesse D *et al.* Ischaemic sciatic neuropathy: An important complication of embolization of a type II endoleak. Eur J Vasc Endovasc Surg 2002; **24**: 462–463.

26 Wisselink W, Cuesta MA, Berends FJ *et al.* Retroperitoneal endoscopic ligation of lumbar and inferior mesenteric arteries as a treatment of persistent endoleak after endoluminal aortic aneurysm repair. J Vasc Surg 2000; **31**: 1240–1244.

27 van Nes JGH, Hendricks JM, Tseng LNL *et al.* Endoscopic aneurysm sac fenestration as a treatment option for growing aneurysms due to type II endoleak or endotension. J Endovasc Ther 2005; **12**: 430–434.

28 Buth J, Laheij RJF, on behalf of the EUROSTAR Collaborators. Early complications and endoleaks after endovascular abdominal aortic aneurysm repair: Report of a multicenter study. J Vasc Surg 2000; **31**: 134–146.

29 Zarins CK, White RA, Schwarter D *et al.* AneuRx stent-graft versus open surgical repair of abdominal aortic aneurysms: Multicenter prospective clinical trial. J Vasc Surg 1999; **29**: 292–308.

CHAPTER 27

Aneurysm sac pressure measurement with a pressure sensor in endovascular aortic aneurysm repair

Lisandro Carnero & Ross Milner

The goal of endovascular abdominal aortic aneurysm repair (EVAR) is to prevent aneurysm rupture by successful exclusion of the aneurysm sac from systemic pressure. Successful exclusion leads to the reduction of pressure inside the residual aneurysm sac and the tension applied to the wall of the aortic aneurysm [1]. Persistent blood flow into the residual aneurysm sac after EVAR is defined as an endoleak. The incidence of endoleak ranges from 12% to 44% [2, 3]. The clinical significance of type 2 endoleaks remains poorly understood and very controversial. Endoleaks, regardless of the size or type, can transmit systemic pressure into the aneurysm sac. Even in an apparently excluded sac by computer tomography angiography scan (CTA), the pressure can still remain increased [4, 5]. The presence of thrombus between the graft and the aortic wall at the neck of an abdominal aortic aneurysm (AAA) may transmit pressure into the aneurysm sac (endotension) [6–8] and could be associated with sac enlargement. This failure of therapy may increase the risk of aneurysm rupture [3, 7, 9].

Unlike conventional repair of an AAA, the branch vessels remain patent in the sac during EVAR and can potentially transmit systemic pressure into the sac [10–13]. The available endografts have evolved since the first implant performed by Dr Parodi [14], in 1991. Despite the improvements in design and engineering, the occurrence of material fatigue, graft migration, limb dislodgment, and fabric tears remain a problem for this technique [15, 16]. The importance of life-long surveillance after EVAR is widely accepted and is, in fact, mandated by the FDA as stipulated in the Instructions for Use of all commercially available stent grafts. Conventional studies focus on migration or contrast leak into the sac and indirectly evaluate residual pressure in the aneurysm sac by measuring sac size [17].

The potential problems mentioned above highlight the need for outstanding surveillance techniques. The current imaging protocols include ultrasound, CTA, or magnetic resonance angiography (MRA). Ultrasound is labor intensive and technologist dependent when attempting to identify endoleaks. CTA exposes the patient to repetitive contrast administration that can be nephrotoxic. MRA is not universally accepted for endoleak detection and can be the most expensive of the techniques. In light of these limitations, invasive pressure sensing has been investigated previously. Numerous publications describe the use of catheters to measure pressure in the residual aneurysm sac [1, 4, 18–21]. Dias *et al.* [18] reported the use of a direct intraaneurysm sac pressure measurement using a tip-pressure sensor attached to a catheter as a useful adjunct to imaging follow-up after EVAR. The authors report a successful EVAR result when the residual pressure in the aneurysm sac is low.

Dr Parodi revolutionized vascular surgery in the early 1990s by creating an endovascular graft capable of excluding an AAA from the systemic circulation [14]. Wireless pressure sensors could likely

Table 27.1 Comparison of AAA Surveillance Modality

Variable	CT/MRI	Pressure Sensing
Location	Hospital	Office/home
Contrast Agents	Yes	No
Parameter Measured	Diameter change, volume change, presence of contrast	Mean Pressure Pulsatile Pressure
Sensitivity	Low	High
Timing	1–2 per year	As needed (hourly – monthly)
Risk to patient	Contrast reaction	None
Pacemaker Compatibility	CT – Compatible MRI – Not compatible	Compatible

revolutionize surveillance after EVAR. This technology can provide an adjunct to the current imaging surveillance protocols or potentially eliminate the current standard of care (Table 27.1). The current status of wireless pressure sensing will be addressed both for AAA and for thoracic aortic aneurysms (TAA).

Abdominal AAA

Endovascular stent-graft repair of AAA has become an alternative to traditional open repair. EVAR has clear benefits in minimizing periprocedural morbidity and potentially reducing mortality [22]. However, complications unique to endovascular repair have been identified; among them the most significant are endoleaks and residual aneurysm sac expansion. The pioneering work on wired pressure measurement after EVAR was performed in the abdominal aorta by trans-lumbar puncture of the aneurysm sac by Chuter *et al.* [1] in 1997. Since Chuter's study, several works have been published using the same approach [18, 19]. This work has shown that a highly pressurized aneurysm sac is associated with AAA expansion and an aneurysm sac with low pressure is associated with shrinkage [23].

Remon impressure AAA sac pressure transducer (Fig. 27.1)
The initial experimental work demonstrating the efficacy of this technology was performed in an adult porcine model of AAA that allowed for creation of endoleaks [24]. The first report highlighted the efficacy of the technology in detecting pressure changes

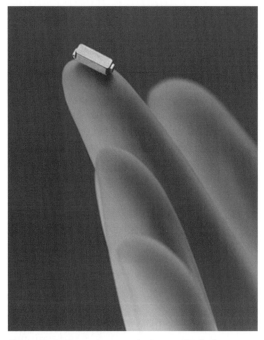

Figure 27.1 Impressure sensor by Remon Medical Technologies. The sensor measures 3 mm × 9 mm × 1.5 mm in size.

with endoleaks as well as the sensor's ability to function while embedded in thrombus [24]. A second report demonstrated the longer-term efficacy in the same experimental model [25].

The first successful wireless pressure sensor placement in man was performed at Mt Sinai Medical Center in New York [26]. The Remon Impressure AAA Sac Pressure Transducer (Remon Medical, Caesaria, Israel) was successfully implanted in 2003. The transducer was handsewn to the outside of the Talent LPS endovascular stent graft (Medtronic AVE, Santa Rosa, CA) and was implanted during the treatment of infrarenal AAA in high-risk patients. The transducer contains a piezoelectric membrane that energizes a capacitor when actuated by ultrasound waves from a hand-held probe. Once charged, a transducer within the device measures ambient pressure and then generates an acoustic signal that is relayed to the hand-held probe. The probe then converts the acoustic signal to a pressure waveform that is presented on computer screen.

The clinical trial [27] enrolled 21 patients. Pressure measurement readings were obtained intraoperatively, at 1 month, 6 months, 1 year, and annually thereafter. Ellozy *et al.* demonstrated the value of long-term wireless sac pressure monitoring. The study confirmed the work performed with invasive pressure monitoring in that patients with aneurysm shrinkage after EVAR have significantly lower pressure when compared to expanding aneurysms [27]. However, the absence of shrinkage does not imply persistent pressurization of the sac. A limitation of this study is that 6 of the 21 sensors did not function appropriately after being implanted. Several explanations are given for the failure of the technology to function in the manuscript. It seems clear that an expensive implant should function appropriately a very high percentage of the time. Interestingly, this sensor is no longer in production for AAA and Remon Medical appears to be focusing the application of their pressure-sensing technology toward the management of heart failure patients.

Cardiomems endosure wireless pressure sensor (Fig. 27.2)

The CardioMems EndoSure Wireless Pressure Sensor (CardioMems, Inc., Atlanta, Georgia) is made of two coils of copper wire within a fused silica matrix with a pressure sensitive surface. An antenna that works both as a transmitter and a receiver emits multiple pulses of radio frequency (RF) energy that activates the coils and makes them vibrate. This vibration generates a resonance frequency that is then received by the antenna. The resonance frequency is related to the ambient pressure in which the sensor is located. Specially-designed software transforms the frequency shift between systolic and diastolic pressures into a wave form and pressure reading.

The initial demonstration of efficacy for this sensor was performed in a canine model by Ohki *et al.* [29]. The initial implant in man was performed by Dr Pierre Silveira in 2004 as a part of the acute pressure measurement to confirm aneurysm sac exclusion (APEX) trial. Seventy evaluable patients were part of the US pivotal study; nine US and three overseas sites participated in this trial. Patients were enrolled in Brazil, Argentina, the United States, and Canada. The initial work was presented at the Society of Vascular Surgery meeting by Dr Ohki [30]. This presentation highlighted the safety of

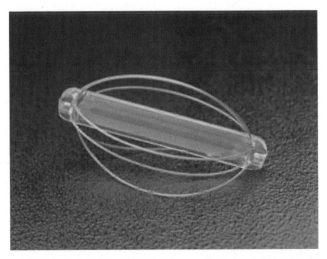

Figure 27.2 EndoSure Wireless AAA Pressure Sensor developed by CardioMems, Inc. This sensor has recently received FDA-clearance for marketing.

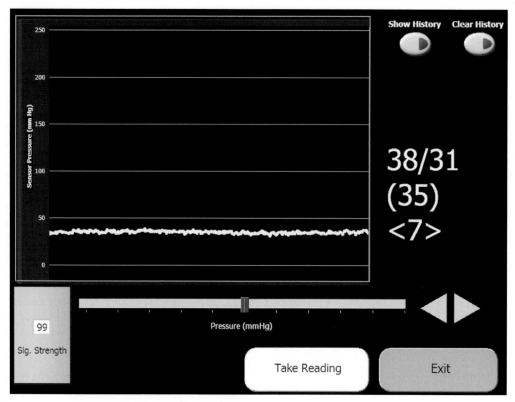

Figure 27.3 Pressure measurement obtained 2 years after endovascular aneurysm repair and placement of a remote pressure sensor. The residual sac pressure is essentially flat-line with a pulse pressure of 7 mmHg.

device implantation; it also demonstrated the efficacy of the EndoSure sensor in confirming AAA sac exclusion during endovascular repair. This data have allowed the EndoSure sensor to gain FDA clearance for acute implantation and initial confirmation of exclusion of an AAA. The sensor is not yet approved for use as a tool for chronic surveillance. However, the first five patients implanted with the EndoSure sensor were successfully interrogated in Brazil at the 2-year time-point with excellent acquisition of pressure measurements (Fig. 27.3). Additional work is in progress to demonstrate the value of pressure sensing as an alternative to radiologic imaging for long-term EVAR surveillance.

Thoracic aortic aneurysm

A decade has passed since the first report of descending thoracic aortic aneurysm (DTA) repair with endografts [31]. FDA-approval of the first thoracic endoprosthesis occurred in the United States in 2005. The results of the phase II multicenter trial of the Gore TAG thoracic endoprosthesis were very promising for the treatment of DTAs, with low mortality, relatively low morbidity, and excellent 2-year freedom from aneurysm-related death [32, 23].

Although, remote pressure sensing remains in its infancy for the thoracic aorta, it may be better suited for postprocedure surveillance in patients with thoracic aneurysms than in patients with AAA. Given the infrequent nature of type II endoleaks with thoracic endografting, any significant increase in intrasac pressure after endovascular thoracic aortic aneurysm repair most likely will be related to a type I or III endoleak which requires expeditious treatment [33].

The first thoracic remote pressure sensor was implanted in 2005 in conjunction with the endovascular repair of a TAA in Florianopolis, Brazil [33]. The implant went well with the standard delivery system used for the abdominal pressure-sensing device. The sensor continues to function well after 6 months of surveillance (Fig. 27.4). The pulse pressure is markedly reduced and the residual aneurysm sac is

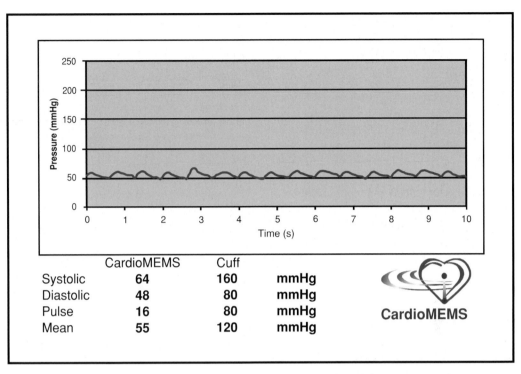

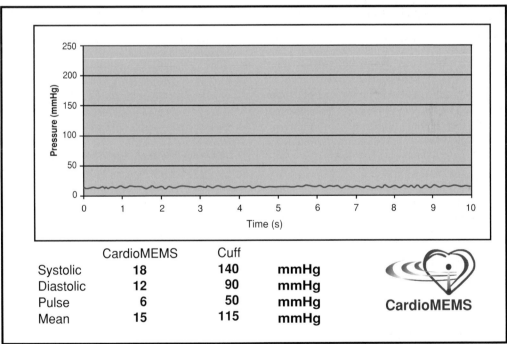

Figure 27.4 Postprocedure pressure measurement (panel A) and 6-month pressure measurement (panel B) after endovascular repair of a thoracic aneurysm. This is the first-in-man thoracic pressure sensor implant.

shrinking. A clinical trial is planned to demonstrate the safety and efficacy of remote pressure sensing in determining acute exclusion of a thoracic aneurysm during endovascular repair. This trial will begin in late, 2006.

Remote pressure sensing may have a substantial role in additional thoracic aortic pathologies. Type B aortic dissection is a likely application for remote pressure sensing when endovascular management is applied to exclude the false lumen from systemic pressure. This treatment modality is being more aggressively utilized and repressurization of the false lumen remains a concern. Remote pressure sensing may assist in confirming exclusion of the false lumen at the time of the initial treatment and assess the durability of treatment during chronic surveillance [33].

Conclusion

Remote pressure sensing in conjunction with endovascular repair of aortic aneurysm disease has been proven to be safe and reliable. More data are needed for pressure sensing to become the standard of care, and perhaps replace contrast CT as the primary modality of endograft surveillance. The preliminary data obtained from the Remon trial and the APEX trial (CardioMems, Inc.) will encourage further research to assess the importance of chronic surveillance with a remote pressure sensor after endovascular repair of an abdominal or thoracic aortic aneurysm. The application of this technology to thoracic aortic pathology is still being investigated and planned.

References

1 Chuter T, Ivancev K, Malina M, Resch T, Brunkwall j, Lindblad B, Risberg B. Aneurysm pressure following endovascular exclusion. Eur J Vasc Endovasc Surg 1997; **13**: 85–87.

2 Fairman RM, Nolte L, Snyder SA, Chuter TA, Greenberg RK. Zenith investigators: Factors predictive of early or late aneurysm sac size change following endovascular repair. J Vasc Surg 2006 Apr; **43**(4): 649–656.

3 Hinnen JW, Koning OH, Visser MJ, Van Bockel HJ. Effect of intraluminal thrombus on pressure transmission in the abdominal aortic aneurysm. J Vasc Surg 2005 Dec; **42**(6): 1176–1182.

4 Chaudhuri A, Ansdell LE, Grass AJ, Adiseshiah M. Intrasac pressure waveforms after endovascular aneurysm repair (EVAR) are a reliable marker of type I endoleaks, but not type II or combined types: An experimental study. Eur J Vasc Endovasc Surg 2004 Oct; **28**(4): 373–378.

5 Imamura A, Koike Y, Iwaki R, Saito T, Ozaki T, Tanaka H, Yamada H, Kamiyama Y. Infrarenal abdominal aortic aneurysm complicated by persistent endotension after endovascular repair: Report of a case. Surg Today 2005; **35**(10): 879–882.

6 Dubenec SR, White GH, Pasenau J, Tzilalis V, Choy E, Erdelez L. Endotension. A review of current views on pathophysiology and treatment. J Cardiovasc Surg (Torino) 2003 Aug; **44**(4): 553–557 (Review).

7 Mehta M, Veith FJ, Ohki T, Lipsitz EC, Cayne NS, Darling RC, 3rd. Significance of endotension, endoleak, and aneurysm pulsatility after endovascular repair. J Vasc Surg 2003 Apr; **37**(4): 842–846.

8 Heikkinen MA, Arko FR, Zarins CK. What is the significance of endoleaks and endotension. Surg Clin North Am 2004 Oct; **84**(5): 1337–1352, vii. Review.

9 Buth J, Harris PL, Van Marrewijk C, Fransen G. Endoleaks during follow-up after endovascular repair of abdominal aortic aneurysm. Are they all dangerous? J Cardiovasc Surg (Torino) 2003 Aug; **44**(4): 559–566 (Review).

10 Dattilo JB, Brewster DC, Fan CM, Geller SC, Cambria RP, Lamuraglia GM, Greenfield AJ, Lauterbach SR, Abbott WM. Clinical failures of endovascular abdominal aortic aneurysm repair: incidence, causes, and management. J Vasc Surg 2002 Jun; **35**(6):1137–1144.

11 Mozes G, Kinnick RR, Gloviczki P, Bruhnke RE, Carmo M, Hoskin TL, Bennet KE, Greenleaf JF. Effect of intraluminal thrombus on pressure transmission in the abdominal aortic aneurysm. J Vasc Surg 2005 Nov; **42**(5): 963–971.

12 Zarins CK, White RA, Hodgson KJ, Schwarten D, Fogarty TJ. Endoleak as a predictor of outcome after endovascular aneurysm repair: AneuRx multicenter clinical trial. J Vasc Surg 2000 Jul; **32**(1): 90–107.

13 Baumr RA, Carpenter JP, Cope C, Golden MA, Velazquez OC, Neschis DG, Mitchell ME, Barker CF, Fairman RM. Aneurysm sac pressure measurements after endovascular repair of abdominal aortic aneurysms. J VAsc Surg 2001; **33**: 32–41.

14 Parodi JC, Palmaz JC, Barone HD. Transfemoral intraluminal graft implantation for abdominal aortic aneurysm. Ann Vasc Surg 1991; **5**: 491–499.

15 Cheng SH, Kato N, Shimono T, Shinpo H, Ishida M, Hirano T, Takeda K. Aneurysm shrinkage after endovascular repair of aortic diseases. Clin Imaging 2006 Jan–Feb; **30**(1): 22–26.

16 Li Z, Kleinstreuer C, Farber M. Computational analysis of biomechanical contributors to possible endovascular

graft failure. Biomech Model Mechanobiol 2005 Dec; **4**(4): 221–234.

17 Elkouri S, Panneton JM, Andrews JC, Lewis BD, McKusick MA, Noel AA, Rowland CM, Bower TC, Cherry KJ, Jr., Gloviczki P. Computed tomography and ultrasound in follow-up of patients after endovascular repair of abdominal aortic aneurysm. Ann Vasc Surg 2004 May; **18**(3): 271–279.

18 Dias NV, Ivancev K, Malina M, Hinnen JW, Visser M, Lindblad B, Sonesson B. Direct intra-aneurysm sac pressure measurement using tip-pressure sensors: *In vivo* and *in vitro* evaluation. J Vasc Surg 2004 Oct; **40**(4): 711–716.

19 Sonesson B, Dias N, Malina M, Olofsson P, Griffin D, Lindblad B, Ivancev K. Intra-aneurysm pressure measurements in successfully excluded abdominal aortic aneurysm after endovascular repair. J Vasc Surg 2003 Apr; **37**(4): 733–738.

20 Baum RA, Carpenter JP, Cope C, Golden MA, Velazquez OC, Neschis DG, Mitchell ME, Barker CF, Fairman RM. Aneurysm sac pressure measurements after endovascular repair of abdominal aortic aneurysms. J Vasc Surg 2001 Jan; **33**(1): 32–41.

21 Sonesson B, Dias N, Malina M, Olofsson P, Griffin D, Lindblad B, Ivancev K. Intra-aneurysm pressure measurements in successfully excluded abdominal aortic aneurysm after endovascular repair. J Vasc Surg 2003; **37**: 733–738.

22 Makaroun MS, Dillavou ED, Kee ST, Sicard G, Chaikof E, Bavaria J, Williams D, Cambria RP, Mitchell RS. Endovascular treatment of thoracic aortic aneurysms: Results of the phase II multicenter trial of the GORE TAG thoracic endoprosthesis. J Vasc Surg 2005 Jan; **41**(1): 1–9.

23 Dias NV, Ivancev K, Malina M, Resch T, Lindblad B, Sonesson B. Intra-aneurysm sac pressure measurements after endovascular aneurysm repair: Differences between shrinking, unchanged, and expanding aneurysms with and without endoleaks. J Vasc Surg 2004 Jun; **39**(6): 1229–1135.

24 Milner R, Verhagen HJ, Prinssen M, Blankensteijn JD. Noninvasive intrasac pressure measurement and the influence of type 2 and type 3 endoleaks in an animal model of abdominal aortic aneurysm. Vascular. 2004 Mar; **12**(2): 99–105.

25 Milner R, Ruurda JP, Blankensteijn JD. Durability and validity of a remote, miniaturized pressure sensor in an animal model of abdominal aortic aneurysm. J Endovasc Ther 2004 Aug; **11**(4): 372–377.

26 Ellozy SH, Carroccio A, Lookstein RA, Minor ME, Sheahan CM, Juta J, Cha A, Valenzuela R, Addis MD, Jacobs TS, Teodorescu VJ, Marin ML. First experience in human beings with a permanently implantable intrasac pressure transducer for monitoring endovascular repair of abdominal aortic aneurysms. J Vasc Surg 2004 Sep; **40**(3): 405–412.

27 Ellozy SH, Carroccio A, Lookstein RA, Jacobs TS, Addis MD, Teodorescu VJ, Marin ML. Abdominal aortic aneurysm sac shrinkage after endovascular aneurysm repair: Correlation with chronic sac pressure measurement. J Vasc Surg 2006 Jan; **43**(1): 2–7.

28 Dias NV, Ivancev K, Malina M, Resch T, Lindblad B, Sonesson B. Intra-aneurysm sac pressure measurements afterendovascular aneurysm repair: Differences between shrinking, unchanged, and expanding aneurysms with and without endoleaks. J Vasc Surg 2004; **39**: 1229–1135.

29 Ohki T, Yadav J, Gargiuolo N *et al.* Preliminary results of implantable wireless aneurysm pressure sensor in a canine model: Will surveillance CT scan following endovascular AAA repair become obsolete? J Endovasc Ther 2003: **10** (Suppl 1): 1–32.

30 Ohki T *et al.* Preliminary outcome of wireless pressure sensing for EVAR (the APEX Trial) Society for Vascular Surgery, Philadelphia, PA. June 18, 2005.

31 Dake MD, Miller DC, Semba CP, Mitchell RS, Walker PJ, Liddell RP. Transluminal placement of endovascular stent-grafts for the treatment of descending thoracic aortic aneurysms. N Engl J Med 1994 Dec 29; **331**(26): 1729–1734.

32 Cho JS, Haider SE, Makaroun MS.Endovascular therapy of thoracic aneurysms: Gore TAG trial results. Semin Vasc Surg 2006 Mar; **19**(1): 18–24.

33 Milner R, Kasirajan K, Chaikof EL. Future of Endograft Surveillance. Sem Vasc Surg 2006 Jun; **19**(2): 75–82.

Index

Note: page numbers in *italics* refer to figures, those in **bold** refer to tables.